Research into Practice

For Baillière Tindall:

Senior Commissioning Editor: Sarena Wolfaard
Project Development Manager: Claire Wilson
Project Manager: Joannah Duncan
Design: Judith Wright

Research into Practice

Essential Skills for Reading and Applying Research in Nursing and Health Care

Edited by

Dr Patrick A. Crookes PhD BSc (Nursing) RGN RNT CertEd

Professor and Head, Department of Nursing,
University of Wollongong, NSW, Australia

Dr Sue Davies PhD MSc BSc RGN RHV

Senior Lecturer in Gerontological Nursing, School of Nursing and Midwifery,
University of Sheffield, UK

Foreword by

Mary Chiarella PhD RN CM DipNEd LLB(Hons)

Chief Nursing Officer, New South Wales Health, North Sydney,
New South Wales, Australia

SECOND EDITION

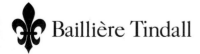 Baillière Tindall

EDINBURGH LONDON NEW YORK OXFORD PHILADELPHIA ST LOUIS SYDNEY TORONTO 2004

BAILLIÈRE TINDALL
An imprint of Elsevier Limited

First published 1998
  Reprinted 2006

ISBN 0 7020 2686 7

British Library Cataloguing in Publication Data
A catalogue record for this book is available from the British Library

Library of Congress Cataloguing in Publication Data
A catalogue record for this book is available from the Library of Congress

Note
Medical knowledge is constantly changing. Standard safety precautions
must be followed, but as new research and clinical experience broaden our
knowledge, changes in treatment and drug therapy may become necessary
or appropriate. Readers are advised to check the most current product
information provided by the manufacturer of each drug to be administered
to verify the recommended dose, the method and duration of administration,
and contraindications. It is the responsibility of the practitioner, relying on
experience and knowledge of the patient, to determine dosages and the best
treatment for each individual patient. Neither the Publisher nor the author
assumes any liability for any injury and/or damage to persons or property
arising from this publication.

The Publisher

ELSEVIER your source for books,
journals and multimedia
in the health sciences
www.elsevierhealth.com

Working together to grow
libraries in developing countries
www.elsevier.com | www.bookaid.org | www.sabre.org
ELSEVIER   BOOK AID International   Sabre Foundation

Printed in China
C/04

The
publisher's
policy is to use
**paper manufactured
from sustainable forests**

Contents

Contributors

Andrew Booth BA MSc DipLib MCLIP
*Senior Lecturer in Evidence Based Healthcare
Information, University of Sheffield, UK*

Peter Bradley MBBS MA MPH MRCGP MFPH
*Acting Head of Section, Pharmaceutical
Reimbursement Section, Norwegian Medicines Agency,
Oslo, Norway*

Esther Chang RN CM BAppSc(Adv. Nur.) DipNEd
MEdAdmin PhD
*Professor of Nursing, School of Nursing, Family and
Community Health, University of Western Sydney,
Sydney, Australia*

Patrick A. Crookes PhD BSc(Nursing) RGN RNT CertEd
*Professor and Head, Department of Nursing,
University of Wollongong, NSW, Australia*

John Daly RN BA BHSc MEd PhD FINE FRCNA
*Professor of Nursing, Head, School of Nursing, Family
and Community Health, University of Western Sydney,
Sydney, Australia*

Sue Davies PhD MSc BSc RGN RHV
*Senior Lecturer in Gerontological Nursing, School of
Nursing and Midwifery, University of Sheffield, UK*

Jan Draper PhD BSc(Hons) RGN
Course Director (Distance Learning), RCN Institute, UK

Lorraine B. Ellis PhD MSc BA(Hons) RGN RNT CertEd
*Senior Lecturer, School of Nursing and Midwifery,
University of Sheffield, Sheffield, UK*

Terry Froggatt BHA MSc RN RMN FAIM
*Regional Manager, Wesley Mission, Sydney, and PhD
Candidate, Department of Nursing, University of
Wollongong, Wollongong, Australia*

Gordon Grant PhD MSc BSc
*Professor of Cognitive Disability, School of
Nursing and Midwifery, University of Sheffield,
Sheffield, UK*

Karen Hancock BSc PhD
*Research Associate, School of Nursing, Family and
Community Health, University of Western Sydney,
Sydney, Australia*

Christine Hibbert RGN RNT CertEd Med
*Nursing Lecturer, School of Nursing, University of
Sheffield, Sheffield, UK*

Yu Chu Huang PhD MMedSci RN
*Associate Professor of Nursing, Department of
Nursing, Fu-Jen Catholic University, Taiwan, Republic
of China*

Christine Ingleton PhD MA BEd(Hons) RGN RNT RCNT
*Senior Lecturer/Head of Department, School of
Nursing, University of Sheffield, Sheffield, UK*

Ulla Lundh PhD RN
*Associate Professor, Department of Welfare and
Care, Linkopings University, Linkopings,
Sweden*

Nigel Mathers PhD BSc MBChB MD MRCGP DCH DipEd
FRSM
*Professor of General Practice, University of Sheffield,
Sheffield, UK*

Liz Matthews BSc(Hons) RGN
*Lecturer in Nursing, School of Nursing, University of
Sheffield, Sheffield, UK*

Ann McDonnell MSc(HSR Technol Assess) MSc(Nursing) BSc RGN RNT
MRC Training Fellow, University of Sheffield, Sheffield, UK

Mike Nolan PhD MSc MA BEd RN
Professor of Gerontological Nursing, Northern General Hospital, Sheffield, UK

David R. Thompson RN BSc MA MBA PhD FRCN FESC
Professor of Clinical Nursing and Director, The Nethersole School of Nursing, The Chinese University of Hong Kong, Shatin NT, Hong Kong

Foreword

When I took up a foundation clinical chair in 2001, a review of the educational needs of the nursing staff indicated that over 50% had no tertiary qualifications. This demographic aside, there was huge enthusiasm for practice development but coupled with a distinct lack of enthusiasm for research (the first research seminar I ran, optimistically entitled 'Let's Do Research' attracted a gathering of three – as opposed to the fifty I often welcomed for other clinical topics!). I realized I needed to rethink my strategies. I needed to find a way to demystify research. I needed to find ways to teach research utilization and critique that was accessible to experienced clinical nurses who were inexperienced in research. I needed to find strategies to link research to practice. I found all of these solutions in the first edition of Crookes and Davies and never looked back.

As the editors state in their introduction, the intention of compiling the book was to:

… encourage, enable and motivate practitioners to:

- *Access, read and understand research reports*
- *Apply research-based knowledge in the practice setting*
- *Influence colleagues on the use of research information*
- *Develop responsibility for their own professional development.*

Crookes and Davies have taken an internationally renowned group of nurse researchers and used their expertise to enable new readers of research to access, comprehend and critique it. The true mark of an expert is to be able to explain difficult concepts relating to their area of expertise in a way that makes the concepts seem easy. This is precisely what has been achieved in this text. The language is user-friendly and there is a range of effective tables and charts to provide helpful overviews of certain topics. There are useful summaries at key points within the chapters and a series of exercises throughout to assist the reader to make sense of the content.

Not every nurse needs to be a researcher. But every nurse needs nursing research. They need it in order to *inform* their nursing practice, and to be able to provide safe and effective nursing care based on the best available evidence. There is now a significant amount of nursing research literature available and increasingly, more clinically based nursing research is being conducted. The desire to provide optimal patient care is the key driver for all nurses, but this is not possible without access to the most current knowledge on what constitutes that care. With decreasing length of stay and increasing patient acuity, our time with the patient is always precious and needs to be focussed on those activities demonstrated to be efficacious.

But equally importantly, nurses need nursing research to *describe* their nursing practice. Nursing research gives language to nursing practice, language that is so needed for us to articulate to others what it is we do as nurses. Without the language that nursing research provides for us, we can neither promote nor explain practice to our patients, our peers, our students, our communities, our fundholders and health care planners.

This book is vitally important because it makes this much-needed language of research more accessible to those who need to speak it and know it – namely, the clinicians who provide patient care. The only purpose for conducting clinical nursing research is to improve practice. The only people who will improve nursing practice are the clinicians practising nursing. The key is to link the clinicians to the research. This book provides that link.

Mary Chiarella, 2004

Introduction

CHAPTER CONTENTS

BACKGROUND

In 1993, the Report of the Taskforce on the Strategy for Research in Nursing, Midwifery and Health Visiting (DoH 1993) emphasized the need for research skills to be more widespread within these professions. The Taskforce was careful, however, to identify that such skills should not be developed via a proliferation of inadequately supervised, small-scale projects. Instead it took a wider perspective of the term 'research skills' to incorporate critical and analytical thinking. It also asserted that information literacy skills – accessing and evaluating literature (in this case research-based literature) – were essential prerequisites for knowledge-based practice.

Shortly after the Taskforce Report was published, we found ourselves working together to develop a new research skills module for qualified nurses and midwives undertaking a 'top-up' degree at the University of Sheffield. Similar modules were being developed around the country as schools and colleges of nursing and health amalgamated with universities. We shared the views of the Taskforce about the need to widen the definition of 'research skills' since our experience of teaching nurses and midwives about research had led us to realize that many see it as of little relevance to their own practice. Many practitioners seem to view research as the concern of 'other people', not least because they associate the term 'research' with the need to actually carry out research themselves. As a result the utilization and implementation of research suffer from a lack of understanding, a lack of motivation and a lack of necessary skills.

We had both attempted to modify this view in our teaching by the use of a model – the 4 A's of research skills (Awareness, Appreciation, Application and Ability). With this model, we were able to differentiate between the skills of understanding available research reports, applying the findings in practice (necessary to all practitioners) and the skills to carry out research (necessary to a few). This philosophy provided the basis for a taught module *Research Appreciation and Application*. Our aim was to produce a programme which did not stop at the development of positive attitudes towards research and its role in clinical practice, but went on to facilitate the skills and knowledge required for the critical appraisal of research-based literature and the application of its findings.

Our experience also told us that 'traditional' methods of teaching research do not typically lead to the development of the skills needed to appreciate and apply research. The content of courses and study days on research is often focused upon steps in the research process, on research methods and writing research proposals, rather than on the identification and evaluation of the characteristics of research which have implications for the application of findings to practice. We feel it is more appropriate to focus *overtly* on the development of skills relevant to research utilization, including skills necessary to initiate and manage change. There are many barriers to research utilization in practice and the research-aware practitioner needs a full repertoire of skills and knowledge to help overcome these barriers.

As a result we developed a new approach to teaching research skills, one which focused on *overtly* developing skills in the critical appraisal of research reports and appropriate implementation of research findings. Our intention was to encourage, enable and motivate practitioners to:

- Access, read and understand research reports
- Apply research-based knowledge in the practice setting
- Influence colleagues on the use of research information
- Develop responsibility for their own professional development.

In other words, to accept research as a normal aspect of professional nursing and health care practice.

The module was also designed to promote the development of important generic skills (such as the use of information technology and writing systematic literature reviews), which could be applied in other contexts, as well as facilitating personal and professional development. In recognition of the findings of the Taskforce Report, we placed an emphasis on the context in which health care research is conducted, disseminated and utilized.

In developing the module, one of the first things we tried to do was identify a text which could support students (and us) through the course. Perusing the texts available at the time identified for us that the practice of equating research activity with 'doing' research had reached the point of ideology or dogma. Furthermore, it was so pervasive that nursing research texts, which were at the time largely North American in origin, covered material in such a way that the reader was taken through the processes of research by considering how to 'do it correctly', rather than by identifying important things to consider when evaluating a research report.

As a result, we decided to develop a text to reflect our own approach to teaching, not least to clearly and strongly assert that there are skills of research appreciation and application, which are distinct from the skills necessary to undertake research. Furthermore, we were keen to demonstrate that the skills of research appreciation and application are not inherently inferior to the skills necessary to 'do' research but that these skills complement each other in the context of modern health care.

In the intervening years, other authors have also recognized that research appraisal and utilization are important issues and so, worth writing about. To date, however, the majority of these have sought to do so via adding chapters on 'Critical Appraisal' and 'Research Utilization' to existing 'doing research' texts. Alternatively, others focus specifically on 'evidence for practice' but have used randomized controlled trials (RCTs) as the principal source of knowledge underpinning health care. As a result, these texts fail to consider the range of research-based literature that health professionals need to underpin and inform their practice.

We wanted, therefore, to further develop a text that would enthuse and excite readers about the potential of research to enhance their practice and which would enable them to develop the skills required both to critically evaluate research and to initiate and manage a problem-based approach to research utilisation. The positive feedback that we received about the first edition of this text suggests that we (together with our contributors) managed to achieve this and we were, therefore, reluctant to 'tinker' with a winning formula. Consequently, we have left the basic structure of the text largely unchanged in the second edition.

However, the context for health and social care practice is continually developing and there was a need to add new material within certain chapters and to update references and examples throughout. In particular, computerized resources and techniques for systematic literature searching have developed apace and thus warranted more detailed consideration within this revised text. A similar comment can be made regarding the policy context that informs the nature of research, how it is funded and who gets the funding to do it, hence the fairly radical changes to Chapter 2. The Evidence-Based Practice (EBP) movement has also developed globally, in particular in relation to the production of evidence-based guidelines. Many such guidelines use as their basis meta-analysis of the data from several research trials, and some have included a new chapter on 'evaluating systematic reviews'. Furthermore, our experience of teaching students to evaluate research-based literature during the years since *Research Into Practice* first appeared has modified our ideas about the best way to present the material included within the text. In this second edition, then, we place greater emphasis on the contribution of research design to decisions about the appropriate interpretation and application of research findings, hence our decision to present two separate chapters on research methods. Our intention is to allow a more detailed examination of key elements of the rigour of quantitative and qualitative research projects and how this should be reflected in the ways in which the process and outcomes of such studies should be reported in the literature.

SCOPE AND PURPOSE

The second edition of *Research Into Practice* thus retains the original intention of the text in that it remains a book designed to prepare the reader to access, critically evaluate, synthesize and utilize research-based literature within professional health care practice. It is aimed at all health care professionals who need to develop skills in the appreciation and utilization of research. However, it should be of particular value to students undertaking educational programmes ranging from Diploma to Masters level, as these all require the development of skills in literature retrieval, analysis and review. We recognise that much of the material is drawn from a midwifery or nursing context, reflecting the backgrounds of the contributors. However, the book is intended to be relevant to all areas of professional health care practice and this reflects the importance of a multidisciplinary approach to research and research utilization.

HOW DOES THIS BOOK DIFFER FROM OTHER BOOKS ON RESEARCH?

As indicated already, this text does not focus on how to *do* research. Instead, it concentrates on the retrieval, analysis and application of existing research in order to identify and develop good practice. The traditional 'order' used in other texts based upon the stages of the research process has been avoided. Instead, we seek to *overtly* develop:

- An appreciation of the range of sources of knowledge which may inform nursing and health care practice
- An awareness of contemporary research and of the context within which health services' research and development takes place
- Appreciation skills using an approach which examines the implications of features of project design and conduct for the critical evaluation of research reports and other research-based literature
- A recognition of the range of skills and insights relevant to the application of research findings and innovation within health care practice.

Throughout, the reader is encouraged to reflect upon the application of these skills within their own practice and that of colleagues.

As you will see, the text is multi-authored to ensure that the content was written by people with particular expertise and insights. However, we have exercised our editorial influence in order to maintain overall coherence. As a result the chapters are presented in a similar style and contain a range of features including ongoing summary of content: reflective exercises, questions for possible discussion and suggestions for further reading. These features are included with the dual intention of making the experience of reading the text as 'interactive' as possible, as well as emphasizing the 'so what?' of key issues covered.

The book is intended to be read in one of two ways, depending on readers' existing knowledge of research. The person new to research will benefit from reading the content as ordered in the text. Those with more knowledge and experience will also find this useful but may prefer to 'dip into' the text at particular points of interest. To make this easier, we now present the 14 Chapters in overview.

CHAPTER 1 KNOWLEDGE FOR PRACTICE-BASED DISCIPLINES: ADVANCING THE DEBATE (MIKE NOLAN, ULLA LUNDH)

This chapter sets the following chapters in context by exploring the role and contribution of different ways of 'knowing' to health and social care practice. The aim is to encourage the reader to recognize the contribution that all types of knowledge can make to effective health care. In particular, the role of users of health care services in developing evidence for practice is explored.

CHAPTER 2 THE CONTEXT OF NURSING AND HEALTH CARE RESEARCH (JOHN DALY, DAVID THOMPSON, ESTHER CHANG, KAREN HANCOCK)

Essentially, this chapter explores the relationship between policy and research. The aim is to alert practitioners to opportunities for utilizing research-based knowledge to inform and develop practice offered by national and local Research and Development strategies. Attention is also paid to the motivating forces which encourage individual researchers and research teams to undertake particular projects, as well as recognizing the effect that researcher and commissioner motivation may have on findings and conclusions. Finally, this chapter provides advice as to how clinicians, especially nurses and midwives, can become more effective in informing health and health research policy in the future.

CHAPTER 3 ACCESSING SOURCES OF KNOWLEDGE (CHRISTINE HIBBERT)

As research activities become more central to nursing and health care practice, the range and volume of resources available to inform practice continue to increase rapidly. The ability to search the literature in a systematic and efficient way is therefore fundamental to the development of a research base to nursing and health care practice. In this chapter, Christine Hibbert seeks to enable the reader to identify and access research-based literature by: suggesting ways of defining and refining topics for successful literature searching; considering different approaches to reading (e.g. skim reading, deep reading); presenting systems for recording and maintaining personal notes and references; and introducing the concept of critical analysis (we see the term regularly but what does it mean?).

CHAPTER 4 MAKING THE MOST OF EXISTING KNOWLEDGE (ANDREW BOOTH)

This chapter identifies the importance of a systematic search of the literature in terms of: helping inform a study's background; its design; the selection of methods and instruments; and conducting the analysis and writing up of conclusions. It does this from the perspective of encouraging you, the reader, to seek for evidence that these processes have been followed, so as to assure you of the strength of the theoretical underpinnings of any given research paper. It introduces techniques for focusing information needs into a searchable question, for filtering a list of potentially relevant references according to study design as well as introducing tools and resources (e.g. CATS and CASP checklists) to support more detailed critical appraisal of study quality.

CHAPTER 5 PHILOSOPHICAL AND THEORETICAL UNDERPINNINGS OF RESEARCH (LORRAINE B. ELLIS, PATRICK A. CROOKES)

The aims of this chapter are to encourage the reader to appreciate the importance of recognizing the philosophical and theoretical perspectives that underpin research and to question and evaluate the theoretical and conceptual bases of individual research reports. To this end, Lorraine Ellis and Patrick Crookes highlight the major components of the relationship between research and theory – most importantly that research should be based upon, and develop, theory and knowledge. The philosophical bases of three broad research paradigms – positivism, naturalism and critical theory – are also explored, along with the processes of inductive and deductive reasoning. The roles of philosophy and reasoning within research processes are then described. Frames of reference (conceptual and theoretical frameworks) are discussed and the contribution made by these frameworks to the development of research methodology and interpretation of findings is considered. In particular, the importance of identifying assumptions underpinning both the research questions and the research process for the study under evaluation is demonstrated.

CHAPTER 6 THE RELATIONSHIP BETWEEN RESEARCH QUESTION AND RESEARCH DESIGN (JAN DRAPER)

Research design is a major factor to be considered when evaluating the appropriate application of research findings. For example, the findings of an ethnographic study are likely to have very different implications for practice, when compared with the findings of a large-scale survey or randomized controlled trial. This chapter will present an overview of the range of research design types commonly used in health care research generally and in nursing and midwifery in particular and discusses the major strengths and limitations of each. The relationship between research design and level of knowledge is also examined. Worked examples, such as the justification for the design used to answer a particular research question, are provided.

CHAPTER 7 EVALUATING QUALITATIVE RESEARCH (NIGEL MATHERS, YU CHU HUANG)

A key issue for the reader of research is the extent to which the research demonstrates rigour. However, the strategies for ensuring rigour will vary depending on the particular methodology used. This chapter will consider how rigour might be evaluated within research that is predominantly qualitative. Discussion will concentrate not only on methods for data collection and analysis, but also on the appropriate interpretation of research findings. Sampling issues are touched upon within this chapter, but are more fully explored in Chapter 9.

CHAPTER 8 EVALUATING QUANTITATIVE RESEARCH (NIGEL MATHERS, YU CHU HUANG)

This chapter follows a similar pattern to Chapter 7, but focuses upon research that is predominantly quantitative.

CHAPTER 9 POPULATIONS AND SAMPLES: IDENTIFYING THE BOUNDARIES OF RESEARCH (CHRISTINE INGLETON)

The intention of this chapter is to make the critical reader of research more aware of the impact of sampling techniques on the implications of any research project. The range of sampling techniques commonly used in nursing and health care research (both quantitative and qualitative) will be described. The implications of using particular sampling techniques for extrapolating research findings to other populations and settings are also considered.

CHAPTER 10 CRITIQUING ETHICAL ISSUES IN PUBLISHED RESEARCH (LIZ MATTHEWS, GORDON GRANT)

This chapter focuses on the ethical implications of research activity in health and social care, both in terms of the conduct of research and its application to practice. Mechanisms for protecting the rights of research participants, such as the research governance framework within the UK, are addressed with the intention of raising awareness of the importance of considering whether such safeguards have been applied within published research.

CHAPTER 11 REVIEWING AND INTERPRETING RESEARCH: IDENTIFYING IMPLICATIONS FOR PRACTICE (SUE DAVIES)

Identifying indicators for practice from research-based literature requires the synthesis of evidence from a number of projects investigating the same area. This may be complicated by the existence of apparently contradictory findings. In this chapter Sue Davies considers the purposes of a literature review and describes a number of tools and techniques which can help the reader to systematically review a body of literature in order to identify implications for practice, education and research. Approaches to structuring and writing different levels of literature review are also presented.

CHAPTER 12 EVIDENCE-BASED PRACTICE AND CRITICAL APPRAISAL OF QUANTITATIVE REVIEW ARTICLES (SYSTEMATIC REVIEWS) (PETER BRADLEY)

Systematic reviews of the literature, some using the process known as metaanalysis, have become key elements of the information base for clinicians wishing to provide evidence-based care. This chapter aims to provide the reader with an introduction to this genre of writing, along with guidelines for the evaluation of systematic reviews and reference to worked examples.

CHAPTER 13 FACTORS WHICH MAY INHIBIT THE APPLICATION OF RESEARCH FINDINGS IN PRACTICE AND SOME SOLUTIONS (ANN McDONNELL)

A number of authors have identified that the utilization of research findings in nursing and health care practice is slow and is hampered by a wide range of factors. Ann McDonnell's chapter reviews the importance of individual and organizational factors. The contribution of organizational culture and the role of facilitative leadership in developing evidence-based practice is considered, in particular.

CHAPTER 14 TECHNIQUES AND STRATEGIES FOR TRANSLATING RESEARCH FINDINGS INTO HEALTH CARE PRACTICES (PATRICK A. CROOKES, TERRY FROGGATT)

A range of methods and strategies have been identified as being effective in maximizing the success of innovation – namely 'models of change'. In this chapter, Patrick Crookes and Terry Froggatt provide the reader with an overview of possible strategies for overcoming barriers to change and inertia within both individuals and organizations. This is an attempt to prepare practitioners wishing to apply the findings of research to the realities of the role of 'change agent'. The key argument of the chapter is that much of the innovation attempted in health care settings fails because people do not approach the management of change in a systematic and planned way. Criteria for the evaluation of previous innovation attempts are presented (those who ignore the mistakes of the past are destined to repeat them), as well as an overview of a number of models for planning change. The nursing context is used for much of the discussion but the principles discussed are relevant to any setting where change is being considered and planned.

We hope that this book will excite readers about the possibilities of using research-based knowledge to inform their practice. We have tried to demystify the terminology, which can seem so off-putting for those new to reading research reports, and hope that the book will enthuse readers to seek to expand their skills of research appreciation and application further. The satisfaction of being able to seek, find and understand research-based literature which provides answers to our questions about practice is the ultimate reward.

Reference

Department of Health 1993 Report of the Taskforce on the Strategy for Research in Nursing, Midwifery and Health Visiting. Department of Health, London

Chapter 1

Knowledge for practice–based disciplines: advancing the debate

Mike Nolan, Ulla Lundh

What constitutes the evidence in evidence-based practice?

(Fawcett et al 2001, p138)

Knowledge, as much as any resource, determines definitions of what is considered as important, as possible, for and by whom. Through access to knowledge and participation in its production, use and dissemination, actors can affect the boundaries and indeed the conceptualization of the possible.

(Gaventa & Cornwall 2001, p72)

Many important policy and practice issues in the fields of health and social care, in the UK and beyond, are reflected in two current and sometimes contradictory debates. The first is captured in the succinct but telling question posed by Fawcett et al (2001) above and concerns the type of 'evidence' that should underpin practice. For as French (2002) notes, 'evidence-based practice' is now very much in 'vogue' and has largely superseded earlier discussions about the relationship between research, theory and practice. Implicit within Fawcett et al's question is the suggestion that there are differing forms of 'evidence' and that it is important to make informed decisions about what 'constitutes' best evidence. A brief overview of the varying forms of evidence (or knowledge) that might be drawn upon to inform practice is one of the main aims of this chapter.

A second major debate prevalent in the policy and practice literatures concerns the relationships between those providing and those receiving services. This is characterized in many ways but is typified in terms such as 'user involvement' and is exemplified in current initiatives such as 'Consumers in the NHS' (DoH 2002) and the 'Expert Patient'

(DoH 2001). As Bernard and Phillips (2000) suggest, the 1990s witnessed a new language of health and social care based on notions of participation and involvement. However, whilst such ideals may now be major policy drivers, achieving greater 'user' involvement poses a 'fundamental challenge' (Barnes 1999) to the taken-for-granted relationship between differing forms of knowledge, especially that held by so called 'experts' and that held by 'lay' people (Barnes 1999). This is not simply an academic debate for if, as is commonly believed, 'knowledge is power' (Park 2001), who defines knowledge and which knowledge is seen as valid are of considerable importance. This is eloquently captured in the second of the two quotations above, for it is not only access to knowledge that matters but also the possibility to influence how it is produced, used and disseminated. Indeed, as Gaventa and Cornwall (2001) argue, such participation largely determines the 'conceptualisation of the possible'. Our second main aim in this chapter is to explore the relationship between the varying types of evidence/knowledge that are available, and to consider who participates in its production, use and dissemination. We will suggest that, while there may have been a move away from a total reliance on 'expert' knowledge (as defined largely by researchers, academics or certain professional groups, notably medicine), coupled with a greater acknowledgement of the value of experiential (or tacit) knowledge, the balance of power still resides with the former. We will further suggest that although greater credence is now given to experiential knowledge, the experiential knowledge in question remains largely that of professionals rather than that of the users of health and social care. We will conclude the chapter by arguing that if initiatives such as the 'Expert Patient' (DoH 2001) are to be successful, then a far broader definition of what 'constitutes the evidence in evidence-based care' (Fawcett et al 2001) is needed that shifts the focus away from the potentially self-serving interests of differing professional groups towards a more genuinely participative approach.

Key issues

- What counts as knowledge?
- Ways of knowing in health and social care practice
- Relationships between different types of knowledge and evidence

WHAT COUNTS AS KNOWLEDGE?

Epistemology, or the theory of knowledge, is concerned with how we know what we know, what justifies us in believing what we do, and what standards of evidence we should use in seeking truths about the world and human experience.

(Audi 1998, p1)

The relationship between research and knowledge is an important one, particularly in practice-based disciplines such as nursing, social work and teaching. Hockey (1996) argues that 'the essential nature of research lies in its intent to create new knowledge in whatever field' (p3), and if we accept such a definition, knowledge and research are inextricably linked. However, the question of what constitutes both research and knowledge is not straightforward and is a highly contested and hotly debated area.

While there is no consensus on what constitutes 'knowledge', there is a broad agreement that there are differing types or forms of knowledge and that practitioners who work in disciplines such as nursing, teaching and social work draw on multiple sources and types of information to inform their practice. If such practitioners are to engage in informed debate about the varying contribution of differing types of knowledge it is important to have an understanding of the commonly used concepts and language that inform differing research approaches or 'paradigms'. According to Denzin and Lincoln (1994) a paradigm is a set of basic beliefs that guide action by providing a worldview, shaping the way we interpret and understand our environment. A paradigm is underpinned by a number of first principles or 'ultimates' (Denzin & Lincoln 1994) which can never be proven to be true but have to be accepted as being correct. Varying research methods reflect differing paradigms and these will be explored in greater detail in subsequent chapters. For our present purpose it is sufficient to know that each paradigm attempts to provide answers to at least three sets of questions. Guba and Lincoln (1989) see these as being ontological, epistemological and methodological questions.

The most abstract of these is the ontological question, concerned with the nature of reality itself. The central issue is whether reality is perceived as something which is fixed and external or whether reality is shaped and influenced by how people interpret and interact with their world. The epistemological question, as the above quote suggests, asks 'what is knowledge?' and seeks to understand the relationships between researchers on the one hand and the 'subjects' of research on the other. Methodological questions are the least abstract and are concerned with the methods and approaches that can be used to generate knowledge. It will readily be seen that although discrete, these questions are nonetheless related in a hierarchical fashion, so that answers to the ontological question influence the answers to the epistemological question, which in turn largely determines the methodological approach that it is considered appropriate to use. Such issues will be considered in more detail elsewhere in this book.

In this chapter we are interested primarily in epistemological questions – those seeking to establish the nature of knowledge. Debates in this area are complex and ultimately there is no way of proving them either right or wrong. Although important, the finer points of such arguments are of more interest to philosophers than to practitioners or researchers. We will therefore deal with them in a manner that some would consider to be superficial. This is inevitable in a book of this nature. The situation is further complicated by the fact that in qualitative research there are currently a number of differing paradigms, each providing a different emphasis. We will not be able to explore these approaches to qualitative research here, and readers who are interested in a more detailed account are advised to consult more advanced texts (Denzin & Lincoln 1994, 2000).

Here we paint a deliberately broad picture highlighting two issues, which seem to us to be particularly relevant. The first reflects traditional debates about the difference between quantitative and qualitative research. The second is a product of more recent concerns about the role and value of scientific knowledge itself and the emerging argument that research should not simply aim to produce knowledge but that it should also actively seek to change and improve the world. From such a perspective, research has a more overtly political and emancipatory agenda – as evidenced in approaches such as participatory action research, feminist research and ethnic research (see Reason & Bradbury 2001 for a detailed account). Although such issues may appear rather academic at this point, an appreciation of them is essential to a better understanding of many of the current debates in the practice literature.

Many readers will already have some familiarity with the long-standing quantitative/qualitative debate, which is still a preoccupation of many researchers and practitioners (see also Chapter 5). Unfortunately arguments are frequently taken to extremes, with people adopting fixed and often inflexible positions. The basis of such disagreements can be traced to the ontological assumptions underpinning qualitative and quantitative research.

The early development of science focused largely on the physical world, involving disciplines such as mathematics, physics and chemistry. Indeed, mathematics is still seen as the 'queen' of sciences (Guba & Lincoln 1994). These disciplines rely heavily – almost exclusively – on quantification, in order to explain the world in terms of equations, statistics and laws. The success of the physical sciences in helping us to understand the world has led to the view that the methods they adopt are the only way to conduct good research. This became widely known as 'the positivist paradigm', which is based on the belief that there is an external reality and that the world is governed by universal laws or laws of nature, which apply at all times and in all places. Because knowledge consists of such laws, researchers can be totally objective and their own beliefs are not considered to influence the results of their research. Within the positivist paradigm, the best way to conduct research is to control and manipulate events, ideally in a laboratory setting.

Whilst such an approach seems reasonable when exploring the physical world, its application to the social world is seen by many as fundamentally flawed. It is argued that people are free agents, not governed by external laws but capable of taking independent decisions. An opposing set of beliefs, 'the qualitative paradigm', therefore emerged. Broadly speaking, those adhering to a qualitative paradigm believe that the social world is not fixed and external, but varies with time and place, and that human behaviour is not dictated by universal laws, but by the shared meanings people hold. As a result, it is not possible for researchers to be objective and value-free. Given these two premises, it is considered inappropriate for researchers to manipulate and control people and events as this alters the way they behave. Qualitative researchers therefore have a commitment to naturalism – studying people in their natural environment. This provides the broad methodological approach within the qualitative paradigm.

It can be seen that in terms of what constitutes knowledge, there is considerable divergence between the qualitative and quantitative paradigms. However, despite such obvious differences both these paradigms have been increasingly criticized by those who believe that they place too much emphasis and importance on the role of the researcher. For example, although qualitative researchers recognize the importance of studying people in a natural setting and acknowledge that their own values can influence their results, ultimately it is still the researcher who takes the lead in deciding what is knowledge.

Critics of both qualitative and quantitative research argue that true power is still vested primarily with the researcher. They further believe that 'telling things as they are' and leaving them unchanged is not sufficient (see Reason & Bradbury 2001). The first set of arguments was summarized by Elliot (1991) as follows:

> *Whether the techniques generate psychometric measures, ethnographies or grounded theories does not matter. They are all symbolic of the power of the researchers to define valid knowledge.*

> (Elliot 1991, p46)

Dissatisfaction with both qualitative and quantitative research has resulted in the emergence of much more radical and political interpretations of research underpinned by the need to empower people and assist them to change their situation. These shifts in ideology about the purpose of research reflect a more general move away from an uncritical acceptance of the value of traditional or scientific knowledge (theory) towards a greater emphasis on personal or experiential knowledge, and action orientated research. This trend is mirrored in much of the recent nursing literature, and attention is now turned to these debates.

WAYS OF KNOWING: AN OVERVIEW

As already indicated, there are generally considered to be several different types of knowledge or 'ways of knowing'. Cohen et al (2000), for example, differentiate between experience, research and reasoning as ways of generating knowledge whereas Moody (1990) talks in terms of folklore, wisdom and scientific knowledge. Broadly speaking, several authors, by implication at least, distinguish the *source* of knowledge and how it is generated from the *type* of knowledge that results. For instance, Burns and Grove (1993) state that you can know a person, comprehend facts, acquire a skill, or master a subject with emphasis here being placed on different ways of knowing. They also suggest that nursing utilizes

knowledge from many different sources such as:

- Tradition (custom and practice – 'it's always been done this way')
- Authority (based on expertise and power)
- Borrowing (from older disciplines such as medicine or sociology)
- Trial and error ('try it and see')
- Experience ('it worked for me')
- A role model or mentor (not dissimilar to authority).

Within the nursing profession much of the debate about the relative value of differing forms of knowledge can be traced to a seminal paper by Carper (1978). She argued that nurses draw upon four types of knowledge to inform their practice and she termed these: empirics; aesthetics, ethics and personal knowledge. The characteristics of these differing forms of knowledge are summarized in Box 1.1.

Chinn and Kramer (1991) contend that all the above types or 'patterns' of knowledge are required by nurses. However, in most disciplines, scientific knowledge (empirics) is traditionally the most highly prized, since possession of a unique 'body of knowledge' is one of the main characteristics of a profession. Indeed the power of a profession lies primarily in its claim to have access to specialist knowledge; the more unique the knowledge and the less it is understandable to lay people, the greater the power (Eraut 1994). It is therefore not surprising that nursing, in its desire to compete with medicine, initially placed great emphasis on scientific knowledge (Burns & Grove 1993, Chinn & Kramer 1991, Meleis 1991, Moody 1990, Rose & Parker 1994). This has also been the case in other disciplines aspiring to professional status such as teaching (Eraut 1994) and social work (Thompson 1995).

During the 1990s many practitioners became increasingly disenchanted with scientific knowledge and sought instead to highlight the value of practical and experiential knowledge. Once again, myriad terms have been used but the essential argument turns on the relationship between knowing *about* something (expressed as facts and theories), knowing *how to do* something (in a practical sense), and how both relate to experience and intuition (Reason 1994).

Kenny (1993), rather prophetically, suggested that the perceived failure of nursing theory would result in an increasing 'reification' of the experiential components of nursing. This was reflected in growing calls to develop the intuitive aspects of nursing (Rose & Parker 1994) in the form of 'personal

Box 1.1 Differing forms of knowledge

Empirics

This is scientific nursing knowledge in the form of theories and models that can be tested against data gathered directly by studying the physical or social world. The purpose of this type of knowledge is to describe, explain and eventually predict events. Empirical knowledge can be written down and learned as a set of ideas or principles constituting a 'body of knowledge'.

Aesthetics

Aesthetics represents the artistic side of nursing, and is made visible through the actions, bearing, conduct and interaction of nurses with others (generally their patients). It involves engaging, interpreting and envisaging. To be engaged requires the direct involvement of self on an experiential rather than a cognitive level. It is about being rather than thinking. Interpretation is the process of making sense of and creating responses arising from interaction or engagement, whilst envisioning is about using knowledge to see or create new possibilities for change and growth. Aesthetics is not expressed in language but rather is experienced (Chinn & Kramer 1991).

Ethics

Ethics is moral knowledge, a matter of what 'ought' to be, what is good or right. It involves having to make difficult decisions for which there are no prescriptive answers. Thus in contrast to scientific knowledge (empirics) ethics cannot be tested against reality as ethical decisions are underpinned by beliefs and values rather than facts.

Personal knowledge

This involves the inner experience of being self aware, the rationale being that in order to know others you have to know yourself first. Personal knowledge is seen as essential for the therapeutic use of self in nursing.

the terms 'know that' and 'know how' to highlight this dichotomy.

These two types of knowledge should be complementary but in the late 1980s and 1990s 'know that', as Kenny (1993) predicted, became increasingly devalued, and 'know how' was seen by many as the way forward for nursing. This resulted in a growing tendency to 'undermine the rational in favour of the intuitive' (Bradshaw 1995), with some arguing that only practitioners can develop legitimate theory (Tolley 1995). Thompson (1995) believes that although appealing, the myth of 'theoryless practice' should be resisted and calls for an appropriate balance to be achieved between propositional (what he terms 'formal') knowledge and practical (informal) knowledge. As Eraut (1994, p42) so cogently points out, 'to recognize that uncodifiable practical knowledge exists need not imply that stored, written knowledge is irrelevant'.

Debates about the value and relative contribution of theoretical and experiential knowledge continue with new concepts and definitions being introduced. For example, Herbig et al (2001) suggest that the notion of 'experience guided working' captures elements of experience in a more tangible form that is more readily taught. Similarly King and Macleod Clark (2002) have recently sought to create closer links between 'intuitive' practice on the one hand and 'analytic thinking' on the other, arguing that intuition is only really useful when used in a symbiotic fashion with a more careful analysis of a situation. Others have taken the debate further by suggesting that intuition is in fact 'lawful, observable, measurable' (Effken 2001). It is the push towards evidence-based practice that has once again raised tensions between 'intuitive' processes and 'measurable research based evidence' (King & Macleod Clark 2002). French (2002), in a thought-provoking review, argues that 'evidence-based' practice is something of a paradox because the term itself is ill-defined and subject to differing interpretations. In a careful consideration of the extensive literature, French (2002) suggests that current conceptualizations of evidence-based practice vary but all comprise differing permutations of five components, these being:

- Research findings
- Information management approaches
- Professional practice development
- Clinical judgement/problem-solving
- Ways of service delivery, for example, managed care.

knowledge' (Sweeny 1994) or 'alternative theoretical frameworks' based on a tacit understanding (Lauder 1994) and 'informal' theories (Pryjmachuk 1996). This development is a facet of the basic tension apparent in most practice disciplines between propositional (theoretical) knowledge and practical (experiential) knowledge, with Ryle (1949) coining

Most definitions still see traditional, largely quantitative, research findings as providing the most robust evidence. Tellingly, while clinical judgement figures in French's (2002) analysis, what is conspicuous by its absence is any reference to the knowledge held by patients themselves being counted as 'evidence'. For Evans (1999), this raises searching questions of an ethical nature about the values and perspectives that inform health care. He calls for a more holistic approach to what constitutes evidence:

> An understanding of illness that reunites the psychological with the experiential will, it has been suggested, require a far richer and more varied conception of evidence than that previously at stake in 'evidence-based' medicine, taking more seriously patients' conceptions of their own value and goals.
>
> (Evans 1999, p19)

Clearly such concerns go to the very heart of debates surrounding the role of 'Consumers in the NHS' (DoH 2002) and the 'Expert Patient' initiative (DoH 2001), which mandate that we adopt a 'far richer and more varied conception of evidence'.

TOWARDS A MORE DIVERSE VIEW OF 'EVIDENCE'

Some of the most telling critiques of the 'traditional' view of evidence (that based either on 'research', whether quantitative or qualitative, or the 'intuition' of professional groups) have come from within critical theory and participatory research paradigms (see also Chapters 5 and 6). Such debates are wide ranging and cannot be given a detailed consideration here. However, one recent example from within the participative inquiry paradigm highlights the potential value of a more holistic orientation.

Park (2001), in a discussion on the relationship between knowledge and participatory research, suggests that there are three broad categories of knowledge. He terms these: representational knowledge; relational knowledge; and reflective knowledge. The purpose of *representational knowledge* is to describe, explain or understand a phenomenon. It comprises two sub-types. Functional knowledge is the equivalent of traditional scientific knowledge associated with the positivist paradigm and seeks to establish correlational or causal relationships. In contrast, interpretive knowledge, as a sub-type of representational knowledge, is primarily concerned with understanding the meanings people bring to situations. Such knowledge is typical of qualitative

methods such as phenomenology. Although there is a difference in emphasis between functional and interpretative knowledge, both, to a greater or lesser extent, are determined by the researcher.

In contrast, *relational knowledge* is primarily concerned with 'knowing' a person, both affectively and cognitively. It is not descriptive, or even about meanings, but more about feelings. Relational knowledge is reciprocal and based on respect, caring, security, authenticity and trust.

Finally, for Park (2001), *reflective knowledge* is concerned with bringing about change by reflecting on and agreeing the values which inform the world in which we live. Park (2001) concludes that:

> We cannot understand knowledge in terms of a narrow definition of rationality that recognizes only the technical. We cannot privilege knowledge inherited from positivist sciences ... we need to be conscious of cultivating all three forms of knowledge.
>
> (Park 2001, p88)

Nursing and other practice-based disciplines have much to learn from such an approach. We would argue that the current conceptualization of evidence-based practice places far too much emphasis on representational, and especially functional, knowledge. Moreover, the 'relationship' between those providing and those receiving care is still viewed as hierarchical, or at best paternalistic, with certain types of 'expertise' (be that based on theoretical knowledge or professional experience) being privileged. Relational knowledge therefore needs to be reconsidered. To compound matters, the values that currently underpin health and social care, such as independence and autonomy, often disadvantage the most deprived and needy members of society.

> Autonomy as an isolated value is incapable of underpinning any shared, societal responsibility for the health of its members, including the least advantaged. As health inequalities widen (both within and between societies) the moral claims for alternative communitarian values become more urgent.
>
> (Evans 1999, p24)

However, there are signs that the emphasis is beginning to shift, at least in terms of the perceived relationship between the professions and those whom they serve. An example of this is the 'Expert Patient Initiative' (DoH 2001), which recognizes that the most significant future challenges to health and welfare systems will be posed by chronic illnesses, and that in such circumstances it is usually the 'patient' (we use the word advisedly) that 'knows' their condition best. There is now recognition that their knowledge and experience have 'for too long been an untapped resource' (DoH 2001, p5). The *Expert Patient* initiative promotes a fundamental shift in the way that diseases are managed so that:

> The era of the patient as a passive recipient of care is changing and being replaced by a new emphasis on the relationship between the NHS and the people whom it serves, one in which health professionals and patients are genuine partners seeking together the best solutions to each patient's problems, one in which patients are empowered with information and contribute ideas to help in their treatment and care.
>
> (DoH 2001, p9)

This is not seen as an 'anti-professional' stance but rather one that acknowledges differing but complementary forms of expertise, one based on the patients' experience of illness, social circumstances, values, preferences and attitudes to risk, the other underpinned by the professionals' skills at diagnosis, treatment options and other forms of specialist knowledge. To be effective, the 'Expert Patient' initiative requires new ways of relating and working. Insights can be found in some of the recent literature.

Liaschenko (1997), for example, provides a potentially useful framework. She believes that, especially in chronic illness, differing kinds of knowledge are required. She identifies three broad types of knowledge that might inform nursing and, we would suggest, health and social care, more widely. These are:

- Case knowledge – This comprises biomedical, disembodied knowledge of a particular condition, for instance stroke
- Patient knowledge – This is best viewed as a 'case in context'. In other words, information about a person's social circumstances, level of support and so on provide a better understanding of the impact of the 'stroke' and the resources that can be mobilized
- Person knowledge – This is based on understanding of an individual's personal circumstances, beliefs and value systems.

Liaschenko (1997) contends that patient and person knowledge are decidedly different and that for 'interventionist' disciplines, that is those which aim to do things to or for people, person knowledge is often essential in order to promote and maintain individual integrity. However, she believes that person knowledge is not appropriate in all contexts.

Eliciting person knowledge may not be relevant in situations where the primary aim is to cure a condition and 'move a person out'. Person knowledge is not therefore intrinsically desirable and may be unacceptably intrusive in certain contexts. Conversely, person knowledge is usually essential where there is an ongoing relationship and its value, but also potentially resource intensive and time consuming nature, has to be recognized. For Liaschenko (1997), this raises political questions, not only for professionals, but also for society more generally, about the type of health care that we 'envision' (requiring Park's reflective knowledge). More holistic care cannot be achieved unless the skills required are seen as not only legitimate but also important. Liaschenko doubts that this is the case as:

> … the kind of attentiveness this (person) knowledge demands is increasingly being seen as fluff, not essential to a vision of health care in which people are cared for only on the basis of case and patient knowledge.
>
> (Liaschenko 1997, p37)

Taking these arguments a step further, Liaschenko and Fisher (1999) contend that if knowledge is to be 'useful' to practitioners then it must be presented in a way that 'makes sense' to them. Citing several studies, they suggest that traditional nursing theories are rarely used unless practitioners are required to do so by a licensing or similar authority. For Liaschenko and Fisher (1999), therefore, neither scientific nor everyday knowledge is entirely appropriate. Rather, they argue nurses need to better understand and thereby to facilitate the 'relational practices' that are required to forge links and connections between case, patient and person knowledge. Patient knowledge is only created, and only relevant, in a health care context and is forged by the fusion of case knowledge with person knowledge so as to highlight the needs of a particular person at a particular point in their health care career. To achieve this requires social knowledge about the preferences, expectations and values of the people involved. Such knowledge enables the 'system' of health care to run smoothly and helps the patient to 'negotiate' their way through a potentially confusing reality.

The idea of 'relational practices' is clearly synonymous with Park's (2001) concept of 'relational knowledge', just as 'case knowledge' can be seen to equate with 'representational knowledge'. We believe that both types of 'knowing' are important, indeed essential, to nursing and health care practice. However, case knowledge, which is largely biomedical in nature, is of itself unlikely to be sufficient and other types of representational knowledge are also needed.

Griffin (Griffin & Ndidi 1997), for example, argues that if individuals are to be empowered and enabled to use service systems to their best advantage, then they need certain forms of understanding. Furthermore, if professionals are to facilitate such an understanding, they too require a thorough grasp of four types of knowledge:

- Structural knowledge – of the way health and social services work
- Communicative knowledge – and the ability to interpret the language used by both patients and professionals
- Cultural knowledge – and the influence of differing ethnic and racial beliefs on the way that health and illness are construed and the expectations individuals have of service systems
- Social knowledge – of the individual, their resources and background.

(after Griffin & Ndidi 1997)

Griffin (Griffin & Ndidi 1997) suggests that practitioners can utilize these four types of knowledge to enable individuals to exert greater control over their situation. However, achieving genuine partnerships between all those involved in health and social care is likely to require a considerable reorientation not only of professional practice, but also of the culture that implicitly underpins the institutions that constitute the 'system'. Such a culture is largely based on the notion of the 'professional as expert', which is deeply embedded in the professional psyche (Qureshi et al 2000). However, Post (2001) contends that there is a need for a shift in values towards an 'epistemology of humility' that explicitly recognizes that the 'constituency' itself, i.e. disabled or ill people and their families, possesses the most important forms of knowledge. This requires the use of what Park (2001) calls 'reflective knowledge', which addresses the morals and values upon which our health and social care institutions are based.

However, despite the rhetoric of empowerment and involvement, when professions 'reflect' upon their value systems, such reflections often belie the ideal of forging genuine partnerships. For example, the 'Colorado Nursing Think Tank' (Fawcett et al 2001) recently identified 'ten unfinished issues' it believed must be addressed in order to 'help save

the discipline from extinction' (p138). The first of these 'what constitutes the evidence in evidence-based practice' was cited at the beginning of this chapter. The other nine are as follows:

- What moral, philosophical, ethical, cultural, conceptual/theoretical, and historical foundations of the discipline are evident in current nursing practices and research?
- Will there be convergence of leadership and scholarship and if so, how?
- What is the interface between discipline and profession and how can we put *nursing* back into clinical practice?
- To what extent is science (theory and research) integrated in nursing; is the integration adequate or is more work needed?
- What is the relationship between scientific and clinical knowledge?
- Is 'theory' part of the other ways of knowing (besides empirics) and what types of theory are important for nursing?
- What, or who, constitutes the scientific community in nursing?
- How can we clarify the paradigms of nursing research (types of research)?
- What are the interrelationships and linkages among nursing research, theory and practice, and which comes first?

All of these questions seem particularly relevant in the context of this chapter, indeed for the book as a whole. Ironically it seems to us that the second question relating to the foundations of the discipline as evidenced in 'current nursing practices and research' (Park's (2001) reflective knowledge) are answered by the authors themselves in the remaining eight questions they pose. All of these are what we might term 'profession-centric' issues and do not mirror Post's (2001) call to move towards an 'epistemology of humility'. Indeed it is likely that none of these issues would be identified as important by those who use the 'system', and it might better advance nursing (or indeed any other profession) if our reflections demonstrated more of the humility that Post (2001) suggests.

CONCLUSION

This chapter began with an increasingly important question about 'what constitutes the evidence in evidence-based practice?' (Fawcett et al 2001).

We are aware that we have not provided a definitive answer, but consider that a single correct answer is neither possible nor desirable. Rather, our goal has been to suggest differing conceptualizations of what is 'possible' (Gaventa & Cornwall 2001). Readers may of course disagree with our analysis but that is the purpose of stimulating debate, and if we have caused you to at least reflect upon and consider the possibilities inherent within partnership working and what this means in terms of 'whose knowledge counts', then we will have achieved our goal.

Exercise 1.1

Think about the parallels between Carper's (1978) definition of empirics, aesthetics and ethics, and Post's

(2001) suggestions of representational, relational and reflective knowledge. What are the similarities and differences between these? How useful are they for informing practice?

Exercise 1.2

Imagine that you were asked to identify 'ten unfinished issues' from the perspectives of users of health and social care. What do you think the issues would be, and how would they differ from the issues identified by Fawcett et al (2001)?

References

Audi R (1998) *Epistemology: A Contemporary Introduction to the Theory of Knowledge*. London: Routledge.

Barnes M (1999) *Public expectations: From paternalism to partnership, changing relationships in health and health services*. Policy Futures for UK Health, No. 10. London: Nuffield Trust.

Bernard M and Phillips J (2000) The challenge of ageing in tomorrow's Britain. *Ageing and Society* 20(1): 33–54.

Bradshaw A (1995) What are nurses doing to patients? A review of theories of nursing past and present. *Journal of Clinical Nursing* 4: 81–92.

Burns N and Grove SK (1993) *The Practice of Nursing Research: Conduct, Critique and Utilization*, 2nd edn. Philadelphia, PA: WB Saunders.

Carper BA (1978) Fundamental patterns of knowing in nursing. *Advances in Nursing Science* 1(1): 13–23.

Chinn PL and Kramer MK (1991) *Theory and Nursing: A Systematic Approach*. St Louis, MO: Mosby Year Book.

Cohen L, Manion L and Morrison K (2000) *Research Methods in Education*. London: Routledge/Falmer.

Denzin NK and Lincoln YS (eds) (1994) *Handbook of Qualitative Research*. Thousand Oaks, CA: Sage.

Denzin NK and Lincoln YS (eds) (2000) *Handbook of Qualitative Research*, 2nd edn. Thousand Oaks, CA: Sage.

Department of Health (2001) *The Expert Patient: A New Approach to Chronic Disease Management for the 21st Century*. London: HMSO.

Department of Health (2002) Consensus in NHS Research: Advisory Group on Consumer Involvement in Research and Development in the Department of Health. Hampshire: Consumers in Research Support Unit.

Effken JA (2001) Informational basis for expert intuition. *Journal of Advanced Nursing* 34(2): 246–255.

Elliot J (1991) *Action Research for Educational Change*. Milton Keynes: Open University Press.

Eraut M (1994) *Developing Professional Knowledge and Competence*. London: The Falmer Press.

Evans M (1999) *Ethics: Reconciling conflicting values in health policy*. Policy futures for UK health, No. 9. London: Nuffield Trust.

Fawcett J, Neuman B, Walker PH et al (2001) Saving the discipline: Top 10 unfinished issues to inform the nursing debate in the new millennium. *Journal of Advanced Nursing* 35(1): 138.

French P (2002) What is evidence on evidence-based nursing? An epistemological concern. *Journal of Advanced Nursing* 37(3): 250–257.

Gaventa J and Cornwall A (2001) Power and knowledge. In: Reason P and Bradbury H (eds) *Handbook of Action Research: Participative Inquiry and Practice*. London: Sage, pp70–80.

Griffin F and Ndidi U (1997) *Discovering Knowledge in Practice Settings*. In: Thorne SE and Hayes VE (eds) *Nursing Praxis: Knowledge and Action*. Thousand Oaks: Sage, pp39–53.

Guba EG and Lincoln YS (1989) *Fourth Generation Evaluation*. Newbury Park, DC: Sage.

Guba EG and Lincoln YS (1994) Competing paradigms in qualitative research. In: Denzin NK and Lincoln YS (eds) *Handbook of Qualitative Research*. Thousand Oaks, CA: Sage, pp105–117.

Herbig B, Büssing A and Ewert T (2001) The role of tacit knowledge in the work context of nursing. *Journal of Advanced Nursing* 34(5): 687–696.

Hockey L (1996) The nature and purpose of research. In: Cormack DFS (ed) *The Research Process in Nursing*, 3rd edn. Oxford: Blackwell Science, pp3–13.

Kenny T (1993) Nursing models fail in practice. *British Journal of Nursing* 2(2): 133–136.

King L and Macleod Clark J (2002) Intuition and the development of expertise in surgical ward and intensive care nurses. *Journal of Advanced Nurisng* 37(4): 322–329.

Lauder W (1994) An exploratory study of the alternative theoretical frameworks of student nurses. *Journal of Clinical Nursing* 3: 185–191.

Liaschenko J (1997) Knowing the patient. In: Thorne SE and Hays VE (eds) *Nursing Praxis: Knowledge and Action.* Thousand Oaks, CA: Sage.

Liaschenko J and Fisher A (1999) Theorising the knowledge that nurses use in the conduct of their work. *Scholarly Inquiry for Nursing Practice: An International Journal* **13**(1): 29–41.

Meleis A (1991) *Theoretical Nursing: Developments and Progress*, 2nd edn. Philadelphia, PA: Lippincott.

Moody LE (1990) *Advancing Nursing Science Through Research*, Vol 1, Newbury Park, DC: Sage.

Park P (2001) Knowledge and Participatory Research. In: Reason P and Bradbury H (eds) *Handbook of Action Research: Participative Inquiry and Practice.* London: Sage, pp81–90.

Post SG (2001) Comments on research in the social sciences pertaining to Alzheimer's Disease: a more humble approach. *Aging and Mental Health*, 5(Supplement 1): S17–S19.

Pryjmachuk S (1996) A nursing perspective on the inter-relationship between theory, research and practice. *Journal of Advanced Nursing* **23**: 679–684.

Qureshi H, Bamford C, Nicholas E et al (2000) *Outcomes in Social Care Practice: Developing an Outcomes Focus in Care Management and User Surveys.* York: Social Policy Research Unit, University of York.

Reason P (ed) (1994) *Participation in Human Inquiry.* London: Sage.

Reason P and Bradbury H (2001) *Handbook of Action Research: Participative Inquiry and Practice.* London: Sage.

Rose P and Parker D (1994) Nursing: an integration of the art and science within the experience of the practitioner. *Journal of Advanced Nursing* **20**: 1004–1010.

Ryle G (1949) *The Concept of Mind.* London: Hutchinson.

Sweeny NM (1994) A concept analysis of personal knowledge: application to nursing education. *Journal of Advanced Nursing* **20**: 917–924.

Thompson N (1995) *Theory and Practice in Health and Social Welfare.* Buckingham: Open University Press.

Tolley KA (1995) Theory from practice for practice: is this reality? *Journal of Advanced Nursing* **21**: 184–190.

Further reading

Carper BA (1978) Fundamental patterns of knowing in nursing. *Advances in Nursing Science* **1**(1): 13–23.

Department of Health (2001) *The Expert Patient: a New Approach to Chronic Disease Management for the 21st Century.* London: Stationery Office.

Liaschenko J and Fisher A (1999) Theorising the knowledge that nurses use in the conduct of their work. *Scholarly Inquiry for Nursing Practice: An International Journal* **13**(1): 29–41.

Reason P and Bradbury H (2001) *Handbook of Action Research: Participative Inquiry and Practice.* London: Sage.

Chapter 2

The context of nursing and health care research

John Daly, David R Thompson, Esther Chang, Karen Hancock

CHAPTER CONTENTS

INTRODUCTION

This chapter explores the relationship between policy and research. It seeks to demonstrate how research is driven by ideological and political factors and how policy is formulated at various levels in society and implemented. Consideration is given to other factors, including professional, political and economic drivers. The way in which these and other motivating forces influence choices about research activity is examined and discussed. In addition, the chapter addresses the way in which research can in turn influence policy. In particular, it discusses strategies that clinicians can use to shape health policy and become more involved in the decision-making process.

Key issues

- The relationship between policy and research
- The formulation and implementation of health policy
- How research can influence health policy
- How clinicians can help share health policy and become more involved in decision-making processes

WHAT IS POLICY?

The word 'policy' is used freely in almost all professional contexts in contemporary society. A policy is 'a purposeful plan of action directed toward an issue of concern in the public or private sector' (Sudduth 1999, p219). In everyday life we hear of the need for policy on a number of levels in society on a regular basis. At the peak level in organized democratic society, government is expected to formulate public policy to ensure equitable and efficient use of resources for the public good. However, one can apply the evidence-based principles of such policy to the private sector, the individual health care setting, a professional organization, a disease/illness, a specific sector of the population by need, or a country's population group (DePalma 2002).

Health policy may be defined as 'those actions of governments and other actors in society that are aimed at improving the health of populations' (Niessen et al 2000, p2). Common themes in health care policy are those of cost control, efficiency, equity and client focus (Commonwealth of Australia 1999, p59). Contextual factors will include political, economic and social climates, demographics and technological development. At a more micro-level, this will also include organizational resources, professional cultures and competing political agendas.

WHO MAKES HEALTH POLICY?

Health policy is formulated and implemented by government and other organizations, including professional and regulatory bodies, but it is also influenced by economic arguments (mainly cost containment or 'value for money') and by changes in public attitudes and expectations. In Western society, although health managers make health policy, doctors are the main influential group in health policy decision-making (Gott 2000a). Indeed, medicine is unique in shaping and constraining health policy. This is largely due to the fact that health care has been primarily practised in the last century in the context of hospitals. Recently, there has been a shift towards community-based health care due to increased institutional health care costs and changing demographics. Thus, there is also a shift in emphasis in health policy as a result, changing from a prevent/cure/care orientation to a community/primary health care emphasis. As a result, other health care providers and consumers can take a more leading role, particularly public health nurses who are community-based.

One way of influencing health policy is to gain the attention of those who make policy, health care consumers and the public who elect governments by media influence (Jennings 2001). The media can be a powerful vehicle for raising awareness and gaining support concerning important issues (Jennings 2001).

NURSING AND HEALTH POLICY

Nurses as a group feel the impact of changes in health policy and systems (Commonwealth of Australia 1999). Despite nurses being the largest group of the health sector workforce, they are not the most influential (Gott 2000a). Nurses tend to carry out health policies decided by governments, who in turn are influenced by doctors. Nurses can experience internal conflict because health policy that is based on meeting economic targets is not congruent with professional beliefs and values surrounding quality health care delivery (Gott 2000a). However, research suggests that nurses' participation in the policy-making process varies over time and over issues (West & Scott 2000). Although nurses and other health professionals are not automatically included in health policy decision-making, there has been a move towards growing consumer participation in policy-making within the health system. In the United Kingdom and Australia, for example, frameworks for managing the quality of health services make explicit the need for opportunities for health consumers to participate collaboratively with health organizations and service providers in health service planning, delivery, monitoring and evaluation at all levels (Department of Health 2000a, New South Wales Health 1999). Thus, rather than dictating health policy, the democratic process in Western societies mandates that governments take account of public concerns and seek to work with people rather than 'at' them (Gott 2000a). However, wide public consultation regarding policy is rarely sought by government, and though rhetoric exhorts participation, it is usually limited to certain interest groups. Nevertheless, Western government health policies are moving from a secondary (hospital) to primary (community-based) care sector focus, and nurses have the capacity and are in a prime position to assist governments' moves in this direction (Gott 2000b).

The push for greater nursing involvement in health policy stems from the belief that health policy is related in an important way to the quality of patient care (West & Scott 2000). Therefore, if clinical care is to be improved, nurses need to take a more active public role in making and implementing health policy at both local and national levels (West & Scott 2000). However, in order for this to occur, nurses need to have political awareness in terms of the range of structural and ideological factors underpinning the emergence of policies (Hannigan & Burnard 2000). Then they can analyse the impact of various policies on nursing and health care. Health policy is an important way in which clinicians can have an impact on their organization's functioning and structure.

Summary

- Health policy refers to actions of governments or other actors in society that are aimed at improving the health of populations.
- Nurses lack influence in policy decision-making.
- Nurses should be more involved in health policy decision-making and influencing the political agenda because policy is related to quality of patient care.

Exercise 2.1

Reflect and make notes on the following question: Why are nurses currently in a good position to increase their influence on health policy?

THE ROLE OF RESEARCH IN INFLUENCING POLICY

In the current climate, research is one of the most important tools for influencing health policy. Policy makers can use research in at least three different ways: as a source of data, as a source of ideas, and as a source of argument that emphasizes the conflictual, collective and incremental nature of the policy (West & Scott 2000). National initiatives such as the NHS research and development strategy in the UK initiated in the early 1990s (Department of Health 1991) aim to ensure that the health service is underpinned by high-quality research, by a framework for the management of research, and by a clarification of the roles and functions of key players within an explicit infrastructure. The strategy aims to create a knowledge-based health service in which clinical, managerial and policy decisions are based on sound information about research findings. Thus, the potential contribution of nursing is now explicitly acknowledged in the research enterprise (Department of Health 2000b).

Research has an important role to play in helping nursing to establish evidence-based practice. The practice of evidence-based care means integrating individual expertise with the best available external evidence from systematic research (Sackett et al

1997). Although there were many developments in nursing research from the 1950s to the 1980s there were still many areas of nursing practice based on tradition rather than practice (Read 1998). The 1990s saw a significant push towards evidence-based research in nursing as well as other health-related areas. In terms of policy, position papers or recommendations to policy makers should report the level of evidence available and enunciate the evidence-based rationale for all recommendations (DePalma 2002).

Although research is important in influencing policy, one reason why research may appear to have little impact on policy is that the timing may not be right. Factors such as election cycles, current public opinion, and the timing of stages of the process by which policy development occurs may be stronger influences than the actual research (West & Scott 2000). However, sometimes despite good timing, influences such as management experience, professional judgement, and statistical and economic information may have a greater impact on decision-making in policy (West & Scott 2000).

Many societal practices are driven by the decisions of government policy makers (Jennings 2001). However, it is argued that in reality, research is not used as much as it should be to affect policy (Jennings 2001). Research is but one of several ingredients that make up policy decisions. Factors such as competing alternatives and conflicting objectives among decision-makers, economic dynamics and emotional overtones affect policy decisions. For example, policies governing breast and prostate cancer were influenced more by persuasive arguments and public attention than research evidence. Thus public demands overwhelmed research in the establishment of policy (Fletcher 1997). Others concur that the link between scientific evidence and formally stated objectives could be stronger (Niessen et al 2000). Policy decisions tend to be the outcome of complicated political processes among parties with different interests (Stronks et al 1997).

Some commentators suggest that it is difficult to conclude that research has had a significant impact on the direction or implementation of government policy (Weller & Veale 1999). However, in the United Kingdom and Australia, for example, governments have acknowledged that health care decisions were not based sufficiently on sound evidence and they have instituted initiatives to improve the situation, including targeted research funding for applying evidence-based clinical practice and evaluating outcomes. In Australia, the Health and Medical Research Strategic Review Implementation Committee in 2001 recommended to the National Health and Medical Research Council (NHMRC) the development of new strategies in public health and health services research. The intention was to facilitate the interaction between research and policy development to ensure that high-quality research is available to inform health policy and practice. In response, a Joint Health Services Research Grants programme was developed. A States and Commonwealth Research issues forum was also developed in 2001 by the NHMRC to determine a range of priorities for research in areas of direct relevance to the provision of health services. Thus, the link between research and policy is increasingly seen as vital among government funding bodies.

Summary

The increased emphasis on evidence-based practice in health care means that research has a great impact on health policy. However, research is not used as much as it could be to affect policy. Other influences include whether the research is timely, conflicting objectives among decision-makers, economic and emotional factors.

Research can affect policy in three ways: as a source of data, ideas and argument.

Exercise 2.2

Jot down as many strategies as you can think of at national level that have been introduced to ensure that evidence-based research is used more in the formulation of policy? How effective have these policies been within your own working environment?

WHAT RESEARCH GETS FUNDED?

Although, as discussed above, public opinion and persuasive lobbying are the major determinants of policy rather than evidence, the priorities of government health policy are also influenced by the burden of disease and injury. Cardiovascular disease, cancer, injuries, mental health problems, diabetes mellitus and asthma are major national health priorities in most Western countries. Health funding distribution is also influenced by societal trends. While advances in medicine and technology have increased survival

for patients with chronic illnesses, unfortunately, increased longevity does not necessarily mean increased quality of life. The increasing burden of chronic disease has led to increased priority in funding research into chronic illnesses. A corollary of increased longevity is that older people represent the largest group of consumers of health care. The fact that this number will continue to grow has resulted in increased funding.

Health services research is a multidisciplinary activity in which collaboration occurs between health professionals, health economists, statisticians, medical sociologists, epidemiologists, information scientists and operational researchers. It involves the identification of the health care needs of communities and the study of the provision, effectiveness and use of health services. Government departments commission research in accordance with policies whereby health services researchers have to compete for funds alongside biomedical researchers with more impressive track records. However, much nursing research does not easily fit within a medical model of research (Department of Health 2000b). Consequently, such research often misses out on competitive funding. Other reasons for lack of nursing research funding are the relative lack of experience and strength as a discipline. The undernourished research base in nursing poorly serves the public, policy makers and members of the health care team. Without targeted investment the health service will fail to deliver the benefits of evidence-based practice (Rafferty et al 2003).

In 2001, the Australian Health Advisory Committee (HAC) identified mental health and biotechnology as priority health issues for research, and these areas receive funding from the Department of Health and Ageing. The HAC deals with the following priority issues: assessing the evidence on socio-economic position and health; preventive health; development of a manual for health workers to deal with violence in rural and remote areas in Australia; conserving Australia's blood supply; and safety and quality in health care (Strategic Research Development Committee 2001).

Nursing research features as one of six of the most rapidly expanding sub fields within biomedicine (Dawson et al 1998). Indeed, compared with Australia and the United States, the UK is the most rapidly expanding producer of nursing publications (Traynor et al 2001). In a bibliometric study of UK nursing research between 1988–1995, Traynor et al distinguished between two types of research: endogenous and exogenous. The former term describes research that tends to be concerned with problems and issues to do with nursing as a profession, and the latter term describes research that is concerned with the nursing of patients (Traynor et al 2001). Interestingly, the endogenous papers when compared to exogenous ones had a more rapid growth in output, fewer authors, appeared in highly esteemed journals but had much less chance of obtaining external funding. Thus, this suggests that although nursing research into professional issues is being increasingly published, it does not appear to be a priority of funding bodies.

Areas of nursing research that are on the agenda of policy makers include primary health care; evidence-based health care and clinical effectiveness; promoting a consumer orientation; the organisation of care in hospitals; recruitment and retention of nurses; quality and clinical governance (West & Scott 2000). Nursing research that is done in areas of national interest, such as cardiovascular disease, cancer and mental health, is probably more likely to be funded by government, research councils, charities or industry. This suggests that access to a stable and sustainable funding source for nursing research has proved elusive (Rafferty 2002). Indeed, there has been debate and intermittent support for the idea of a nursing research council, in the UK at least (Rafferty et al 2000). Although some have argued that a dedicated fund may lead to marginalization from mainstream funding sources, a more secure funding base for nursing research could strengthen the position of nursing. However, positive developments are occurring in the UK, for example, where increased funding has occurred as a result of alignment of political and professional research agendas, as well as, importantly, the availability of resources for investment alongside the political will to do so. Arguments for this investment were justified with research evidence: although nursing research has been growing at a rapid rate, as judged by the generation of research income and output, it was significantly underfunded in relation to other comparable professions such as teaching and social work, and benchmarked poorly against government investment in North America (Rafferty 2002, Rafferty et al 2003).

In addition to topical issues being more likely to be taken up by the policy-making community, quality of research is also important. Davis and Howden-Chapman (1996) found that factors detracting from success included: a poorly defined research question; inadequate consideration and piloting of methods;

lack of experience and low morale among researchers; inadequate funding and unrealistic timescales. In terms of the type of research that has the greatest impact on policy, research in Australia found that researchers appointed to full-time research positions in the biological sciences, irrespective of their source of funds, achieved higher visibility for their research than researchers who also had undergraduate teaching or clinical practice obligations (Bourke & Butler 1999). However, there is now more of a push away from the traditional university-based model of research to one characterized by the involvement of employers, practitioners and patients (Scott & West 2001). Such a strategy may provide an avenue for clinicians to have more of an impact on the research agenda and to conduct research in evaluation of health policy (Scott & West 2001).

Summary

- Health services research is a multidisciplinary activity in which collaboration occurs between health professionals, health economists, statisticians, medical sociologists, epidemiologists, information scientists and operational researchers.
- Reasons for lack of nursing research funding are the relative lack of experience and strength as a discipline as well as the fact that much of nursing research does not fit easily within a medical model.
- Areas of nursing research that are on the agenda of policy makers include primary health care; evidence-based health care and clinical effectiveness; promoting a consumer orientation; the organization of care in hospitals; recruitment and retention of nurses; quality and clinical governance.

Exercise 2.3

- What areas of health research are more or less likely to receive funding?
- Why do you think this is?

THE SHAPING OF RESEARCH POLICY

Nurses (including researchers) and nursing have generally responded to changes in the political environment and been less successful at shaping it. It has to be acknowledged that nurses and nursing must bear some of the responsibility for this situation. Much of the research conducted in nursing has been limited in terms of scale, quality and impact. Also, there has been no collective nursing voice within the health research policy arena and neither has nursing been clear in establishing and articulating research priorities. Further, much of the research agenda has been dominated by a biomedical paradigm, though a broader methodological perspective is increasingly being assumed. There may also have been reluctance among nurses to engage in the public policy arena because of a perceived lack of knowledge in areas such as political science and economics (Scott & West 2001).

Most health research priorities are aligned to major diseases and health concerns. Although high-quality primary research is being done by nurses in areas of national priority – such as cancer, heart disease and mental health – comparatively little of this work is being done across multiple centres, using a range of expertise, and developing systematically over many years into coherent national or international programmes. Neither is it done in collaboration with other disciplines. Rather depressingly, much research activity in nursing is still typified by small-scale projects, conducted in a single ward by a lone individual with limited or no resources. If nursing research is to have a significant impact in terms of health policy, it needs to move towards large-scale, thematic programmes of research in order to develop depth in the knowledge base and focus attention on real priorities (Thompson 2003).

For research to have an immediate impact on policy, it needs to be timed so that it is high on the political agenda (West & Scott 2000). Thus, important contemporary themes include primary care, evidence-based health care, service organization and delivery. Researchers and practitioners need to collaborate much more so as to influence the research agenda. There is a strong case for additional investment to develop a number of designated national centres of expertise (Department of Health 2000b). Certainly, a clear, coherent and sustained strategy is needed to ensure that the nursing contribution to key health priorities is realized and that the research agenda is properly informed by nursing expertise.

Because of the role that policy making has in influencing quality of nursing care, nurses should be involved in the decision-making policy process. Health professionals have great potential to influence health policy. As well as direct input into the policy-making process, they have the power to define needs and problems, to allocate resources and to control their own work as well as having power over people (West & Scott 2000). Not only are health professionals important in producing and disseminating knowledge related to policy, they also apply it to practice, thereby influencing the policy agenda (West & Scott 2000). Although health professionals, particularly nurses, are in theory in a powerful position, they need to apply strategies (discussed below) to increase the policy impact of their work.

THE ROLE OF NURSING LEADERS IN INFLUENCING NURSING RESEARCH POLICY

Nurses offer a unique contribution to health care due to their numbers, flexibility and the work they do (Commonwealth of Australia 2001). A World Health Organization (WHO) expert committee on nursing practice noted that because of their in-depth knowledge and experience, nurses have much to offer in the areas of health care assessment and policy development (WHO 1996). However, as leaders, nurses tend to lack a clear professional identity (Commonwealth of Australia 2001, Duffield & Franks 2001), often being seen as an invisible body (Price et al 2001). They tend to be excluded from health care decision- and policy-making fora (Borman & Biordi 1992, Duffield & Franks 2001).

It has been argued that one of the reasons for lack of clear leadership and visibility is that nurses lack confidence and represent themselves as an oppressed group (Fulton 1997). Nursing needs to face and deal with its insecurity, be more competent in dealing with change and market its skills more confidently (Fulton 1997). It also needs individuals in senior nursing positions to attain even more senior positions in the wider health care arena where policy and funding decisions are made that influence nursing practice (Duffield & Franks 2001). There seems little doubt that nurses need to be more forthcoming in contributing to health debates, and to express the important role that they play in positive patient outcomes (Duffield & Franks 2001). The nursing profession has often been divided and fragmented in its deliberations on policy issues and there is undoubtedly a need for the profession to have a unified voice and to provide leadership and strategic planning for research. Antrobus and Kitson (1999) propose the development of nursing policy units to develop the expertise necessary to analyse health policy, to assess the implications for clients and to communicate a professional response representing nursing as a body. They also suggest such a unit would need to portray itself as 'a credible research agency and "think tank" in its relationship to and influence with the government of the time' (Antrobus & Kitson 1999, p752).

To enable nurse leaders to operate effectively as both practice and policy shapers, Antrobus and Kitson (1999) argue that restructuring of career pathways for nurses is needed. This would involve bringing together central aspects of nursing practice and knowledge, combining this with roles which enable leaders to influence and shape policy and practice. However, the lack of consensus on nursing leadership has led to leadership development programmes for nurses that have overlooked nursing knowledge in favour of corporate and political skills (Antrobus & Kitson 1999).

While health policy to date has lacked input from nursing, some positive developments have taken place to help improve the situation. For example, in the UK, a Centre for Policy in Nursing Research has been established. Also within the UK, the Royal College of Nursing has established a research committee to advise on research policy matters, a chief officer to direct research activities and a professional adviser to coordinate efforts. At government level the Department of Health has a nursing research advisor who is responsible for influencing the research agenda. The RCN has developed a voice on the value of nursing which has credibility in the political sphere. However, there is a need for a strategic alliance of all key players representing the broad constituency of nursing, including government and the professional organizations.

There is much to learn from experiences in the United States where the establishment of the National Institute for Nursing Research has helped to identify priorities as part of a national nursing research agenda. These priorities include quality of care outcomes and their measurement, effectiveness of nursing interventions, symptom assessment and management, health care delivery systems, and health promotion and risk reduction (Hinshaw 2000).

Antrobus and Kitson (1999) conducted an ethnographic study of the role of nursing leadership in influencing and shaping health policy and nursing practice. They found a divide between the ideology and language used by nurses in practice and those of policy makers. The research data suggested that nursing leaders play an important role in providing an intermediary nursing voice between practitioners and policy-makers.

Summary

- Much of the research conducted in nursing has been limited in terms of scale, quality and impact. Also, there has been no collective nursing voice within the health research policy arena and neither has nursing been clear in establishing and articulating research priorities.
- Health professionals are in a good position to influence health policy because of the power (eg defining needs and problems, allocating resources etc), skills and knowledge they possess.
- Nurses and other health professionals indirectly shape policy by applying policy to day-to-day practice. However, they need to apply strategies to increase the policy impact of their work.

Exercise 2.4

Make notes on the reasons why nurse leaders lack a clear professional identity and representation as a visible body.

HOW DOES NURSING INFLUENCE POLICY?

Nurses can influence policy by demonstrating good nursing practice that is effective and sustainable (Gott 2000b). However, strategies other than evidence-based research are needed to influence policy decisions, such as educating and informing interested parties, and participating in policy debates (Buerhaus & Needleman 2000). This assumes that nurses are invited to these fora to enable them to have a presence, and deliver an articulate point of view. In the clinical setting, nurses must often 'jockey for a seat at the boardroom table'. Then nurses need to overcome their insecurities and raise controversial issues in a way that encourages discussion. In the area of policy, nurses also need to 'persuade disinterested parties who prefer the status quo' (Jennings 2001, p114). Part of the nurse's role is to educate other health service decision makers about the many roles of nurses. Salvage (1999) identified the following roles: expert clinicians, counsellors, managers, teachers, researchers, professors, policy-makers, civil servants and trade union leaders. Enhancing this awareness may increase decision-makers' under-standing of the role nurses play in the health and well-being of society, thereby influencing policy.

Although nursing as a representative body lacks visibility in the policy arena, national bodies such as the Royal College of Nursing of the United Kingdom and the Royal College of Nursing of Australia report that increasingly government and health care bodies are seeking their views on a wide range of nursing/health care related policy development issues. The Colleges respond to submissions, analyse draft pol-icy documents, attend public inquiries, and develop and circulate position statements on nursing and health care related issues to nurses, government, health care bodies and consumer organizations. They also raise issues of nursing importance to the national health agenda by publishing discussion documents. The aim of these documents is to stimu-late debate on the issues presented to assist in the informed development of policies and practices relating to nursing and health care (Royal College of Nursing Australia 2000).

OTHER STRATEGIES TO INCREASE THE IMPACT OF NURSING RESEARCH ON HEALTH POLICY

As discussed above, for research to have an immedi-ate impact on policy, an important prerequisite is that the topic is timely. Important current themes have been covered. Nurses and clinicians therefore need to be socially and politically aware of themes that are on the political agenda before planning research.

Evidence-based nursing research can make a significant contribution to policy by offering unique and incisive evidence-based information. Because nursing lacks large numbers of researchers with the experience to design and conduct large randomized controlled studies upon which evidence-based medi-cine is premised, nurses may 'get a foot in the door' by developing an interdisciplinary team that includes nurse researchers. By developing a research profile, nurses can become leaders in research studies.

West and Scott (2000) suggest that nurses should develop social networks that involve both policy makers and researchers to allow them a greater impact on policy. However, they note that one of the drawbacks is that it may be more difficult to initiate research that is critical of current policy. They also suggest that the nursing profession could be more proactive in shaping public and political awareness of issues related to nursing care given that social problems are socially constructed and influenced

by interest groups as well as policy-makers (West & Scott 2000). However,this requires greater collabo-ration between nurse researchers and practitioners. As mentioned, research and development agencies (e.g. NHMRC) have implemented strategies to increase collaboration.

Another way in which nurses could improve their 'marketing' of research and influence policy is to explain to the policy makers how the research is connected to priorities on the political agenda. Nursing researchers should be more direct in mak-ing policy recommendations in ways such as pub-lishing summaries of scientific papers in journals that policy makers are likely to read and including 'health policy' as key words on academic publica-tions (West & Scott 2000). This may raise policy makers' awareness of such research.

As well as focusing on topics of immediate relevance to nursing, nurses should contribute to multidisciplinary, multiprofessional health ser-vices research to increase their impact on policy (Department of Health 2000b). Belonging or having links with the health policy research community locally and internationally may also assist in increas-ing clinicians' impact on policy decision making (Scott & West 2000).

Summary

- Nurses can influence policy by overcoming their insecurities and raise controversial issues in a way that encourages discussion. They may need to be persuasive of disinterested parties who resist change.
- Educating decision makers of the many roles nurses play in the health and well-being of society may increase their understanding and thereby influence policy.
- Nurses may need to 'spell out' how their research is related to research policy.
- Government departments commission research in accordance with policies whereby health services researchers have to compete for funds alongside biomedical researchers with more impressive track records. However, much nursing research does not easily fit within a medical model of research.
- Nurses should develop social networks that involve both policy makers and researchers to have a greater impact on policy. They would benefit from having links with the local and

> international research policy-making community.
> - Nursing researchers should be more direct in making policy recommendations (e.g. publishing implications in journals).

Exercise 2.5

- What are the current themes on the political agenda in nursing research?
- How do nursing bodies such as the Royal College of Nursing influence policy?

UTILIZING RESEARCH-BASED PRACTICE TO INFORM AND DEVELOP PRACTICE

As discussed above, the concept of evidence-based practice is continuing to gain widespread acceptance within most Western health care systems. Nurses can serve as catalysts for optimizing patient care through evidence-based practice. In a study of the utilization of research in practice and the influence of education, nurses who read at least one journal regularly, had had more study leave, or had attended research courses also had a higher level of research utilization (Rodgers 2000). The study concluded that in order for utilization of research to occur, other prerequisites apart from education must be in place (Rodgers 2000). Not only must nurses have the skills and knowledge to critique the research, they must have a positive attitude that the barriers to utilizing research can be overcome, and that others value its implementation. Other researchers have found that nurses needed organizational support to apply research-based information to their practice (Bryar et al 2003, McCaughan et al 2002, Retsas 2000, Thompson et al 2001a, b). It has been argued that 'resistance from professional groups and structural barriers to change will only be overcome if evidence-based health care can demonstrate positive effects in clinical practice, research, evaluation and policy development' (Stronks et al 1997, p331).

Clinical guidelines are one way of translating evidence to practice. Clinical guidelines are defined as 'systematically developed statements to assist clinicians and patients' decisions about appropriate health care in specific clinical circumstances' (Niessen et al 2000). If they are based upon evidence, their value is in improving health care quality and the health of individuals as well as resource efficiency. However, guidelines are only effective if properly monitored and evaluated. In the policy arena there are a growing number of advocates for improving the health of the population, and evidence-based approaches are a valuable tool to help set priorities in this area (Niessen et al 2000). Clinical guidelines are further discussed in Chapter 13.

PARTNERSHIPS AND COLLABORATION

Most health care systems are moving towards an interdisciplinary approach to providing care, with health care professionals working interchangeably (Glen 2000). Given this worldwide emphasis on collaborative development of evidence-based practice, health professionals need to work together effectively to influence policy.

Many innovative approaches and developments have occurred to consolidate the relationship between education, research and practice, including clinical professors, consultant nurses, clinical research fellows and lecturer-practitioners. Universities and health authorities fund most of these posts jointly and the staff who occupy them work in both institutions.

The importance of collaboration in research is emphasized in the literature as a way of reducing barriers to research utilization (Clifford & Murray 2001). Barriers to using research evidence in nursing practice include accessibility of research findings, anticipated outcomes of using research, organizational support to use research, and support from others to use research (Bryar et al 2003, McCaughan et al 2002, Retsas 2000, Thompson et al 2001a, b). An example of the role of collaboration in reducing barriers is that of a project leader working closely with staff in clinical areas to ensure they have ownership of the work (Clifford & Murray 2001). This may result in increased motivation to participate in the research and utilize research evidence in practice.

Contemporary government health policy in terms of research and research training is focussed on linkage and collaboration within and across disciplines and institutions, to foster close alliances, avoid duplication and adopt a more strategic and managed approach. Nursing has a crucial role to play in this endeavour but a coherent and sustained strategy is needed to ensure the nursing contribution to key health priorities is properly researched, evaluated and supported by robust evidence, and that the research and development agenda is properly informed by nursing expertise (Department of Health 2000b).

The NHMRC in Australia is working closely with other agencies to develop links that will foster collaborative projects on quality and evidence-based practices in clinical and public health areas. Links are being further developed with the National Institute of Clinical Studies, the National Health Priorities Action Council, the National Health Information Management Advisory Committee, the Australian Council for Safety and Quality and Health Care, and the National Public Health Partnership (Annual Report of the National Health and Medical Research Council, Chairperson's report).

The Medical Research Council (MRC) of the United Kingdom is also developing a more international focus to its strategic policy. There is potential for the NHMRC and the MRC to develop new partnership arrangements, with a particular focus on the development of personnel capacity in areas such as clinical trials, antibiotic resistance, bioinformatics and the assessment of grants (Annual Report of the National Health and Medical Research Council 2001, CEO's Annual Report).

Summary

- In order for utilization of research in practice to occur, nurses need the skills and knowledge to critique the research, a positive attitude that the barriers to utilizing research can be overcome, and to feel that others value its implementation. Nurses also need organizational support to apply research-based information to their practice.
- The importance of collaboration in research is emphasized in the literature as a way of reducing barriers to research utilization.
- Given the worldwide emphasis on collaborative development of evidence-based practice, nurses and other health professionals need to work together effectively to influence policy.

- Linkage and collaboration within and across disciplines and institutions foster close alliances, avoid duplication and assist in adopting a more strategic and managed approach.

Exercise 2.6

- List some innovative approaches and developments that have occurred to consolidate the relationship between education, research and practice in nursing.
- What role does nursing have in fostering collaboration in research?

CONCLUSION

Nurses have made an important contribution to collaborative multidisciplinary research. However, they have been less successful at influencing government policy regarding the research agenda, including priorities and funding. The majority of nurses traditionally work as direct caregivers within clinical practice and the stereotypical view, reinforced by the media, is that nurses are solely concerned with care delivery and have no interest or role in policy decision making. Nurses need to be more politically 'savvy' and to improve their leadership and entrepreneurial skills so that they can be more influential in terms of health policy decision making. Part of that role may be to educate other decision makers about the value of nurses and nursing. If nursing research is to thrive, nursing leaders must engage more actively with appropriate funding bodies and contribute more effectively in consultations about priorities (Department of Health 2000b). Given nurses' increasing role in collaborative research, and the shift from secondary and hospital-based care settings to primary and community-based care settings, the future role of nurses in influencing health research policy could be promising.

References

Annual Report of the National Health and Medical Research Council. 2001. NHMRC: Canberra.

Antrobus S and Kitson A (1999) Nursing leadership: influencing and shaping health policy and nursing practice. *Journal of Advanced Nursing* 29: 746–753.

Borman J and Biordi D (1992) Female nurse executives, finally at an advantage? *Journal of Nursing Administration* 22(9): 37–41.

Bourke P and Butler L (1999) The efficacy of different modes of funding research: perspectives from Australian data on the biological sciences. *Research Policy* **28**: 489–499.

Bryar RM, Closs JC, Baum G et al (2003) The Yorkshire BARRIERS project: diagnostic analysis of barriers to research utilization. *International Journal of Nursing Studies* **40**: 73–84.

Buerhaus P and Needleman J (2000) Policy implications of research on nurse staffing and quality of patient care. *Policy, Politics and Nursing Practice* **1**(1): 5–15.

Clifford C and Murray S (2001) Pre- and post-test evaluation of a project to facilitate research development in practice in a hospital setting. *Journal of Advanced Nursing* **36**: 685–695.

Commonwealth of Australia (1999) Knowledge and innovation: a policy statement on research and research training. Canberra: Commonwealth of Australia.

Commonwealth of Australia (2001) National review of nursing education discussion paper. Canberra: Commonwealth of Australia.

Davis P and Howden-Chapman P (1996) Translating research findings into health policy. *Social Science and Medicine* **43**: 865–872.

Dawson G, Lucocq B, Cottrell R and Lewison G (1998) Mapping the landscape: National biomedical research outputs 1988–1995. London: The Wellcome Trust.

DePalma J (2002) Proposing an evidence-based policy process. *Nursing Administration Quarterly* **26**(4): 55–61.

Department of Health (1991) Research for health. London: HMSO.

Department of Health (2000a) The NHS plan. London: Department of Health.

Department of Health (2000b) Towards a strategy for nursing research and development. London: Department of Health.

Duffield C and Franks H (2001) The role and preparation of first-line nurse managers in Australia: where are we going and how do we get there? *Journal of Nursing Management* **9**: 78–91.

Fletcher S (1997) Whither scientific deliberation in health policy recommendations? Alice in the Wonderland of breast-cancer screening. *New England Journal of Medicine* **336**: 1180–1183.

Fulton S (1997) Nurses' views on empowerment: a critical social theory perspective. *Journal of Advanced Nursing* **26**: 529–536.

Glen S (2000) Partnerships: the way forward? *Nurse Education Today* **20**: 229–340.

Gott M (2000a) Nursing practice, policy and change. In: Gott M (ed) *Nursing practice, policy and change*. Oxford: Radcliffe Medical Press, pp3–21.

Gott M (2000b) Nursing practice, policy and change: the future. In: Gott M (ed) *Nursing practice, policy and change*. Oxford: Radcliffe Medical Press, pp195–213.

Hannigan B and Burnard P (2000) Nursing, politics and policy: a response to Clifford ... 'International politics and nursing education: power and control'. *Nurse Education Today* **20**: 519–23.

Hinshaw AS (2000) Nursing knowledge for the 21st century: opportunities and challenges. *Journal of Nursing Scholarship* **32**: 117–123.

Jennings B (2001) The role of research in the policy puzzle: Nurse staffing research as a case in point. *Research Nursing and Health* **24**: 443–445.

McCaughan D, Thompson C, Cullum N et al (2002) Acute care nurses' perceptions of barriers to using research information in clinical decision-making. *Journal of Advanced Nursing* **39**: 46–60.

New South Wales Health (1999) A framework for managing the quality of health services in New South Wales. Sydney: NSW Health.

Niessen L, Grijseels E and Rutten F (2000) The evidence-based approach in health policy and health care delivery. *Social Science and Medicine* **51**: 859–869.

Price K, Heartfield M and Gibson T (2001) Nursing career pathways project. Report 01/16 to the Evaluations and Investigations Programme, Higher Education Division, Department of Education, Science and Training, Canberra. www.dest.gov.au/highered/eippubs/eip01_16/default.htm

Rafferty AM (2002) Sustainable funding for nursing research in higher education. *Nursing Inquiry* **9**: 219–220.

Rafferty AM, Bond S and Traynor M (2000) Does nursing, midwifery and health visiting need a research council? *NT Research* **5**: 325–335.

Rafferty AM, Traynor M, Thompson DR et al (2003) Research in nursing, midwifery, and the allied health professions. *British Medical Journal* **326**: 833–834.

Read S (1998) The context of nursing and health care research. In: Crookes P, Davies S (eds) *Research into practice*. Edinburgh: Baillière Tindall, pp23–42.

Retsas A (2000) Barriers to using research evidence in nursing practice. *Journal of Advanced Nursing* **31**: 599–607.

Rodgers S (2000) A study of the utilization of research in practice and the influence of education. *Nurse Education Today* **20**: 279–287.

Royal College of Nursing Australia (2000) Role in Health Care Policy. www.rcna.org.au/RCNApolicies/Role%20in%health%20care%20policy.html. Accessed 28 April 2003.

Sackett DL, Richardson WS, Rosenberg W et al (1997) *Evidence-based medicine: how to practice and teach EBM*. Edinburgh: Churchill Livingstone.

Salvage J (1999) Carry on, nurse. NHS 50th Anniversary Lecture Series. Leeds: National Health Service Executive.

Scott C and West E (2001) Nursing in the public sphere: health policy research in a changing world. *Journal of Advanced Nursing* **33**: 387–395.

Strategic Research Development Committee (2001) Annual Report of the National Health and Medical Research Council. NHMRC: Canberra.

Stronks K, Strijbis A, Wendte J et al (1997) Who should decide? Qualitative analysis of panel data from public, patients, health care professionals, and insurers on priorities in health care. *British Medical Bulletin* **315**: 92–96.

Sudduth A (1999) Policy evaluation. In: Milstead JA (ed) *Health policy and politics*. Gaithersburg, MD: Aspen Publishers, pp219–256.

Thompson C, McCaughan D, Cullum N et al (2001a) The accessibility of research-based knowledge for nurses in United Kingdom acute care settings. *Journal of Advanced Nursing* **36**: 11–22.

Thompson C, McCaughan D, Cullum N et al (2001b) Research information in nurses' clinical decision-making: what is useful? *Journal of Advanced Nursing* **36**: 376–388.

Thompson DR (2003) Thinking bigger about research. *Journal of Advanced Nursing* **43**: 1–2.

Traynor M, Rafferty AM and Lewison G (2001) Endogenous and exogenous research? Findings from a bibliometric study of UK nursing research. *Journal of Advanced Nursing* **34**: 212–222.

Weller D and Veale B (1999) Changing clinical practice: evidence-based primary health care in Australia. *Health and Social Care in the Community* **7**: 324–332.

West E and Scott C (2000) Nursing in the public sphere: breaching the boundary between research and policy. *Journal of Advanced Nursing* **32**: 817–824.

World Health Organization (1996) Nursing Practice. Report of a WHO Expert Committee. Technical Report No 860. Geneva: World Health Organization.

Further reading

Antrobus S and Kitson A (1999) Nursing leadership: influencing and shaping health policy and nursing practice. *Journal of Advanced Nursing* **29**: 746–753.

Gott M (2000) Nursing practice, policy and change. In: Gott M (ed) *Nursing practice, policy and change.* Oxford: Radcliffe Medical Press, pp3–21.

Gott M (2000) Nursing practice, policy and change: the future. In: Gott M (ed) *Nursing practice, policy and change.* Oxford: Radcliffe Medical Press, pp195–213.

Scott C and West E (2001) Nursing in the public sphere: health policy research in a changing world. *Journal of Advanced Nursing* **33**: 387–395.

West E and Scott C (2000) Nursing in the public sphere: breaching the boundary between research and policy. *Journal of Advanced Nursing* **32**: 817–824.

Chapter **3**

Accessing sources of knowledge

Christine Hibbert

INTRODUCTION

The aim of this chapter is to examine the practicalities of literature searching and to introduce the idea of generic critical reading skills, which are applicable when reading both research and non-research based literature. The chapter is divided into three sections. The first section is about searching for literature, defining and refining topics for consideration and reflecting upon ways of putting boundaries around search areas. Strategies for successful literature searching are outlined, along with the use of resources additional to the library, such as subject authorities and relevant organizations. The second part of the chapter commences with a discussion of speed reading techniques which can help you to quickly ascertain the relevance of books and articles, without necessarily having to read them in depth. Pointers for practising 'skim reading' of both texts and journal articles are presented. This section of the chapter ends with a discussion of various systems for recording and maintaining personal notes and references. Examples of a selection of reference storage systems are presented. The third part of the chapter introduces the idea of critical analysis. The meaning of this term is discussed and a distinction is made between 'critical analysis' and 'critique' which is perceived as a higher order skill and not expected of those new to research. A simple exercise is then used to enable you to practise making balanced decisions about written work and writing about such decisions. References and suggested further reading are offered throughout the chapter and summarized at the end.

This chapter links closely with Chapter 11 in this book. Whilst this chapter looks at accessing and evaluating literature at a basic level, Chapter 11 presents more advanced criteria for evaluating the rigour of research-based literature, before moving on to the processes of collating information (synthesis) from a variety of sources to produce systematic, critical literature reviews.

Key issues

- Strategies for defining and refining topics to facilitate successful literature searching
- Techniques to allow rapid evaluation of the usefulness of literature
- Methods for developing skills in critical analysis

SUCCESSFUL LITERATURE SEARCHING

Starting to look for literature can seem a huge task. It can be frustrating, but if the search is fruitful, very satisfying and useful. This section of the chapter is intended to help you to maximize the chances of success in any searches you may undertake.

Why carry out a search in the first place? Polit et al (2001) identify two reasons for undertaking literature searches and reviews:

- To develop a picture of what is known – perhaps as a preparation for undertaking research
- Searching and reviewing may result in 'a critical summary of the state of the art of a topic, which may be an end in itself'.

The latter is the focus of Sue Davies' chapter later in this book, as she discusses the synthesis of a range of material, then explores the constituents of critical literature reviews. Many health professionals undertake literature searches to complete an element of a course, whilst others have a specific question or area that they wish to explore, either for interest or perhaps as part of their work. This text as a whole seeks to further develop the skills needed to do these things more successfully.

WHERE TO START?

The first section of this chapter contains suggestions and hints from experienced searchers about using different approaches to searching. These apply to searching both for journal articles and books. The first myth to dispel about searching is that it must start in a library. Many initial discussions about the focus of a search take place with peers and teachers. Resources can be shared and – in the initial stages particularly – it is worth talking to as many relevant and interested people as possible. Ideas and information can come from the most surprising sources and settings. Informal discussions with colleagues can be useful in helping to broaden or focus a topic area and may even yield specific articles and references. For example, if the topic area is pain relief, advice from colleagues may be that this is too broad and that to focus on pain assessment tools might be more appropriate. Someone may have undertaken courses where this was discussed and have reference lists associated with it, whilst others may have examined the topic in some depth and have specific research papers that they are willing to share. Meanwhile, supervisors and teachers often have a variety of resources, not necessarily associated with their specialist area, or they may know of others who may be able to help. Adequate discussion and consideration about the intended focus of a literature search should take place before even setting foot in a library.

SEARCHING NEEDS TO BE SYSTEMATIC

A second myth to dispel about searching the literature is that as many references as possible should be collected on the topic in question. Burnard (1993) calls this the 'broad brush approach' to literature searching. However, this usually results in the collection of masses of references which then have to be sifted through to identify the ones which are, or appear to be, most relevant. Such an approach can be costly in terms of time and photocopying or printing, not least because it is not always possible to be sure of the usefulness or quality of an article without reading it in full. There are times when this approach is particularly useful, for example when the (re)searcher has limited knowledge about the topic area and wishes to ensure that they are at least familiar with the range of material that is available on a topic. It can also help to verify or refute a perception that very little is known or has been written about a particular topic.

DEFINING AND REFINING THE TOPIC

If the broad-brush approach is used, the best place to start is somewhere quiet, not necessarily a library and not in front of a computer. Time and space to concentrate are very important, as beginning a search is a creative exercise which may require a degree of lateral thinking. A blank piece of paper and a pen are essential, while a dictionary and a thesaurus are useful. A sensible starting point is to write a sentence which encompasses all the important points or concepts within your topic area. If the reason you are doing the search is to write an essay, then split the essay title up into its constituent parts. If the reason is to find out more about a topic, then think through exactly *what* it is you want to know more about. As previously suggested, refining your topic may be helped by discussing things with experts and/or colleagues.

Having defined the search area, the next task is to refine it. Start by writing down as many words as possible that mean the same as the concepts within the title or topic area identified. More than one word can be used, for example 'nursing care' instead of just 'care'. These are called key words or subject terms. Having done this, write down as many words as possible connected with the key words (the dictionary and thesaurus are again useful for this). These are called associated key words. Once the key words have been worked through and refined in this way, it does not matter how many words there are or how the page is organized. Some people find it easier to make lists because they prefer to work with words on paper; others find it easier to use spider diagrams, conceptual maps or 'mind maps'. Buzan (1981) discusses this at great length and makes many suggestions about how much easier planning a topic is, if such methods are used. Figure 3.1 shows an example of a spider diagram, whilst Figure 3.2 shows a linear key word presentation for the same topic area – pressure area care. As you can see the end-product is essentially the same – it is purely a matter of choice.

FURTHER REFINING OF SEARCH TERMS

Once key words have been identified it is appropriate to turn to the indexes. Indexes are citations to journal articles, listed under subject headings and placed in alphabetical order. They may be either in a printed form or computer based. These can be searched for references by simply entering keywords into the electronic databases or by hand searching printed indexes. This would be termed a 'free text' search of the index or database. Such a strategy may be the reason that some people fail to find as much material as they would like or perhaps expect, and may explain why many become disheartened and disillusioned. I suggest that you take an extra step to refine the key words you intend to search on within a particular index.

To do this, you first need to identify which index you intend to access. Let us say that you decide to use the electronic database CINAHL (Cumulative Index of Nursing and Allied Health Literature). This database has a thesaurus within its programme, allowing you to check if the word(s) or term(s) you have identified actually appear in that database. An obvious issue is differences in spelling depending on where the index originates, e.g. 'oesophagus' (English) and 'esophagus' (American). On the other hand, those who construct the index may not have categorized the term in the same way you do. For example, you may use the term 'pressure sores' while the index refers to these as 'decubitus ulcers', or you may use 'cancer' while the index lists such material under 'neoplasia'. The terms decubitus ulcers and neoplasia would therefore constitute 'subject headings' within that index. If you entered the term 'pressure sore' you would identify few (if any) references. However, if you entered 'decubitus ulcers' you would find far more references because you have used the correct subject heading *for that index*.

Each index has its own list of subject headings. Within CINAHL the online thesaurus fulfils this role and so refining your key words would involve applying the thesaurus option to each of them, to see if they appear in the database, or to suggest other terms which should be used in their place. If the online index you intend to use has no thesaurus facility *or* you are using a printed index, then the same process would apply, except that you would have to consult the printed 'subject heading index' (typically found in the reference section of libraries) for that particular index. It is important to recognize that because of the variation in subject headings between indexes, this process of refining and identifying terms needs to be repeated for each individual index. A successful search using key words refined from the CINAHL subject heading index *may not* be as successful when using the MEDLINE database. As a result, it is important that you record the indexes *and* the search terms you use for any search you undertake.

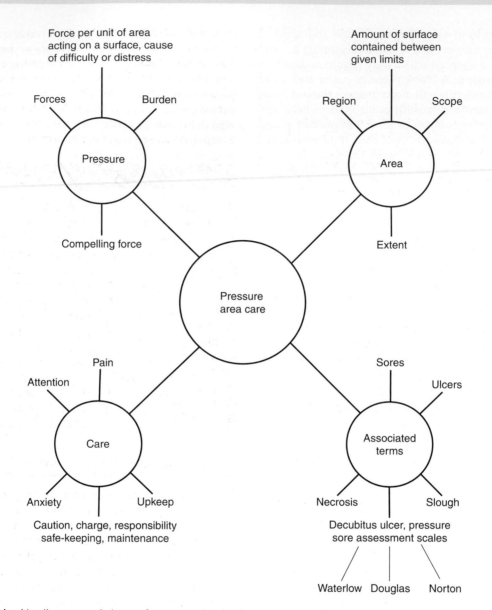

Figure 3.1   A spider diagram or mind map of concepts related to 'pressure area care'.

Many libraries now provide a full text service within a database that can often be accessed remotely from a home computer. This is most useful as it means that it is not necessary to visit a library or photocopy material. The downside is that printer costs are usually higher than photocopies and extra costs are incurred if searching takes place on line from a home computer. This is all the more reason to ensure that your search strategy is refined *before* attempting any on line searching.

Whilst a full text database is useful, the tendency is to use only the information provided which can dramatically limit the search. One of the ways to reduce missing information is to do an incremental search to ensure that relevant references and articles are included. If this is carried out on line then there are usually indications in the reference list at the end as to whether the references are also available as full text. Look carefully at the articles that are not available to ensure that no relevant or seminal works are missed.

Key words or terms – pressure, area, care
Pressure: pressure, pressing, press, presses, force, forces, compulsion, compelling force, burden, cause of difficulty or distress
Area: area, region, scope, extent, amount of surface contained between given limits
Care: care, heedfulness, attention, caution, charge, responsibility, upkeep, maintenance, look after

Associated key words or terms – Sores, ulcers, necrosis, granulation, slough, decubitus ulcer, turning, pressure aids, mattress, pressure sore assessment tools, pressure sore assessment scales, Waterlow, Norton, Douglas

Figure 3.2   A linear presentation of the same brainstorming exercise as in Figure 3.1.

Exercise 3.1

Either choose a topic area relevant to your practice or use the heading 'management of acute pain', then brainstorm and list key words and present either as a mind map or a linear list. Access the library either remotely or on foot to locate and consult the subject heading index for an electronic database relevant to your discipline. Then refine your key words into the subject headings used by that database. After this, search the index using those terms and note the results. You may find it interesting to do another search using your 'unrefined' terms to see just how many potentially useful references you might have missed.

USING THE INTERNET

The Internet has become a very popular way of accessing information and can be useful in litera- ture searching. However, this often encourages a broad-brush approach which can produce so much information that it can be daunting in terms of look- ing for specific information about an aspect of care. Some people with little experience of searching might only look on the Internet and not elsewhere and then assume that the only information available is that which is shown. For example, if you put the words 'pressure area care' into a general informa- tion request on the World Wide Web, the informa- tion provided is generally about how to buy special beds. This could lead to an assumption that there is little information available when in fact, this is not the case. Specific information and in particular pri- mary sources of information can only be accessed via

specialist databases. On the other hand, where little is known or for a general idea about the state of knowledge about a specific area, starting to search in this way can help. Most libraries have guidelines and advice about which search engines to use, which databases are useful and how to refine a search. It is well worth taking a little time to check these out and ensure that you can find the information.

Summary

It is important to appreciate that you need to put time and effort into the literature searching process *before* you are ready to peruse written or electronic indexes for references. Important and useful data can be missed, simply because inadequate preparation has gone into developing the search strategy. To draw an analogy with another systematic approach to problem-solving – medical diagnosis by doctors – inadequate preparation in developing a search strategy and moving straight to indexes is akin to a doctor deciding to operate on a patient with abdominal pain without first carrying out a detailed history and examination and reaching a diagnosis.

REFINING A SEARCH IS AN ONGOING PROCESS

Key words generated in this way enable you to search systematically through a printed or electronic index. However, the process does not necessarily end with looking for the terms in the printed index or feeding them into the search field of the electronic database and then recording the results. To be most successful, you need to be prepared to revise the search terms or use combinations of them. This is particularly true of searching using electronic data- bases as they have facilities for widening or nar- rowing searches depending on results. To return to the example of pressure area care, having searched the terms 'pressure' and 'nursing care' individually and found literally hundreds of references, you might then reasonably combine the results of the two using the 'and' option (i.e. references including the term pressure *'and'* nursing care) so as to narrow the search down to a more reasonable number. If, however, you had found only a few references, you might have used the *'or'* option (pressure *'or'* nurs- ing care references). If you find too many or only a few references, the search terms themselves may also need modifying, though this should not be the case if the above refining process has been carried out. There may also be some merit in examining the citations you get a little further. Rather than merely reading the reference and the abstract, you will find that somewhere in the citation is a list of other subject headings related to the topic area concerned. Extending the original search to include these terms *may* elicit further useful material. There are a number of these more advanced searching techniques. My advice is to practise those I have discussed and then build upon them by consulting with library staff and undertaking training courses available at your library.

WHICH INDEX?

A number of printed and electronic indexes are available. An index is a list of references organized under subject and author headings. An electronic index usually organizes references using a number of such 'fields', for example the related subject headings identified earlier. Some indexes even provide a short summary or abstract of the article, so that decisions can be made about whether or not they will be useful to the search at this point. This is very helpful as it can minimize time wasted retrieving items which appear to be relevant from their title, yet are of little value when the content is considered. Time can also be spent searching through the library catalogue system or the relevant section of the library to find books on the subject of interest.

With many indexes available, a number of other factors need to be considered when choosing which to search. Perhaps most obvious are that the index should be readily available to you and contains relevant material. With time and experience you will find that you come to prefer certain indexes more than others.

It is not only important to consider the scope of the literature indexed, but also the coverage in terms of years. For example, CINAHL and MEDLINE do not index and review all nursing and health-related journals, even some that are quite well known to practitioners. Some indexes are only available for recent years, while others have extensive retrospective coverage. In your search strategy it is therefore worth including some indication of the years which you feel will be useful, as well as checking which journals are included in the indexes available to you. Decisions of this sort may be informed by the topic in question. For example, 'research governance', 'single

assessment process' and 'midwifery-led care' are relatively recent phenomena so a search covering the last 5 or 6 years would probably identify the most relevant material. In time, you will become increasingly familiar with the index(es) that relate to material which is most relevant and useful to you.

LITERATURE SEARCHING CAN BE TIME CONSUMING

At this point another myth should be dispelled. It is not usually possible to 'nip into the library at lunch time' to do a 'quick search', nor indeed to spend 10 minutes in front of a computer finding what you need. Searching thoroughly usually takes some time. Time spent in the library or in front of a computer should be allocated to three distinct tasks:

- Searching the indexes
- Finding the journal(s) or book(s)
- Photocopying or printing the article(s).

First, allow time for searching in the indexes (electronic and print) for relevant references. Having found the references it may be necessary to find the specific journal on the shelves and check that the relevant item is included or order it from another library. Alternatively it may be necessary to try and find an electronic version of the journal that holds full text articles. Herein lies one of the biggest frustrations, particularly of using electronic indexes – they invariably identify numerous references to articles which appear very useful, but which are very difficult or expensive to access. Even if the journal title is held in the library, the particular issue or article you need may not be on the shelves. Also, if the journal is available on the Web, it may be the latest issue only or only hold abstracts of certain articles. If books are identified as having possible use, then they should be quickly checked for their relevance (see Exercise 3.2) and borrowed using the appropriate system. Finally, you should allow time to photocopy or print specific articles using library or computer facilities. Queues can form at busy times and so additional time may be necessary to use the photocopier, printer or see the librarian. In view of the above, the process of literature searching, collecting and reviewing, invariably takes more time than initially planned for.

Time is also a consideration because it is very easy to become sidetracked by looking at other interesting topic areas. Whilst searching on a particular topic, you need to be single-minded and focused to keep

Table 3.1 A search strategy record for using CINAHL (research and governance)

No	Records	Search requirement
#1	25	1995–1997
#2	35	1996–1999
#3	81	2000–2003

the process up to speed. The key word plan should help with this. It is also recommended that you keep a record of the key words used, the searches that have been carried out and the outcome(s) achieved, otherwise you will find yourself going over the same ground again and again. Using a systematic recording system reduces the likelihood of repeating searches and wasting time. This is especially useful if the searches are carried out on a part-time basis and over a longer period of time. If you are concerned that you will forget about material which *might* be useful at some later date, then keep a separate list for such references. A simple example of a search strategy record for the topic of 'research governance' is presented as Table 3.1. It is useful to note that electronic databases will allow you to print out a copy of the strategy you use, for your records.

INCREMENTAL SEARCHING

Burnard (1993) also identifies the *incremental* approach to literature searching. This involves initially finding one or two pieces of literature on the chosen topic area, which may be chapters in books as well as articles (though it is worth remembering that books quickly become dated), and then following up the references listed at the end of the piece. This strategy is particularly useful when examining a topic on which little has been written, or when working in a very specialist or narrow field of study. An ideal place to start is with seminal texts on the subject. Which texts can be considered seminal is information which can be usefully sought from experts in the field, as discussed earlier. Literature retrieved from this exercise can then, in turn, be examined for further references to see if there are any which might prove useful. Searching for literature in this way can be as detailed as necessary. In practice, this depends on what the aim of the search is. If it is merely to find out a little more about a topic then a few articles may suffice. However, if the intention is to find out what is known, then the search would

continue to a point where little or no new information was being identified by ongoing searches.

There are problems associated with incremental literature searching. Perhaps the most obvious is that it can be very time consuming, particularly as reference lists are not always as accurate or detailed as they should be. There is nothing the searcher can do about this, other than be prepared for the time that will have to be spent 'chasing' references. The benefits of developing good working relationships with library staff should be reiterated here, as there are a number of techniques and short cuts which can help in tracking down such material quickly.

Other problems include the fact that important pieces of work can be missed since they have not been cited by a particular author (who may not have been systematic in their search!). There is also the possibility of introducing a cultural bias, because authors tend to cite work from their own country. Some writers tend to use sources from their own reprint collections which means that they may omit more recent material. All of these problems can be limited by continuing the incremental searching process through as many references as possible, until it becomes apparent that no new writers, references or material are being identified. Properly done, the process can be seen as self-limiting, the end having been reached at this point of 'saturation'. Obviously other factors – most notably time, may curtail the search before this point is reached. The important thing is to recognize that such a search *may* be limited in terms of both scope and depth (one cannot be sure as saturation will not have been reached). Furthermore, if the outcome of the search is a written review, then this potential limitation should be shared with the reader (see Chapter 11).

CITATION INDEXES

Is incremental searching cheating? The simple answer to this is 'no'. It is a well-recognized method of searching the literature. In fact the *citation indexes* found in most libraries are actually lists of references presented by authors at the end of their articles. The best known nursing citation index is produced by the *American Journal of Nursing* and presented in its International Nursing Index. Such indexes are useful in several ways when searching for literature, including:

- Verifying journal citations inadequately cited elsewhere

- Following the progress of a theory or topic through publications
- Checking what other works an author has produced
- Getting some idea of who is writing in a particular field and perhaps who is being cited the most.

Exercise 3.2

Use the references at the end of this chapter to identify a book that you think might be useful for learning more about study skills. Write down the reference in full and during your next library visit, try to find it. Then make a decision about whether it is currently relevant to you. It may be useful to scan it to see if it is readable and easily understandable by picking pages at random and reading short abstracts. If the answer to the above questions is 'yes', then borrow it and read it in more detail.

Exercise 3.3

Find an article in a current journal on an area of interest to you, then check the references at the end and identify two that look useful. Note the journal titles and find out whether they are readily available in the library(ies) to which you have access. Write down the references in full and during your next library visit, or when you are next on line, try to find them. Again, make a decision about whether the articles are currently relevant to you. Also scan them to see if they are readable and easily understandable. If the answer to the above questions is 'yes', then read the article in detail and perhaps copy it, if it is going to be of use to you in the future. Techniques for improving 'scanning' are discussed in 'Reading the literature' (page 31).

INTEGRATED APPROACH

There is a third approach which is used frequently by experienced searchers. This is a combination of the two approaches discussed so far which I call the *integrated approach* to literature searching. When following this approach, the first thing is to find a good review article on the topic in question and follow the incremental approach already discussed. Again, the advice and counsel of someone knowledgeable in the field will be invaluable. Note that the suggestion is to find a *review* article, not a research article. This is because reviews are designed to do

just that – to provide an overview of what has been written about a particular issue or topic. The references listed in the review (which will probably include empirical *and* review literature) can then be examined in more detail and useful material collected. Following this and whilst awaiting any papers which have had to be ordered from elsewhere, the broad-brush approach can be used to identify whether there are any omissions in the citations accrued from the incremental search. Once the articles and books are retrieved, these can also be incrementally cross-checked for further references. Additional material can then be requested while the original sources are being read and analysed. In this way, the time available can be used most effectively. It is important to reiterate here a point made earlier, that is, the need to keep a record of the search strategy followed and its results.

OTHER SOURCES OF INFORMATION

Local sources

Using one or a combination of these approaches is possible in any professional library context independent of the topic area. The size of the library is immaterial. However, there are other sources of information. Searching for additional material outside the library should begin at a local level. Friends and colleagues often prove useful in this instance, as do clinical specialists within the various disciplines in practice settings. There are many other local sources of information, for example:

- Specialist departments (e.g. intensive care unit or coronary care unit)
- Health promotion units
- Voluntary organizations (e.g. The British Heart Foundation and the Stroke Association)
- Citizens Advice Bureau

A telephone directory is a useful tool for identifying and locating such groups in your locality.

National sources

In Britain, as in other countries, there are a number of national organizations willing to search for references, provided that they have a specific set of key words. Some require payment for this service, but the turnaround time from request to a list of available references delivered to the door can be very speedy. The British Reference Library holds many journals and books and will provide an international service.

However, a search for a specific article for an individual is very expensive and it is recommended that one of the professional libraries with whom they hold contractual arrangements should request the items. The Royal College of Nursing and the King's Fund also have extensive library resources. Many professional libraries will offer this or similar facilities. In the 'real world' therefore, a searcher needs to make a decision about the required depth of the search, as this will determine the need and practicality for using these invaluable but sometimes expensive resources.

World Wide Web

Access to the World Wide Web via Internet facilities is becoming increasingly available in many resource centres and at home. This opens up access to a whole new dimension of world wide information. Using such facilities successfully can, however, be rather time consuming, particularly if you have not had a formal introduction to at least the rudiments of the system. It is very easy to spend several hours 'surfing the net' with little or no useful material to show for it at the end of the day. The various search engines and web site directories are helpful but, as with electronic databases, perhaps the best advice is to get some training in their use before you waste a lot of time and are perhaps 'switched off' to the technology because of early failure. Most libraries equipped with such facilities will provide training programmes.

This text is not intended to provide detailed advice on searching the Internet, not least because there are a number of texts which already do this. My suggestion is that you take a look at some of these, to help develop your skills in the area. One example of such a text is *Guide to the Internet: an Introduction for Healthcare Professionals* (2nd edition, 1988) by Mark Pallen.

A final point to be made here is that the results of systematic reviews of evidence-based medical and nursing literature are increasingly available via traditional means (reports and circulars such as Oxford Health Authorities' *Bandolier* publication) and via the Internet (e.g. The Cochrane Collaboration Database and various Internet discussion groups).

Summary

Plan search strategies carefully. Get as much information as possible and define the search area as clearly as possible before you even access an index or database. Refine your search terms using thesauri and subject headings, remembering that subject headings vary from index to index. A combination of broad-brush and incremental searching is often necessary. Recognize that a lot of information and advice can come from 'experts in the field'. These may be subject authorities, helpful library staff, or information specialists. Once you start searching, keep records of the search steps followed and the resources examined. Try not to get sidetracked with material that looks interesting but is irrelevant to the task in hand. Remember that searching for references often takes more time than you originally thought. Expect to get frustrated as items are often missing or out on loan. Seek assistance from library staff, particularly about how to get the best from resources and training opportunities.

READING THE LITERATURE

Once literature has been obtained, the first step is to check it for relevance to the subject area and what you particularly want to know. With practice, this can take very little time, provided that there are no distractions. This requires the skill of *skim reading*. This is an important skill because it means that you will not waste time reading material which is of little use to you. This section of the chapter is concerned with how to speed up the reading process and consists of suggestions about the usefulness of speed reading when trying to quickly evaluate the relevance of articles and books to a particular topic or line of research. There are also two exercises designed to help you to practise these skills of scanning and skimming. Maslin-Prothero (2002) suggests that there are three different levels of reading:

- Scanning/skimming
- In depth reading/re-reading
- Inferring.

Whilst scanning and skimming literature help you to make decisions about whether it is relevant for your specific purpose, deep reading is required for understanding and considering the possible application of the literature to the 'real world'. The exercises below include the use of these strategies and highlight the fact that reading is an active process, that skills such as skim reading need to be seen as learned skills (rather than a natural ability) and finally that they have to be worked at, developed and practised. Deeper reading techniques are not discussed specifically here, since this text as a whole is designed to provide insight into research, and enable deeper reading of research-based literature.

'SKIMMING' A JOURNAL ARTICLE

To check the relevance of a journal article it is worth reading the abstract. An abstract is a brief summary of the article and usually identifies what type of information is being presented. If there is no abstract then read the introduction and the conclusion. Reading these sections will give an indication of relevance to the subject area and to the paper's readability. The task is to check for relevance, not to read the document in its entirety or be diverted by interesting sections of it. There will be an opportunity for deeper reading at a later stage, if the piece is relevant. A decision can then be made about what type and what level of knowledge are reflected in the piece and thus whether it should be marked for further examination.

At this stage, the references should also be examined. Well-referenced pieces tend to carry more credibility. On the whole, they should consist of up-to-date citations, unless classic pieces of research are cited. The references may also usefully contribute to further incremental searching. The following exercise summarizes particular points to consider when skimming an article or book to decide whether to read it in more detail at a later time.

Exercise 3.4

Choose a recent journal article on a topic you are interested in and read the abstract or the introduction and conclusion. Look at the list of references but do not read any further. Try to answer the following questions.

- Is it currently relevant to you?
- What is the level of knowledge? (after DePoy and Gitlin 1998, Ch. 16)
- Does it look easy to read?
- Is it detailed or superficial?
- Is it well referenced?
- Are the references recent publications?

- Would you read the article in more detail if the opportunity arose?

'SKIMMING' A BOOK

To check a book for relevance would seem initially to be a more difficult process. However, with a little practice it can take only a few minutes. In many ways, checking a book for relevance is a similar process to checking a journal article.

The first task is to check when the book was published. Many books on specific subject areas quickly become dated. This is particularly the case for books that discuss clinical practice, which changes rapidly – though incrementally – all the time. Deciding whether a book should be considered current requires quite complex judgment, basically because you need some knowledge of the topic to know that the material has been superseded. If you do not have such knowledge, you should seek advice from specialists in the area, or possibly librarians, before continuing.

If the book is considered current, the next task is to decide whether you think the author has credibility in the field. Points to consider in making this decision include relevant qualifications and any professional and academic positions held. Both of these will give some indication of the author's standing as an authority in the field about which they are writing.

Having decided that the author(s) appears credible, read the contents page(s). The chapter headings should give an overall picture of the book. Following this, read the introduction (sometimes called a preface) as in this section authors tend to give an overview of the reasons for writing the text and what they hope(d) to achieve by writing it. They often expand on chapter headings and how various aspects of the text tie together. It is recommended that you use this section to make a judgment on a book, rather than using the comments on the dust-jacket which is invariably advertising material. Finally the references should be checked. There are usually two places to search for these. In edited books, references are often placed at the end of each chapter (as in this book). In other books they are placed after the text, before the main index. The reason for checking the references is the same as with a journal article – in case they are useful as primary sources and to make sure that they are concurrent with the publication date of the book. They should also be sufficient in number to suggest that a range of material has been considered.

Exercise 3.5

Choose a book and time yourself while you check the publication date, contents pages, introduction/preface and the references, then answer the following questions.

- Is it relevant to the work you are currently doing?
- Is the book relevant in terms of publication date?
- Does the author appear to be a credible authority on the subject in question?
- Which chapter(s) would you look at first?
- Were the intentions of the book stated at the beginning of the introduction or preface?
- Were there ample references and did any look interesting?
- Would you examine this book more closely if given the opportunity?
- How long did it take you to do this exercise?

The key to success with skim reading is practice. I therefore recommend that you repeat these exercises until you are satisfied that the answers to the above questions can be found quickly, for any article or book you choose to peruse. It is important to develop the confidence to feel that you will not miss useful information by checking books and journals in this way. From my experience, I have noted that in high-standard scholarly work, key issues are clearly identified at the start of any piece of writing, before being discussed in detail in the body of the work. Approach the task confidently.

Deep reading is also a skill that should be developed and practised. This is explored in some detail in Sue Davies' Chapter 11, where more advanced skills of critical analysis are discussed.

Summary

Skim reading skills are important because they help you to avoid wasting time reading material which is of little relevance to the task in hand. The key to success with skim reading is practice. Work through the exercises provided to help you structure this practice.

MAKING RECORDS AND KEEPING NOTES

Having searched for and found appropriate literature, the next step is to consider how to organize and record the material (references for articles/books and notes). Bell (1999) and Greetham (2001) offer some very useful suggestions about using card indexes and boxes. Basically these systems involve making a record of each reference on a computer card. As most academic writing in the health and behavioural sciences uses the Harvard (author–date) system of referencing, it is sensible to record, on card or computer, information according to this system. Each card should include details of the author, date, title, publisher and source. For a journal article, the journal and page numbers should also be recorded. Additional information about where the piece of literature is kept can also be quite useful, especially if it is a book which has to be returned to the library. Finally, brief notes about the particular piece may prove useful, especially when using a computer card file, as this will assist in the retrieval of information. With increasing knowledge of both research methodology and the topic under consideration, these notes may extend to discussions of the rigour of research, the theoretical bases of arguments used and any recommendations made. Sue Davies provides an excellent framework for structuring such notes in Chapter 11.

Most computer database applications will contain some form of card file recording system. Essentially these differ from manual recording in that instead of writing the information on a card, it is recorded on a computer screen. An example of an entry in a computer card file index is presented in Figure 3.3.

There are advantages and disadvantages to using either system (card or computer). Both require that you adopt a systematic approach to collating information and that it is an ongoing process. Both methods are quite time consuming at first, but time spent early on will save many hours of hunting for previously read documents and references in the future. Computer card files do have an advantage in that they often have a key word (text search) facility for searching through the collected references for a particular topic area. Card indexes need to be quite elaborately colour coded to achieve similar results.

There are a number of more advanced bibliographic software packages (e.g. EndNote and

Mordiffi, Siti Zubaidah; Tan, Seo Peng; Wong, Mei Kin (2003) Information Provided to Surgical Patients Versus Information Needed. *AORN*. Volume 77(3) pp 546–549, 552–554, 556–558, 561–562

- A detailed and lengthy report of a study
- Identifies that a thorough literature search has been undertaken
- Methodological discussion, and conceptual framework described
- Study identifies detailed methods, number of participants, ethical approval.
- Only seems to have been carried out in one area
- Detailed discussion about changes in practice as a result of this study
- Discusses limitations
- Looks initially very detailed but need to examine methods of data collection

Held in HOME LIBRARY

Figure 3.3   Example of an entry in a computer card file index.

Author	: C A Takman, E I Severinsson
Year	: 1999
Title	: A description of health care professionals' experiences of encounters with patients in clinical settings
Source	: Journal of Advanced Nursing
Volume	: 30
Issue	: 6
Pages	: 1368–1374
Publisher	:
Place	:
Summary	: A study carried out in an acute medical setting to describe health care professionals' way of experiencing their encounters with in- or outpatients, while working in acute medical care hospitals.
Themes	: Communication skills Learning skills Reflective skills
Boundaries	: One hospital 11 participants 3 enrolled nurses 5 staff nurses 3 physicians
Methods	: Individual interviews Phenomenological approach
Findings	: Encounters between health care professionals and patients can be complex in nature and health care professionals might need support in trying to understand those patients whose 'way' of expressing experienced suffering is unknown to the health care professional.
Critique	: Limited literature search Overuse of jargonistic language Some discussion of ethical considerations Limitations discussed Best seen as a useful exploratory study

Figure 3.4   An example of an entry in a bibliographic software package.

ProCite) which offer more than merely a computer screen version of a card. More detailed information of interest from references can be entered under headings (also known as 'fields') such as 'themes', 'boundaries' and 'methods'. Key word searching is also available. Such packages can not only store references, but can also place them within text in a word-processed document *and* generate a reference list at the end. Developing such a database from the outset of any project or essay can save much of the time and effort which normally goes into the generation of reference lists. Figure 3.4 shows an example of a more detailed reference entry, typical of EndNote.

Computers can be expensive, they are prone to breaking down and are not always portable – though all three aspects are rapidly changing. Using a paper system means that spare cards can be completed in the library and used wherever study takes place. Unfortunately, once the paper card system increases in size, it can be tedious to search for specific topic areas and increasingly loses its portability. Perhaps a combination of the two is best, where information is initially collated on cards then entered on the computer when accessible. Alternatively, a laptop may be used to note down information and a back-up system put in place to make sure that information is not lost.

The importance of systematically reading and recording useful references as essential aspects of the process of searching for and analysing literature cannot be emphasized enough. However, as with recording search strategies and their outcomes, these steps are often missed or dealt with in a haphazard manner because they are time consuming, laborious and appear to delay getting on with the 'real work'. Yet, when properly set up and maintained, they provide a useful and ongoing resource. As a potential 'life-long' learner, I encourage you to consider these suggestions for developing your own information database.

Summary

A system for recording references and literature is an important feature of any strategy for collecting and storing information. Paper card files are portable and reliable but retrieving topic information from them can be a slow process. Computer card files facilitate quick topic retrieval, but they are less portable and not always available. The Harvard system is usually required for academic writing so it is worth recording references in this style. Computer-based bibliographic packages are useful as they not only retain reference material but also aid in the laborious task of writing reference lists. A combination of paper notes and computer files is perhaps the best way forward.

CRITICALLY ANALYSING THE LITERATURE

This final section of the chapter focuses on the analysis of material retrieved from literature searches. This book as a whole is designed to facilitate insight into research processes, to allow readers to make reasoned decisions about the credibility (or otherwise) of research reports. However, at this point I wish to make general points about the processes of being critical and analytical, which can be exercised by anyone when reading or writing scholarly work. More detailed knowledge can then be brought to bear as it is assimilated.

It is difficult to articulate the difference between description, analysis and critical analysis. These terms invariably appear in the learning objectives for academic courses, but what do they mean? Description entails giving a narrative account of something, a statement of how something is, rather than what it could or should be. The word 'analyse' is defined as: 'to examine minutely, so as to determine the essential constitution, nature, or form' and as 'The investigation of any production of the intellect, as a poem, tale, argument, philosophical system, so as to exhibit its component elements in simple form' (*Oxford English Dictionary* 2003).

In any analysis of a piece or a body of literature, there will always be an element of description to identify for the reader what the work is about. However, excessive description means that the reader would be better reading the original than your précis of it. Unfortunately, many people new to the art of

scholarly or 'academic' writing have a tendency towards description rather than analysis.

WHAT IS CRITICAL ANALYSIS?

To be critical often implies that fault must be found with whatever is being reviewed. However, *The Oxford English Dictionary* (2003) defines a critic as 'Skilful in judging, *esp.* about literary or artistic work'. It also states that to be critical means 'involving or exercising careful judgement or observation' and goes on to define criticism as being 'so as to determine or decide; decisively; critically'. It can be seen from these definitions that being critical in its true sense involves making decisions about the worth or value of a piece of literature or other art. Furthermore, by referring to 'careful judgment', the definition indicates that in being critical, a person should consider both the good and bad points of the work in question. This is perhaps a departure from the popular use of the term 'to criticize', with its typically negative connotations. If you put this together with 'analyse', the term to 'critically analyse' a piece of literature can be seen to encompass breaking it down in some way (perhaps along the lines of ideas presented, or the research process) and examining it in detail, both in terms of its parts and how they fit together. It also includes an imperative to make decisions about the work – about what is good and bad about it; whether on balance it has merit; and whether it is of use to the reader. As no piece of literature is all good or all bad, it follows that having 'critically analysed' it, a reader will end up with a balanced view of the material presented and will have reached decisions about its value.

It is perhaps worth noting at this point that there is a difference between critical analysis and *critique*. To critique a piece of literature is a high-order skill requiring advanced knowledge of research ethics and methodologies. One would not expect those new to research to be able to work at this level. Try this next exercise, taken from the news page in a popular nursing journal, to see if you can come up with a critical analysis of the following paragraph. You are encouraged to think in terms of what the item is about (description) and its merits (positive and negative).

Exercise 3.6

Nurses cannot eliminate all hospital-acquired infections (HAIs) and need training on their prevention, according to a news report. The report, from Health Service Watchdog

NHS Quality Improvement, Scotland, found that more than 33 000 patients a year in Scotland contract HAIs (News 2003).

Take a blank piece of paper and write a sentence describing what the paragraph is about. There are any number of variations in this sentence but the key is to narrow it down so that the description is as short as possible. Next, draw a line down the middle of the paper and write two headings 'positive' and 'negative', one at the top of each half. Read the paragraph again, identifying what you think are the 'merits' (including positives and negatives) of the piece. Write your thoughts under the appropriate heading.

The next task is to construct some sentences. In each sentence put in the positive and the negative comments. Remember to avoid unsubstantiated, overly argumentative or provocative statements. Words like 'must', 'should' and 'will' should be replaced with words like 'might', 'perhaps', 'suggest' and 'maybe'. An example of an unsubstantiated statement would be 'nurses do not understand research'. This could be replaced by 'the literature suggests that many nurses do not understand research'.

When describing a piece of literature, a good word to use at the start is 'this'. For example, you could say: 'This paragraph is about the need for better training for nurses in order to prevent hospital acquired infections (HAIs)'. In analysing it, most people find it easier to find fault with the literature but you are encouraged to try to reach a balanced decision. For every negative point that you make, try to think of a positive as well. In some cases you may find that the negative is the same as the positive – being brief and to the point can lead to a lack of detail, but also provide emphasis. Below are some examples of the kind of things you might write.

POSITIVE	NEGATIVE
It raises awareness	It could be alarming for patients
It is short	There is not enough information
It is easy to read	There is not enough detail
The report is identified	Not sure what credibility they have
The report comes up with a solution	It does not appear enough to solve the problem
It identifies that research has been carried out	There is no information about the scope and depth of the research

Examples of the kind of sentences you could construct about the article are as follows:

This paragraph raises awareness about the need to be vigilant with hospital acquired infections, however it could be unnecessarily alarming. The paragraph is short but there is not enough information to make a decision about whether it is valuable. It is also easy to read but unfortunately there does not appear to be enough detail. Although this information is supported by a report from the Health Service Watchdog, there is no information about the credibility of this organization. In addition, whilst there is acknowledgment that research has been carried out, there does not appear to be any information in the article about how the statistics were compiled.

By using the key words in the initial analysis, it is quite easy to construct the sentences and already there is nearly as much written in the analysis as in the original article. Another point is that if all the sentences start with a positive and end with a negative it can become quite tedious, therefore it is worth considering varying the format. For example, 'It could be said that this information is unnecessarily alarming but at least it raises awareness about this issue'. The final step is to use the last sentence to leave the reader of the analysis with a lasting impression of your overall decision. If you think that overall, it was a good piece, it is worth considering ending with a positive comment. If, on the other hand, you think that it was a poor piece overall, you should consider ending with a negative comment.

You might like to consider using this exercise as a basic structure for making notes from material you read. As you learn more about research, this structure will naturally become more complex – as suggested by the criteria for evaluating research and non-research based literature presented in Chapter 11 later in this text. The techniques demonstrated for attempting to ensure balanced analysis are also relevant when writing literature reviews – an issue also returned to in Chapter 11.

Summary

Critical analysis of research literature involves judging the merits of the research and coming to a balanced decision about it. It is *not* merely the identification of what the researcher did wrong. No literature is all good or all bad. Therefore, when taking notes or when writing yourself, try to retain a balanced view. In particular, avoid unsubstantiated statements as they can detract from the argument being presented. An unsubstantiated statement is one for which the origin of the opinion is unknown. Finally, critiquing research is a very high order cognitive skill. It requires knowledge of the conceptual, methodological and ethical components of research. This book is intended to help you move towards this goal.

CONCLUSION

In this chapter I have examined skills and knowledge which will enable you to be more effective in finding literature about any subject you have an interest in, and from there to make fairly quick decisions about its quality and relevance to you. To do this, I described strategies for making index searching (paper and electronic) more effective – essentially by encouraging you to be systematic and perhaps putting a little more effort into preparing a search strategy before examining databases. Next, I described approaches to reading the literature discovered as a result of such searches. I particularly concentrated on techniques you can use to enable

you to make quick decisions about the content – and therefore relevance – of texts and articles you find. This is important because, invariably, literature searching unearths far more information than you can actually use. Any mechanism which helps you to sort out 'need to know' from 'nice to know', without having to read it all in depth, is very useful, not least because of the time it saves.

Being able to critically analyse and to demonstrate this ability in scholarly writing is an important skill, not least because it is typically required for academic studies, as well as by credible professional journals. Critical analysis of research is also a basic requirement of the clinician who wishes to be actively involved in evidence-based practice. However, it should be acknowledged that these 'generic' aspects of critical analysis need to be combined with an insight into research methodology, if you are intending to critically analyse scholarly (i.e. research and/or theoretically-based) literature. Furthermore, this book as a whole seeks to inform you, the reader, about key aspects of this knowledge base. Fairly advanced criteria for evaluating research and theoretically-based literature are presented by Sue Davies in Chapter 11.

References

Bell J (1999) *Doing Your Research Project*, 3rd edn. Buckingham: Open University Press.
Burnard P (1993) Facilities for searching the literature and storing references. *Nurse Researcher* **1**(1): 56–63.
Buzan T (1981) *Make the Most of Your Mind*. London: Pan Books.
Carper BA (1978) Fundamental patterns of knowing in nursing. *Advances in Nursing Science* **1**(1): 13–23.
Depoy E and Gitlin LN (1998) *Introduction to Research: Understanding and applying Multiple Strategies*, 2nd edn. St Louis: Mosby.

Greetham B (2001) *How to Write Better Essays*. Basingstoke: Palgrave.
Maslin-Prothero S (2002) *Baillière's Study Skills for Nurses*, 2nd edn. London: Baillière Tindall.
News (2003) Report aims to improve infection control. *Nursing Times*. 4 February. Vol 99. No 5. p.8.
Oxford English Dictionary (2003) Oxford: Oxford University Press.
Polit DF, Beck CT and Hungler BP (2001) *Essentials of Nursing Research: Methods, Appraisal, and Utilization*, 5th edn. Philadelphia, PA: Lippincott.

Further reading

Buzan T (1991) *Speed Reading*. Newton Abbot: David and Charles.
   Very detailed information about reading and planning, there is even information about the ambient temperature of a room. In-depth exercises also presented in a popular style.
Cuba L (1993) *A Short Guide to Writing About Social Science*, 2nd edn. New York: Harper Collins.
   Good section on writing an essay.

Powell S (1999) *Returning to Study: A guide for professionals*. Buckingham: Open University Press.
   Detailed information on reading, writing and expectations at different academic levels.

Chapter 4

Making the most of existing knowledge

Andrew Booth

INTRODUCTION

This chapter aims to go beyond accessing published sources of literature towards learning how to make the most of the existing knowledge base. In doing so, the chapter will focus on three specific techniques: focusing the question, filtering the literature and using products that have been preappraised (preassessed) for quality (Booth & O'Rourke 1999). To illustrate complementary sources of knowledge, the chapter will focus in detail on two quite different, yet important, types of research – randomized controlled trials and qualitative research. However, it is recognized that existing knowledge is embodied in a wide range of research designs and brief suggestions are also given for other common types of question.

Key issues

- Making the most of the existing knowledge base
- Focusing questions effectively
- Filtering the literature
- Using resources that have been preappraised (preassessed) for quality

FOCUSING THE QUESTION

We have already seen that the published literature is an important resource in identifying and defining the scope of your clinical or research question (McKibbon & Marks 1998, Hibbert; Chapter 3). It helps you to narrow down the bewildering variety of options open to you when faced with a perplexing decision. You certainly do not want to 'reinvent the wheel', spending your precious time, energy and resources on a research question that has already been well covered or a therapy that has been proven to be ineffective. It would be a mistake, however, to think of the literature as merely a means for avoiding repetition. In a positive sense, it can help to shape and direct not only *what* you will do (as in the previous chapter) but also *how* you might do it. In contrast to the *scoping* search, covered in the previous chapter, which aims to give you a 'flavour' of the topic area, this chapter focuses on the idea of a comprehensive and systematic search of the literature. Here the analogy is of 'immersing yourself' in the topic you have selected.

There are many benefits to be gained from surveying the literature in such a comprehensive way. Broadly speaking, these benefits fall into two categories. The first is to help increase our knowledge of *what is already known* (which may inform our planning of patient care). The second is in informing *what is needed to generate new knowledge* (which may contribute to a researcher's preparation for research). Both of these are important issues when evaluating the conceptual basis of all forms of research-based literature. This is because we need to assure ourselves that any researcher has based their project on what is already known and that they have developed a rigorous method for clarifying their research question and then going about answering it.

The former (*identifying what is known*), therefore, includes being able to:

• Use the published literature to *obtain a broad overview of alternatives and choices when making clinical decisions*, identifying what may work and what has been tried and proved ineffective.
• *Resolve differences in practice among clinical colleagues* and dispel myths and rituals that have persisted in the absence of evidence (e.g. preoperative fasting, certain topical wound agents and prenatal pubic shaving).
• *Identify more economic treatments* that have been demonstrated to be equally effective to current practice.

The latter (*generating new knowledge*) may include:

• Using previously published literature in 'deciding whether any new research is required on an issue, by *exposing the main gaps in knowledge [and] identifying the principal areas of dispute and uncertainty*' (Mays et al 2001).

• The opportunity to consider multiple examples of research in the same area *to look for general patterns to findings in that topic area*. The mere act of bringing together studies with apparently conflicting findings helps a researcher to explore potential explanations for such discrepancies.
• Using existing literature to *define terminology or identify variations of definitions* used by researchers or practitioners.
• Using previous research in the area to help *identify appropriate research methodologies* (even a study with inconclusive results may yield valuable insights into how research might be conducted). It may particularly help a researcher to *identify validated scales and instruments* for use in a new study.
• Using existing literature to help a researcher *conduct their pilot study more efficiently and effectively*. Pilot studies, even if only for questionnaires or interviews, are necessary but also time-consuming and costly. The published experiences of previous researchers may inform a pilot and provide insights a researcher would only gain had they conducted multiple pilot studies.
• Identifying from previous research *existing theories or models* that may have a bearing on study design.
• Establishing from previous research *that any proposal is relevant and timely*. The supporting literature can demonstrate that the question is worth asking and answering.
• A systematic approach to tackling the published literature which may help in *establishing your credentials as an investigator* as you demonstrate skills in identifying, synthesizing and critiquing materials (Shojania & Olmsted 2002).

Summary

The case study in Box 4.1 illustrates how these various beneficial elements of literature searching and reviewing can come together to ensure that a sound research project is developed.

With multiple potential uses of the literature, not to mention sub-topics and supplementary searches, even such a simplified scenario demonstrates how a comprehensive and systematic search of the literature is central to the successful outcome of research. Note how the midwife makes connections between her own clinical practice, what she retrieves from

Box 4.1 Case study: attitudes of different professions to hand washing in a delivery suite

A midwife is taking part in a New Researcher Training Programme and is conducting a research project on the attitudes of different staff to hand washing. Her topic firstly requires a literature search to *focus the scope* of the original question. Although the literature on hand washing is vast she needs to discover whether there is a significant body of published research conducted specifically in obstetrics and gynaecology settings. Indeed, has anyone researched the topic specifically in a delivery suite?

Second, she discovers that her original concept of hand washing has many more definitions than she had envisaged. Does her idea of hand washing include papers describing the use of a hand rub? Does it constitute use of water only? What is the minimum period of time that the procedure takes place before it is classed as 'hand washing'? The literature search enables her to *explore different definitions* of her main concepts.

Another role of the literature is in *cross-fertilization of ideas* between similar, but not directly related, research. For example, a study initially carried out among surgeons may assist in *selecting an appropriate methodology*. Should her research use questionnaires or interviews, group interviews or focus groups? Would it be appropriate to combine investigation of attitudes with a period of observation of what actually happens? This discovery might lead the midwife to review the literature to see whether any *validated instruments* have been developed specifically to measure attitudes to hand washing or, failing that, to routine hospital hygiene. The literature review process may also inform *selection of appropriate outcomes* – these might include those employed in previous studies (literary warrant) or those considered appropriate by the relevant clinical community (user warrant). For example, is she focusing solely on attitudes or will she also investigate knowledge and/or behaviour?

the literature and her own planned research. You should look for evidence of such processes, when critically appraising the literature review section of any research paper.

Exercise 4.1

Consider a question that you may wish to investigate from your own clinical practice. In which ways, perhaps similar to those in Box 4.1 above, might the literature potentially contribute to successfully providing an answer to your question?

SYSTEMATIC LITERATURE REVIEWS

A particularly useful product of a systematic and comprehensive search of the literature is the systematic literature review (Wood 2003). Although these are covered in more detail, by Sue Davies in Chapter 11 they are worth mentioning at this point, because they can particularly help you to make the most of the literature. A well-conducted systematic review helps practitioners avoid being overwhelmed by the volume of literature (French 1998, Hewitt-Taylor 2002). Review articles help you keep up-to-date, define the boundaries of what is known and what is not known and can help you

avoid knowing less than has been proven. Systematic reviews add to these virtues, mentioned above, by addressing clearly defined questions, searching exhaustively (over ten or more databases) and presenting the results in a standardized and highly structured format. By critically examining and then collating the findings of a number of primary studies, systematic reviews also improve our understanding of inconsistencies within diverse pieces of research evidence. By quantitatively combining the results of several small studies, a particular type of systematic review incorporating meta-analysis (see Chapters 11 and 12) can create more precise, powerful, and convincing conclusions (Khan et al 2003). Alternatively, there are other methods for synthesis involving the outcomes of qualitative research projects.

Exercise 4.2

Identify a recent example of a systematic review from within your area of interest. Answer the following questions:

– How many data sources (databases, websites, etc.) did the reviewers use in order to identify relevant material?
– What steps did they take to make sure that their search strategy identified relevant material?

- How did they bring all the included studies together? Did they use tabulation? Graphical presentation of results? Textual or thematic analysis?
- How do your answers to the above questions affect your confidence in the quality of the review?

Summary

Researchers can use systematic reviews to summarize existing data, refine hypotheses and help define future research agendas. Without systematic reviews, researchers may miss promising leads or may embark on studies of questions that have already been answered.

AS EASY AS PIE

It may have been sufficient for the purposes of your scoping search to have typed a few broad concepts such as 'hand washing' and 'obstetrics' into a bibliographic database such as CINAHL or MEDLINE and seen what came up. However, this will not be suitable if you want to make sure that you do not miss anything relevant. Chris Hibbert has already identified, in the previous chapter, the importance of brainstorming various concepts for variations in terminology or spelling. This can be made even easier if you break your original question into its component parts. A helpful framework or 'anatomy' for doing this is by using the Problem-Intervention-Evaluation (PIE) model to help focus your search term(s).

The *Problem* includes the patient or population being studied and the setting in which they are found. It also includes any details of their age, condition and specific illnesses or symptoms. As we have seen, our population may, in fact, be a group of staff as in our delivery suite scenario.

The *Intervention* is anything that we plan to do to address the problem. It can therefore be a treatment, a diagnostic test, an aspect of nursing care or an educational or health promotion technique.

The *Evaluation* involves what we plan to measure and how we are planning to measure it. We want to know if the intervention we have chosen has made a difference. We are therefore interested in outcomes (such as pain relief or reduction in blood pressure) and outcome measures (such as the Melzack Pain Scale or mmHg).

FOCUSING QUESTIONS FURTHER

Breaking a question into its component concepts will help you to think of search terms and to define all aspects of your question (Booth & Fry-Smith 2001). This is what is known as a focused question (Richardson, 1995). You will occasionally see this PIE approach referred to, particularly in the medical literature, in a fuller form as PICO (Patient/Population, Intervention, Comparison, Outcomes) (Anonymous 2002, Flemming 1998). This is because it is often helpful to have a comparison in your question, especially if you want to see whether one intervention works better than another. This comparison may be between two similar types of treatment (e.g. aspirin versus paracetamol), two different modalities (behaviour therapy versus acupuncture) or between some new intervention and the existing way of doing things (standard care). 'Outcome(s)' is, of course, similar to Evaluation but conveys a narrower range of measures than the full spectrum of effects you may be interested in.

Exercise 4.3

Attempt to separate your question (from the previous experience) into the Problem-Intervention-Evaluation components. If you have a comparison in mind, you might wish to go further and attempt the components of the PICO anatomy.

PROBLEM (Who am I doing it with/to?)
INTERVENTION (What am I doing/thinking of doing?)
EVALUATION (How will I measure it? How can I know that I have made the difference I intended?)

Of course, if your question does contain a Comparison also, it is well on its way to indicating what type of study you will need to find or do, to answer it (McKibbon 1999). For example, a comparative study between one treatment and another is a 'controlled trial'. If it has been conducted in a rigorous way then it will have *randomized* a population [POPULATION] into two (or more) groups – one into the control group [COMPARISON] and the other(s) into the treatment or experimental group(s) [INTERVENTION]. Both groups will be assessed using the same outcome measures [OUTCOMES] (Stevens 2002). Minimizing bias in this way and ensuring that both groups are treated equally, both before and during the trial, are just some of the reasons why randomized controlled trials are regarded as the 'gold standard' for studies of outcomes.

Exercise 4.4

Take a question from your own area of practice that you would be able to answer using a randomized controlled trial design. *Remember that it needs a group of people with the same problem or condition. They need to be randomly allocated between two alternative treatment options (or one active treatment and a placebo) and to be measured against the same outcomes.*

Summary

The chances of successful literature searching can be enhanced, by framing good quality questions. When searching for outcomes-related material, the PIE model is an extremely useful tool.

FILTERING LITERATURE SEARCHES

Once it becomes apparent that you need a particular type of literature to answer your question (for example, randomized controlled trial literature), then you can start to restrict (or filter) your results to retrieve only research that has employed that specific study design (Haynes et al 1994). You can do this in two ways. The first relates to the fact that in a database such as MEDLINE, you can search for your topic as described previously and then use the 'Limit' command to limit your results to the publication type 'randomized controlled trial'. This can be likened to using a fishing net with holes so large that you only 'net' the larger, better-quality fish. To employ a slightly finer 'net' would be to use the 'Limit' command but this time to restrict your results to the publication type 'clinical trial' (all randomized controlled trials are indexed with the publication type 'clinical trial' but not all 'clinical trials' are indexed as randomized controlled trial). Using 'clinical trial' as a publication type admits a broader range of research articles into the results of the search.

The second relates to the fact that you can search a database that has been specifically designed to contain only a certain type of study – in other words, someone has already filtered off the higher study designs for you. The Cochrane Library, a compendium database made of several components,

Table 4.1 Effect of clinical trial and randomized controlled trial publication types on MEDLINE (May 2003)

Total number of MEDLINE articles	12,525 345
Total number of clinical trials	350 182
Total number of randomized controlled trials	171 277

Box 4.2 Approaches to answering a therapy question

Searching for a therapy (or intervention) question?

- When searching MEDLINE, limit your search to 'randomized controlled trial' in the publication type field or, more liberally, to 'clinical trial' in the publication type field, or
- Search the Cochrane Library

contains the 'Cochrane Controlled Trials Register' which details randomized controlled trials or clinical trials suspected of being such (see Appendix 4.1). Because it is made up from articles that have not only been identified from MEDLINE but from other databases such as EMBASE and CINAHL, and from systematic hand searches through the world's journal literature, it contains even more clinical trials than MEDLINE.

FILTERS FOR OTHER TYPES OF RESEARCH PROJECTS

Of course, not all questions can be answered by studies using a randomized controlled trial design. Our midwife's question was not about whether one method of hand washing is more effective than another. It was about different attitudes to hand washing. Attitudes and feelings are frequently (and rightly) examined using qualitative research methods. The question therefore arises – 'are there filters, comparable to the above instance for "clinical trial", that can be used to retrieve qualitative research?'. The answer to this is, at the same time, both yes and no! Yes there are certain words or phrases that you can look for in the MEDLINE database that are more likely to indicate that a study is qualitative. However, these research studies are not coded as a specific publication type. Instead, the optimal strategy includes terms that are contained either in the title, abstract or subject terms of relevant papers. Such search terms are therefore 'noisier' than the 'clinical trial' filter, in the sense that they may retrieve more inappropriate articles along with the appropriate ones. Nevertheless, they may prove very useful.

You will notice that none of the terms suggested above are approved Medical Subject Heading (MeSH) subject terms. Instead, as indicated by the abbreviated command 'tw', after each term, they are based on textwords – that is, words from the authors' title or abstract. This reflects the notoriously poor coverage of qualitative studies by the indexing language of MEDLINE. Instead we use three terms: one general term for the type of study (i.e. 'qualitative'); one term that frequently (but by no means exclusively) is used to describe a method of eliciting qualitative data (i.e. 'interview'); and one term that characterizes the 'results' of qualitative research (i.e. 'findings').

In addition to randomized controlled trials (for outcomes or effectiveness studies) and qualitative research (for attitudes, opinions and feelings) there are numerous other study types, depending on the question you are seeking to answer. Such other types of studies have their own versions of filters. These use either the 'publication type' field (as with 'randomized controlled trial'), subject indexing terms (such as 'explode sensitivity-and-specificity' to find high-quality diagnosis studies) or textwords in the titles or abstracts of articles. Longer versions of the filters may even combine two or more of these approaches. Filters will not only vary according to the database you use (for example, filters on MEDLINE are different from those on CINAHL) but even between different versions of the same database (for example, MEDLINE PubMed will use different commands from MEDLINE via the Ovid service provider). Filters also differ according to whether you wish to run a quick 'one-line' filter for rapid results, to maximize your chances of retrieving something relevant (so-called 'maximum sensitivity filters'), or to minimize your chances of retrieving something irrelevant (so-called 'maximum specificity filters'). It will therefore be well worth your time contacting

a librarian for details of strategies that might apply to locally available databases. Further to this, a very useful book by a librarian and colleagues *PDQ Evidence Based Principles and Practice* (McKibbon et al 1999), contains details of the most important filters, for a range of studies on the MEDLINE, EMBASE, CINAHL and PsycLit databases. Box 4.4, meanwhile, lists useful 'one-line' strategies for different types of research study on MEDLINE.

Summary

Search filters can be very useful, once you know that you want a particular type of literature. Such filters vary between databases and designs so librarians can be useful in helping you to structure searches using such tools.

Exercise 4.5

What types of studies would be most appropriate for answering your own research question? Is there an appropriate filter for identifying this type of study from MEDLINE or other databases?

USING PREAPPRAISED MATERIALS

Up to this point we have focused on issues concerned primarily with search quantity (the number of 'hits' from a search) rather than the quality (in this case, relevance) of the papers found. We want to design a search strategy that will maximize our chances of finding material that is relevant to our research question. From within a broad 'pool' of potentially relevant materials we aim to filter those that are most likely to address the research question, according to their study design. However, the fact that a research study has an appropriate study design does not automatically mean that it is of sufficient quality. For example, is the study that you have identified, a good randomized controlled trial or a poor one; a good qualitative research study or a poor one? Here you have two choices: you can either assess the study yourself (the knowledge and skills to do so, form the basis of this entire text), perhaps using an appropriately selected checklist, or you can look for a commentary on that literature, produced by someone else (Guyatt et al 2000). Here it is important that the commentator judges the study according to how good its design is, not according to largely irrelevant factors such as the author's credentials, the status of the source journal or the prestige enjoyed by the hosting organization.

Obviously, as it is time consuming to appraise or evaluate an article from scratch, it is preferable for the busy practitioner to look for a 'preappraised' source first. If such a source does not exist, or alternatively if reading such a source indicates that a research study will likely prove useful (if that is the intention), then you would undertake the entire process of appraisal yourself.

Three main sources of preappraised resources offer commentaries on the quality of individual research studies:

- Publishers
- Database producers
- Enthusiastic individuals, usually clinicians.

These will be considered in turn.

PUBLISHERS

It has been increasingly recognized that the volume of health literature is too great for any practitioner to navigate successfully in its entirety. Certain publishers have therefore developed a genre of so-called 'secondary' journal literature that seeks to summarize and appraise approximately 30 of the highest quality research studies produced over a 2-month period. This 'cream' is then showcased in journals with titles such as *Evidence Based Nursing*, *Evidence Based Medicine*, *Evidence Based Mental Health* and

Evidence Based Healthcare. Each secondary journal has a similar one-page format:

- An indicative title that summarizes the findings of the research study in one sentence
- A two-thirds of a page summary of the design of the study, its main features and its principal results
- A brief one-third of a page summary of the implications of the article for practice written by an acknowledged expert in the field.

Of course, it is the summary of the research design that is most useful for you as you will no doubt wish to examine the implications of the article for yourself, within the context of your specific research question.

DATABASE PRODUCERS

Organizations such as the NHS Centre for Reviews and Dissemination (NHS CRD) at the University of York, have realized that key articles will be examined by numerous health practitioners, within a culture of evidence-based practice. They have therefore decided to offer more than the traditional informative abstract provided by bibliographic databases such as MEDLINE. NHS CRD has therefore identified particular types of studies for inclusion in specific databases:

- Systematic reviews – detailed in the Database of Abstracts of Reviews of Effects (formerly Effectiveness) (DARE)
- Cost studies or economic evaluations – itemized in the NHS Economic Evaluations Database (NHS EED).

In both cases experienced researchers use a standardized template with set questions to judge the quality of a published article. The results of their appraisals are then made available within a database, where each record is structured into a number of common paragraphs addressing aspects such as the design, outcome measures used and results. These databases are available free to the international research community via the Internet and are also included in the Cochrane Library (see Appendix 4.1). By such means a researcher or practitioner can identify the major reviews (or economic evaluations) in their topic area and gain an instant assessment of their quality.

As already implied, critical appraisal can only really be carried out on a selective basis, so the numbers of articles covered by the *Evidence Based …* journals, or the NHS CRD databases, are but a small fraction of the published output. Fortunately,

Box 4.5 Some examples of CAT-banks

Centre for Evidence-Based Medicine
  http://www.minervation.com/cebm2/
  cats/allcats.html
University of Rochester
  http://www.urmc.rochester.edu/MEDICINE/
  RES/CATS/index.html
University of Michigan
  http://www.med.umich.edu/pediatrics/ebm/
  Cat.htm
University of North Carolina
  http://www.med.unc.edu/medicine/edursrc/
  !catlist.htm
Canadian College of Naturopathic Medicine
  http://www.ccnm.edu/catbank/
Best-BETS (Emergency Medicine)
  http://www.bestbets.org/

however, there are clinicians, typically associated with major specialties or research centres, who have identified key questions in their area of expertise and then systematically combed the published literature for a research study that addresses their question. They then produce a critically appraised topic (CAT) report, summarizing the rigour and findings of this study (Sauve et al 1995). This approach has the advantage of being determined by clinical questions that matter (i.e. they are consumer-driven) rather than the published research outputs of major journals (production-led). The products of their appraisal are often made available to other users on the World Wide Web in the form of banks of such resources – so-called CAT-banks. Box 4.5 presents a list of some of these CAT-banks.

Such approaches to interpreting the literature are not without their critics, however (Coomarasamy et al 2001). Typically the searcher has a finite amount of time to spend on answering their question. They may not have the skills or the resources to access all the major databases and their selection may be completely arbitrary or even intentionally skewed to a certain point of view. The answer(s) that they derive will often be very specific to the patient or clinical setting that initiated the question and therefore may not be generalizable to a broad range of patients or settings. You will, therefore, obviously want to ensure that you have been energetic in tracking down all the relevant literature even if a CAT-bank

or, for that matter, an evidence-based journal or appraised database, offers you a handy shortcut to some of the major studies in your research area, before changing your practice or embarking upon a course of research.

Exercise 4.6

Using the evidence-based journals, the NHS CRD databases and the CAT-banks listed above try to identify a preappraised article that may address your clinical or research question.

For example accessing the NHS CRD Web page at http://nhscrd.york.ac.uk and typing the word 'handwashing' yields articles such as:

> (Record 4)
>
> Assessment of two hand hygiene regimens for intensive care unit personnel.
>
> Larson E L, Aiello A E, Bastyr J, Lyle C, Stahl J, Cronquist A, Lai L, Della-Latta P. Critical Care Medicine 2001; 29(5): 944–951.

While accessing the Evidence-Based Nursing site at http://ebn.bmjjournals.com/ reveals:

> Handrubbing with an alcohol based solution reduced healthcare workers' hand contamination more than handwashing with antiseptic soap
>
> Donna Moralejo and Andrew Jull (commentator) Evid Based Nurs 2003 6: 54

DO-IT-YOURSELF APPRAISAL

Although Chapter 3 has identified some general principles and techniques for reading any type of literature, we have already seen that certain types of research study may prove more fruitful when asking particular types of question. Obviously, if we have identified a study with an appropriate design it will be helpful to use criteria, in the form of a checklist, that specifically address this type of study. 'Critical Appraisal' is described as:

To weigh up the evidence critically to assess its validity (closeness to the truth) and usefulness (clinical applicability).

(Sackett & Haynes 1995)

Table 4.2   Sources of Appraisal Checklists

Tool	Source	Location
Critical appraisal tool for systematic reviews	Critical Appraisal Skills Programme	*http://www.phru.org.uk/~casp/reviews.htm*
Critical appraisal tool for randomized controlled trials	Critical Appraisal Skills Programme	*http://www.phru.org.uk/~casp/rcts.htm*
Critical appraisal tool for qualitative research studies	Critical Appraisal Skills Programme	*http://www.phru.org.uk/~casp/qualitat.htm*
Critical appraisal tool for quantitative studies	University of Salford	*http://www.fhsc.salford.ac.uk/hcprdu/tools/quantitative.htm*
Critical appraisal tool for qualitative studies	University of Salford	*http://www.fhsc.salford.ac.uk/hcprdu/tools/qualitative.htm*
Critical appraisal tool for mixed-method studies	University of Salford	*http://www.fhsc.salford.ac.uk/hcprdu/tools/mixed.htm*
Critical appraisal tools for diagnostic, etiology, prognosis, therapy, clinical guidelines,economic evaluations and systematic reviews	University of Alberta (EBM Toolbox)	*http://www.med.ualberta.ca/ebm/ebm.htm*

A whole series of checklists have been developed to meet this need. These were originally in the form of User Guides to the Medical Literature (Guyatt & Rennie 2002). The use of critical appraisal checklists for assessing the relevance and rigour of research findings is established in disciplines that pursue evidence-based practice and has led to development of guidelines for surveys, cohort studies, clinical trials and case-control studies (Crombie, 1996). Qualitative research, economic analyses and systematic reviews have also been targeted for a checklist approach. In recent years, these have been modified by leading groups, such as the Critical Appraisal Skills Programme (CASP) in Oxford, to be more user-friendly and accessible to busy practitioners (Mulhall et al 1998, Bradley, see Chapter 12). Much of this text is designed to provide the reader with key insights and skills, to enable them to meaningfully and correctly appraise the research literature. It will suffice here, therefore, to identify the major resources that are available (Table 4.2) and thereby provide an insight into how the above-mentioned preappraised products are actually produced.

Regardless of the source from which you choose to obtain a checklist for appraising the literature you retrieve, you should seek to ensure that it covers the validity of the article, the reliability of its results and its applicability to the setting in which you plan to use it.

Exercise 4.7

For one of the research studies that you have previously identified for your topic, attempt to identify a relevant checklist for use in appraising the study. Keep research study and checklist together for use when you have considered Chapters 7 and 8.

Summary

Sometimes hard-pressed clinicians need quick evidence-based answers to clinical questions. Pre-appraised literature with implications for practice can provide such answers. There is, however, a hierarchy of credibility of these sources, with highly regarded journals and database producers at the top. CATs produced by enthusiastic individuals or groups need to be viewed rather more sceptically, though they are nonetheless useful and important sources of evidence-based material.

CONCLUSION

This chapter has attempted to provide a bridge between the fundamental principles of accessing sources, described in Chapter 3, and the more rigorous principles of critical reading (critical appraisal) covered in Chapters 7 and 8. Value-added ways of using existing knowledge include:

- *Focusing your initial question*, breaking it down into its main components
- *Filtering the results* from databases so that you concentrate on those study designs that are most likely to answer your question
- *Appraising retrieved articles for validity, reliability and applicability*, either by doing it for yourself (using the checklists commonly available on the

Web) or by looking at a summary that someone (publisher, database producer or international colleague) has already produced.

It is hoped that these techniques will help you to manage the large volumes of published and unpublished literature that exist around clinical and educational topics in an efficient manner and to harness your limited time to good effect in pursuit of your research question.

References

Anonymous (2002) Ask an expert. Popping the (PICO) question in research and evidence-based practice. *Applied Nursing Research* **15**(3): 197–198.

Booth A and Fry-Smith A (2001) Developing the Research Question. In: Auston I (ed) Electronic Textbook on Health Technology Assessment (HTA) Information Resources. Bethesda: National Library of Medicine, www.nlmnihgov/nichsr/ebooks/hta/chapter11drafthtml

Booth A and O'Rourke AJ (1999) EBM Notebook: Searching for evidence: principles and practice. *Evidence-Based Medicine* **4**(5): 133–136.

Coomarasamy A, Latthe P, Papaioannou S et al (2001) Critical appraisal in clinical practice: sometimes irrelevant, occasionally invalid. *Journal of the Royal Society of Medicine* **94**(11): 573–577.

Crombie IK (1996) *The Pocket Guide to Critical Appraisal*. London: BMJ Books.

Flemming K (1998) EBN notebook. Asking answerable questions. *Evidence-Based Nursing* **1**(2): 36–37.

French B (1998) Developing the skills required for evidence-based practice. *Nurse Education Today* **18**(1): 46–51.

Guyatt G and Rennie D (2002) *Users' Guides to the Medical Literature: A Manual for Evidence-Based Clinical Practice*. Chicago: AMA Press.

Guyatt GH, Meade MO, Jaeschke RZ et al (2000) Practitioners of evidence based care. *British Medical Journal* **320**: 954–955.

Haynes RB, Wilczynski NL, McKibbon KA et al (1994) Developing optimal search strategies for detecting clinically sound studies in MEDLINE. *Journal of the American Medical Information Association* **1**: 447–458.

Hewitt-Taylor J (2002) Continuing professional development: clinical development of evidence-based practice. *Nursing Standard* **17**(14/15): 47–52, 54–55.

Khan KS, Kunz R, Kleijnen J et al (2003) Systematic reviews to support evidence-based medicine: how to apply the findings of healthcare research. London: RSM Press.

Mays N, Roberts E and Popay J (2001) Synthesising research evidence. In: Fulop N et al (eds) *Studying the Organization and Delivery of Health Services: Research Methods*. London: Routledge: pp188–220.

McKibbon KA (1999) EBM Notebook: Finding answers to well-built questions. *Evidence Based Medicine* **4**(6): 164–167.

McKibbon KA and Marks S (1998) Searching for the best evidence. Part 1: where to look. *Evidence Based Nursing* **1**: 68–70.

McKibbon KA, Eddy A and Marks S (1999) PDQ: evidence-based principles and practice. Hamilton, Ontario: BC Decker.

Mulhall A, Alexander C and Le May A (1998) Appraising the evidence for practice: what do nurses need? *Journal of Clinical Effectiveness* **3**(2): 54–58.

Richardson WS (1995) The well built clinical question: a key to evidence based decisions. *ACP Journal Club* **123**(3): A12–13.

Sackett DL and Haynes RB (1995) On the need for evidence-based medicine. *Evidence-Based Medicine* **1**(1): 5–6.

Sauve S, Lee HN, Meade MO et al (1995) The critically-appraised topic (CAT): a resident-initiated tactic for applying users' guides at the bedside. *Annals of the Royal College of Physicians and Surgeons of Canada* **28**(7): 396–398.

Shojania KG and Olmsted RN (2002) Current methodological concepts. Searching the health care literature efficiently: from clinical decision-making to continuing education. *American Journal of Infection Control* **30**(3): 187–195.

Stevens KR (2002) Research issues. The truth about EBP and RCTs. *Journal of Nursing Administration* **32**(5): 232–233.

Wood MJ (2003) Systematic literature reviews. *Clinical Nursing Research* **12**(1): 3–7.

Further reading

Ajetunmobi O (2002) *Making Sense of Critical Appraisal*. London: Arnold.

Bowers D, House A and Owens D (2001) *Understanding Clinical Papers*. Chichester: Wiley.

Greenhalgh T (2000) *How to Read a Paper: The Basics of Evidence Based Medicine*, 2nd edn. London: BMJ Books.

Khan KS, Kunz R, Kleijnen J et al (2003) *Systematic Reviews to Support Evidence-Based Medicine: How to Apply the Findings of Healthcare Research*. London: RSM Press.

APPENDIX 4.1 – THE COCHRANE LIBRARY

The Cochrane Library is the main output of the Cochrane Collaboration, an international organization devoted to identifying and summarizing the results of clinical trials conducted in health care, This resource includes:

- **Cochrane Database of Systematic Reviews.** A regularly updated electronic text of systematic reviews of research on the effects of health care. Each systematic review seeks to address a precisely formulated review question, defined in terms of the PICO anatomy.
- **Database of Abstracts of Reviews of Effects [formerly Effectiveness] (DARE).** Produced by the NHS Centre for Reviews and Dissemination, University of York. A collection of bibliographic references with structured abstracts reporting and quality assessing the findings of systematic reviews published in the journal literature.

- **NHS Economic Evaluations Database (NHS EED).** Produced by the NHS Centre for Reviews and Dissemination, University of York. A collection of bibliographic references with structured abstracts reporting and quality assessing the findings of economic evaluations (e.g. cost-benefit studies) published in the journal literature.
- **Cochrane Controlled Trials Register.** A master index of all the controlled clinical trials that have been identified in the research literature, including items identified from bibliographic databases, hand-searching and the unpublished literature. The largest collection of bibliographic details of clinical trials in the world.
- **Cochrane Review Methodology Database.** A classified register of books, journal articles and other resources to support the production of systematic reviews.

Chapter **5**

Philosophical and theoretical underpinnings of research

Lorraine B. Ellis, Patrick A. Crookes

INTRODUCTION

If there was a word more likely to engender a swift turning of the page or a drift into the arms of Morpheus than 'research', then for many people it would be 'philosophy'. For others it would be 'theory'. Perhaps this is because these are terms that people do not perceive to have everyday relevance. However, they are terms which are of fundamental importance when considering research. In this chapter we cover these topics with the intention of explaining what they are and describing how a researcher's philosophical standpoint or 'world view' can impinge on the research they undertake and *how* they undertake it. This builds on material touched on in Chapter 1. We will then go on to discuss why any research study needs to relate to what is already known (theory). By developing an understanding of the philosophical bases of research paradigms and their associated methods, and by appreciating the relationship that *should* exist between theory and research, the critical reader of research will be well placed to evaluate research papers. You will be able to do so with regard to the appropriateness of the research design and research methods, the suitability of the research question and the compatibility between the research methods, findings and conclusions.

We will first examine some of the assumptions and beliefs which underpin the traditional philosophical 'camps' of experimental-type (variously called quantitative, scientific or positivist) and naturalistic (qualitative or non-positivist) designs of research, then briefly compare these with a third research philosophy – critical theory. We will then revisit the idea first raised in Chapter 1, that no research philosophy or 'paradigm' (an example or model used as a standard) should be viewed necessarily as having the ascendancy over another, but rather that researchers should choose methods which reflect the level of knowledge on the topic in question and which will meaningfully add to that knowledge base.

From this starting point we will consider theory – what it is and how it can be generated or tested – including a brief explanation of inductive and deductive reasoning. This will lead on to a discussion of the relationships which (should) exist between theory and research. This is important because, as indicated already, being able to judge whether the right questions have been asked by a researcher, is an important aspect of critically reading research reports.

Finally we will discuss how researchers use frames of reference in an attempt to share their 'world view' with the critical reader and indicate how they perceive their research builds upon what is already known. This will include the identification of key points to consider when evaluating the conceptual bases of research studies. The most important thing to consider when reading research is whether or not it builds upon the existing body of knowledge, which in most cases will be indicated via links which can be drawn between the literature review and the research design. However, there are some researchers who attempt to clearly and overtly identify the theoretical bases of their research. They do so through the presentation of a frame of reference. The final section of this chapter therefore concentrates on 'frames of reference in research'.

Key issues

- The relationship between philosophy and research design
- Paradigms in research
- Processes linking theory and research: induction and deduction
- Theories as mechanisms for explaining and predicting phenomena
- Conceptual and theoretical frameworks

PHILOSOPHY AND RESEARCH

The term 'philosophy' has many definitions, as a brief perusal of any comprehensive dictionary will illustrate. Invariably such definitions refer to the pursuit of wisdom, allude to the system of values by which we live and acknowledge that general principles underlie all branches of study, fields of activity or approaches to solving practical problems. Definitions suggest that philosophy is about the generation and development of knowledge, including an indication of what we, as human beings, *need* to know. Furthermore, these definitions emphasize that adherence to a particular philosophy can require a person to follow particular rules of conduct. Christian philosophy, for example, encourages forgiveness and love of fellow man. Philosophy also helps make explicit the general principles and beliefs which underpin particular fields of activity or study. For example, the philosophy of many medical practitioners, commonly termed the 'medical model' (or paradigm) of care, is said to be characterized by a concentration on the diagnosis and treatment of symptoms, rather than the implications of disease and its treatment for the patient.

In the same way, the various philosophies underpinning research can be seen to attend to these issues, for example by helping researchers:

- Identify issues 'worthy' of study – what do we *need* to know?
- Decide what it is *possible* to 'know' about such issues
- Identify a *process* to follow to ensure that they can be seen to have been systematic and rigorous in their work.

These underpinning philosophies help us to make decisions about the 'ontological', 'epistemological' and 'methodological' questions discussed by Mike Nolan and Ulla Lundh in Chapter 1.

Research paradigms reflect value systems which impinge on research design, data collection methods and the nature of researcher involvement in the field of study. By examining the philosophical traditions of positivism, naturalism and critical theory and how those traditions manifest in the research process, you as a consumer of research should be more able to discern and appreciate rigorous and valuable research studies.

Some researchers and authors may not make their philosophical viewpoint explicit. This may be because they see it as either unnecessary or unquestionable or because they are simply unaware of it. The following discussion is intended to indicate key points of similarity and difference between the two traditional research philosophies, along with a consideration of a third research paradigm – critical theory. The intention is to help the critical reader to consider the philosophical underpinnings of research studies they read. Detailed discussions of the limitations of each paradigm are not presented, not least because this has been eloquently done before. These references are offered as suggested readings in the text.

PARADIGMS IN RESEARCH

THE POSITIVIST PARADIGM

This can be seen as representing the traditional 'scientific' view of research and underpins what is commonly known as experimental research. As with any paradigm or worldview, the positivist paradigm (also called quantitative and scientific, amongst other things) represents a particular way of viewing the world – in this case the world of research and knowledge, what can be known and how such knowledge should be discovered and verified. The researcher operating in this paradigm believes that anything that is worth knowing can be known objectively (i.e. measured or quantified and typically represented numerically) and verified by independent observers. The positivist perceives that the object of research or study can only be truly understood by reducing it into parts and examining them in detail. Relationships between the parts considered important by the researcher can then be identified by repeated observation and measurement, leading finally to a point where it is considered reasonable to make predictions, based upon mathematical verification of the 'facts' (statistics). Positivism is based on the tenet that valid knowledge can only be discovered when the researcher occupies a position of detached observer (in other words, unbiased and value free). This is considered possible if certain 'universally' accepted research techniques or processes (essentially researcher as non-participant) are followed and reflect the stages of 'the' research process alluded to in most research texts. DePoy and Gitlin (1994) eloquently outline this approach as:

> ... [having accepted] a theory or set of principles as holding true. Specific areas of inquiry (sic) are defined and hypotheses, or expected outcomes of an inquiry, are posed and tested ... data are then collected and mathematically analysed to support or refute hypotheses. Through incremental deductive reasoning ... 'reality' can become predictable
>
> (DePoy & Gitlin 1994: 17)

A practical example of this approach to knowledge development would be an attempt by a 'researcher' to learn about the workings of a car engine by systematically dismantling and rebuilding it. Working in this paradigm, he or she would seek to establish the *relationship(s)* between the component parts, e.g. cylinders, valves and pistons. The logical and structural principles that inform the relationship(s), such as combustion and emission, would also be discovered and through the collection and analysis of data, a theory would be tested which would allow us to *predict* phenomena from that which is already known. In this case, perhaps a way for improving the performance of this and other car engines in the future could be established.

Table 5.1, adapted from Leininger (1985), summarizes key characteristics of the positivist research paradigm or worldview. It also presents comparisons of this paradigm with the naturalistic and critical theory paradigms, which will be discussed shortly. Leininger (1985) could be said to be one of the authors who seek to undermine positivism to validate their use of naturalistic or 'non-scientific' research methods. Nevertheless, she presents an excellent exposition of the philosophical underpinnings of both quantitative and qualitative research paradigms, along with her views of the strengths and weaknesses of the two approaches with regard to research and knowledge development. You are recommended to read this text to supplement the necessarily basic discussion in this book. Table 5.1 summarizes these comparisons.

THE NATURALISTIC PARADIGM

The naturalistic paradigm also has several different labels including qualitative, interpretive and phenomenological research and non-positivism. It has also been termed 'holistic'. As with positivism, the naturalistic paradigm reflects a particular school of thought on the nature of knowledge, including: what we need to know; what can actually *be* known; and how best to find out or generate that knowledge. Meaningful parallels end at this point.

Unlike positivists, researchers in the naturalistic paradigm operate from the fundamental belief that humans need to know far more about themselves and the world in which they live than can be 'measured' objectively. It is for this reason that it is considered by some to be 'unscientific'. The kind of knowledge that is considered valid and useful

Table 5.1   A contrast of quantitative, qualitative and critical theory paradigms (adapted from Leininger 1985)

Domains	Quantitative methods	Qualitative methods	Critical theory (action research)
Definitional focus	*Quantity*: Measurement focus of a thing, object or subject (how much)	*Quality*: Nature, essence, meaning and attributes (what it is and characteristics)	*Quality*: Meaning, perspectives and appreciation of issues
Orientation	Reductionist and deductive	Open discovery and inductive	Inductive, reflections on the phenomena of interest
Data sought	Measurable/quantifiable/numerical	Seek interpretive (subjective) and objective data. Emphasizes subject's personal interpretation of events	Context-specific, emphasizes subject's personal interpretation of events Pluralistic emphasis
Relation to people being studied	Detached observation, generally non-involvement, non-participation	Frequently direct involvement and participation with people. Close relationship between knower (researcher) and known (participant)	Role integral to the research setting, close involvement with participants, emphasizes collaboration and democracy
Research goal	Hypothesis testing/emphasizes cause and effect/prediction	Development of understandings and meanings of what one sees, hears, experiences and discovers. Access participants' experiences of *their* reality	Planning and taking action to change practice, introduce change to conditions to improve a situation. Problem resolution
Reliability indicators	Repeated measures, generalizability to other cases, reproducibility	Recurrent themes, patterns, lifestyles and behaviours	Patterns of behaviour
Domains of analysis	Predetermined, prejudgements and *a priori* position taken, non-dynamic, fixed and planned research design	Can reformulate and expand focus of study as one proceeds, no predetermined *a priori* judgements	*A priori* position taken, dynamic and flexible, participants involved in the process of analysis, dialectic critique

therefore differs between the two paradigms. To expand, positivism is based on the assumption that there is one truth and that this truth can be established objectively, i.e. *measured* in some way in a value-free manner. Naturalistic philosophy, however, reflects a belief that the meaning of human experience is affected by the interpretation placed on it by individuals, based on such things as previous experience and personal beliefs and that therefore those who have experiences are the most knowledgeable about them. As a result, this philosophy allows for the fact that in certain circumstances there may be any number of 'realities' or truths regarding a particular research question, not least because the 'answers' are generated *post facto* from data derived from those who have had an experience – rather than being determined in advance by a researcher.

There is also an explicit acceptance within the naturalistic research paradigm that the role of researcher can never be one of neutrality or being value free, as is expected of the 'scientific' researcher. This is not least because the mere act of choosing to research something indicates that a value has been placed on it. Also, whilst the researcher may seek to be objective and detached, they cannot control whether the research subject(s) view them as neutral and value free. It is because of the necessity of acquainting themselves with the research area and the subjects within it that naturalistic researchers actually see merit in being 'subjective' and participating in the research context, to tune into what people are saying and doing *within the natural context.*

Those adopting a naturalistic perspective also believe that, because positivist research methods require that the object of study be reduced into its constituent parts for closer examination, preferably in controlled and replicable conditions, then such approaches must be found wanting when attempting to explore and explain complex issues such as human motivation and behaviour. In other words, qualitative researchers believe that human experience and an individual's reactions to that experience are so complex that it is only possible to understand them by considering them holistically and in the 'real-life' setting, *not* by examining those aspects viewed as being of particular importance or relevance by researchers. This has been termed the 'gestalt' perspective, where the assembled parts are considered to accumulate to form a reality bigger or more complex than the sum of the individual parts would indicate. The goal of a naturalistic approach to research is therefore to interpret, as fully as possible, the totality of whatever is being studied from the research subject's viewpoint (Leininger 1985, Meerabeau 1992). Research based in the naturalistic paradigm is generally described as being diametrically opposed to reductionist positivism, as essentially it underlines the need to consider everything in its entirety, on the basis that in the social sciences everything influences everything else.

To explain this further, the researcher operating in a naturalistic paradigm might be interested in the concept of homeostasis from the point of view of the individual's *experiences* of blood pressure control and fluid balance. The researcher would be interested in the ways in which the quality of human life is affected by hypertension and fluid restrictions. Naturalistic inquiry seeks to capture the reality of these issues through the perceptions of those experiencing a raised blood pressure and restrictions in drinking fluid. The inter-relatedness of altered physiology (reality or the known), and the *experience* of altered physiology (the knower) underpins the research throughout. The researcher would not only be interested in predicting phenomena but also in *describing* and *exploring* the ways in which hypertension and a restricted fluid intake affect the lifestyle of research participants. The researcher attempts to tell it as it is, the 'is' being the participant's perspective. The different characteristics and emphases of the positivist (quantitative) and the naturalistic (qualitative) paradigms are contained in Table 5.1.

Like positivism, naturalistic inquiry has strengths and limitations. Qualitative research often produces large volumes of textual data, which the researcher must analyse (Leininger 1985). For example, describing and exploring the participants' experiences of fluid restrictions and how this affects their quality of life would involve the researcher in encouraging participants to talk about themselves, perhaps using semi-structured or unstructured interviews with several open-ended questions. The potential variety of responses makes handling the data difficult and introduces the possibility of bias in its interpretation. Conversely, this open and very flexible approach is a real strength of naturalistic inquiry, as it allows the researcher to explore the *complexities* and therefore the *completeness* (holism) of human experience. For

example, the effects of a restricted fluid intake on the lifestyle and self-image of someone for whom drinking enhances a social occasion can only be effectively examined within a qualitative research design. In these terms naturalistic inquiry lends itself to researching new, obscure and uncharted areas (Leininger 1985) leading to the generation of new theories.

CRITICAL THEORY

Critical theory or critical social theory is an alternative research paradigm, which reflects yet another particular worldview. It is similar in many ways to the naturalistic paradigm in emphasizing the informant as knower, the creative nature of knowing, and a belief in the existence of multiple realities. However, critical theory is distinct from positivism and naturalistic inquiry in two key respects: the purpose of the research per se and the role of the researcher in achieving that purpose.

Critical theorists aim to change the world by empowering the subject(s) of inquiry to enact social change. In this sense critical theory can be seen as a form of change management. Indeed Titchen (1995) makes the suggestion that critical theory reflects the philosophy of realism, as opposed to the 'objectivity' of 'science' and the idealism of naturalistic enquiry, neither of which appear to have an imperative for action to take place within their schema. Within this pragmatic paradigm the researcher's part in the research process is to act as a change agent (which may take many forms), the research itself being the vehicle through which change is enacted. Accordingly, the principal aim of this approach is to improve practical situations. This is where the role of the researcher comes in. Underpinning the critical theory paradigm is a fundamental belief that when a power imbalance exists between one party and another, this has the effect of disempowering at least one of the parties.

Traditionally, in both quantitative and qualitative research, the role of researcher is one of outsider looking in. Webb (1990) refers to this as the 'smash and grab' approach to research, where researchers come into situations, grab data and then disappear again, without ever necessarily fully explaining what is going on to the 'subjects'. It is not uncommon for little or no personalized feedback to be given to them, though they may in due course read about themselves in a professional journal! In such circumstances it is not surprising that many subjects feel little or no ownership of the research and may fail to accept the findings or apply recommendations 'in practice'.

The researcher working within the critical theory paradigm – often termed an 'action researcher', seeks to avoid such problems by involving subjects throughout the research process (including identifying what needs to be researched) in such a way that the researched are also the researchers. There is also a tendency for the researcher to be an active participant within the context in question so that they too are 'the researched'. In addressing the imbalance of power in these ways, it is considered that the people involved in the research will develop and maintain a sense of ownership for the research findings and seek to make use of them, whilst the researcher will be firmly grounded in 'reality' and so generate reasonable and realistic solutions to problems identified. Action research does not therefore sit easily in either the qualitative or quantitative camp, not least because it stems from a different, more pragmatic philosophical standpoint than more traditional paradigms. However, building on Leininger's (1985) work, it is possible to highlight some of the characteristics of this philosophy and indicate some of the major differences between paradigms, as in Table 5.1.

As with other paradigms, critical theory has strengths and limitations. A major strength of action research is its ability to empower subjects through participation (Hart 1995). However, as one might imagine, the success of this approach is heavily dependent on the accessibility of the research setting and the role of the researcher in what may be a politically sensitive area, as well as the researcher's communication and research skills. The researcher must take account, for example, of participants' traditional view of their role in the overall plan of care and in the decision-making process. Acting as an agent of change, the researcher must be sensitive to participants' agendas and consider the perceived impact of events, developing, where necessary, an ongoing strategy to enact change. Creativity is characteristic of this paradigm, with the action researcher acting as an imaginative diplomat introducing change. In contrast to positivistic approaches, the action researcher forms an integral part of the research setting, which, whilst crucial to the success of action research, poses questions of validity. The action researcher establishes validity by processes of self-validity, participant validity and peer validation (Titchen 1995). Whilst this process establishes the rigour of the research, it is extremely time consuming and is therefore a disadvantage of researching within

this paradigm. Nevertheless, checking out multiple realities across participants also serves to highlight differences in orientation and potential barriers to change. Titchen (1995) presents an excellent discussion of all three research paradigms. You are encouraged to read this in addition to Leininger's work.

Summary

We hope we have shown that the 'quantitative versus qualitative' debate is somewhat redundant, not only because there is another paradigm to consider, but also because all three possess strengths and weaknesses which depend very much on how they are used. Different research methods need not compete as what we need to understand is that they tell us different things. The real issue for a researcher should therefore be 'how can I best go about answering the research question?', rather than basing design selection on a view that some methods are more 'scientific' than others.

Another issue to consider is your own philosophical viewpoint. It may be that, knowingly or otherwise, you are of the view that some research methods, based on the various theoretical perspectives discussed, hold an ascendancy over others. If this discussion has made you reconsider that mindset, then it has been useful.

THEORY AND ITS RELATIONSHIP TO RESEARCH

THE MEANING AND CHARACTERISTICS OF THEORY

Numerous definitions of theory can be found in research texts and in books on nursing theory. For example, theory is defined as a set of concepts (Burns & Grove 1993, Polit & Hungler 1991), a set of constructs (Kerlinger 1973) and a set of related ideas (DePoy & Gitlin 1994). Despite such incongruities it is possible to discern commonalities among these definitions. Most authors refer to theory as an abstraction consisting of a set of interrelated components. Kerlinger (1973) suggests that theory is a set of constructs, definitions and propositions, while McKay (1969) defines nursing theory as logically interrelated sets of confirmed hypotheses. Taken together, such definitions suggest that theories *are representations of reality comprising a combination of concepts and/or constructs that are in some way related*. The nature of these concepts and the relationships between them can be determined and verified through research.

THE PURPOSE OF THEORY

Theory forms an inherent and arguably necessary component of professional practice and everyday life. Theories inform and guide how we think and how we behave though we may not be consciously aware of this. Theories may allow us to predict what might happen in a given set of circumstances (via deductive reasoning) or they may provide a means for us to interpret and explain reality (via inductive reasoning). Without theory we would be in the position of trying to comprehend what goes on every day as if everything was a new and novel experience, as well as being unable to anticipate what the effects of our actions will be. For the most part we are not aware of our use of theories, yet we use them constantly. For example, the theory of meteorology seeks to predict the likelihood of sunshine or rain, whilst the theory of probability allows us to decide whether or not it is wise to believe the weather forecast, based on the perception that it is often wrong!

The theory of meteorology is a theory of the physical sciences. Other theories belonging to this category include Einstein's theory of relativity and Newton's law of gravity. Theories generated or developed in the context of health services research are often associated with the human and social sciences. They include, for example, Becker's theory of health-seeking behaviour or the 'Health Belief Model' (Becker 1978), and Orem's 'Self Care Model' (Orem 1985). Whether a theory is of the physical or social sciences, the purpose is still to interpret and explain reality (Benoliel 1977) or to predict human experiences (DePoy & Gitlin 1994), and so provide information to guide everyday and professional life. This is none the less so in the world of research, and as such, theories perform similar functions within research projects. Given our reliance on theory, we need to have confidence in its approximation to reality. This requires that we are able to examine the premise(s) on which any theory is based. It is critical that we consider the underlying processes which may have led to the generation and/or testing of theory.

HOW RESEARCH PROCESSES CONTRIBUTE TO THEORY DEVELOPMENT

This section is concerned with the underlying conceptual processes that guide and may drive a research project. Research design is the outcome of a variety of important factors that have helped shape and determine the overall research approach and the methods selected. Factors include practical issues such as funding and time constraints, personal preferences and past experiences of particular methodologies. Equally important, the researcher will be asking himself or herself, two important questions:

- What is already known on the subject?
- What am I trying to find out?

In answering these questions, the researcher goes through particular thought processes that are indicative of different ways of reasoning known as induction and deduction. Induction and deduction pervade everyday thinking and help us make sense of our experiences. At a basic level, induction and deduction can be thought of as problem-solving mechanisms that help us to make sense of our observations in the real world, through a logical and ordered process to eventually arrive at a conclusion. One of the most distinguishing characteristics of deduction and induction are their respective starting points or 'take on reality'. They are very different. The researcher using deductive forms of reasoning adopts a more generalist perspective and views the world through a wide-angle lens, gradually working towards the specifics or particulars of a given situation or context. The reverse is true of the researcher who uses inductive forms of reasoning who starts with the specific and moves to the general or whole.

Induction and deduction, therefore, are processes involved in problem solving and arriving at a conclusion. The same is true for the researcher, who, depending on the problem to be solved, either begins at the generalist level or focuses on the specifics. Inductive and deductive processes provide the route taken by a researcher in problem solving, from the type of research question selected through to the sample size and the forms of data collection and analysis. Thus, induction and deduction suffuse the entire research process and manifest at the various stages of the research, from its inception in the formulation of a research question or hypothesis through to its findings. With reference to the stages of the research process, the critical reviewer of research may discern the forms of reasoning associated with an overall research design and the forms of methodology.

In general, the inductive researcher begins with an individual case or cases, out of which general rules evolve, processes normally associated with *theory generation*. The reverse is true of the deductive researcher who begins with a belief or general principle, which is then applied to a specific case, a process normally associated with *theory testing*. Research processes allow for such lines of thinking and argument to be tested and validated in some way, and then shared with the reader. Inductive and deductive reasoning processes therefore have varying parts to play in any research project. The degree to which they do so depends on the intention of the research itself, whether it is to explore, explain or allow predictions to be made.

Summary

The thoughtful researcher uses inductive or deductive reasoning depending on their approach to the problem or question under investigation, as well as how much is already known about the topic. As a critical reader of research, you should search for evidence of such processes throughout any research report.

WHAT SHOULD BE THE RELATIONSHIP BETWEEN THEORY AND RESEARCH?

Perhaps the most important point to be made about the relationship between theory and research is that research studies should build upon the existing body of knowledge. Ascertaining what is already known about a topic in order to identify a focus for new research constitutes vital early work in the process of any research project. Such insight ensures that the work is placed within a theoretical context and consequently that the research is informed by – and indeed adds to – the existing body of knowledge. This notion of research growing from and building upon what is already known is explained further by the following example of how you might go about researching something as commonplace as a garden.

Researching a garden

Suppose we asked you, a visitor from Mars, to research a garden. In the first instance you would presumably describe it: the size and shape of the ground covered; the presence of walls or fences; perhaps areas of light and shade, wet and dry. This could be followed by a description of the plants within the garden – trees, shrubs, flowers, weeds and grass. Such descriptions would usefully include reference to sizes, shapes and colours of the plants. At this stage, however, you would be unable to name them owing to a lack of knowledge of earth vegetation. If you wished to pursue your interest further, you could consult experts or access books on earth flora and from your initial descriptions begin to identify the various species of plant in the garden. This would be possible because the existing knowledge of earth flora is such that others have already examined and classified all the *known* plants growing on the planet. The plants have probably been photographed and presented in texts. As a result you would soon be in a position to differentiate between trees, shrubs, flowers and vegetables and probably name all the vegetation to be found in the garden under research. You would therefore be operating at the *exploratory* level of knowledge by attempting to describe, clarify and name objects (concepts) you have seen.

Ongoing observation of the garden would, however, indicate that you are not aware of all the information which could be useful to you, such as changes to the plants occurring through the seasons. You might also become aware from your observations that some plants tend to flourish in certain areas of the garden but not in others. This could be seen as reflecting knowledge at the descriptive level as, having clarified the objects and issues involved (such as the various plants, light/shade, wet/dry conditions), you have begun to consider possible relationships between things like the rapid growth of certain plants in particular areas of the garden. However, you would not be sure of the *nature* of the relationships identified, that is, whether they are cause-and-effect relationships.

Suppose, then, that you had noticed that there was a relationship between the strong growth of azaleas and the acidity of the soil, i.e. these plants appeared to flourish in such soils. It would be easy to jump to the conclusion that azaleas prefer acidic soils – but could it not also be the case that azaleas make the soils around them more acidic? For your knowledge to be at the level of *explanation or prediction*, you would have to carry out some sort of trial to establish the true cause and effect of this apparent relationship. Having done so, you would be able to state with some certainty that azaleas do indeed prefer acidic soils and, as a result, be able to recommend certain sites for planting them – in other words, to make predictions.

Basing research on what is already known has other benefits

- Minimizing the chances of repeating the past mistakes of others and unnecessarily duplicating work.
- Informing decisions regarding research methodology such as: What level of questioning is indicated? What level of data will be collected? What methods of data analysis will be used?
- Maximizing the chances that conclusions reached and any recommendations made will be realistic and based on the findings.

Identifying the relationship between what is known (theory) and empirical knowledge which is sought (research), is therefore an imperative for a researcher in the development of their research methodology. There is also a need to share the links between theory and research, as viewed by the researcher, with the research consumer.

Implications for the reader of research

We should recognize that theories are not merely abstract notions but useful mechanisms for explaining and predicting phenomena. They are representations of reality and as such they are as useful in 'real-life' as they are in research.

In research, theories are particularly useful because they offer a means of articulating to the reviewer of research (as well as clarifying for the researcher) just how the researcher believes a particular set of concepts or constructs are related, so allowing them to follow lines of argument and reasoning (inductive and/or deductive), as well as the evaluation of results (explanations and/or predictions) and any recommendations made.

The most important thing to consider when reading research is whether or not it builds upon the existing body of knowledge, which in most cases will be indicated via links which can be drawn between the literature review and the research design.

There are some researchers, however, who attempt to clearly and overtly identify the theoretical bases of their research. They do so by presenting a 'frame of reference'.

FRAMES OF REFERENCE IN RESEARCH

In this section we will examine frames of reference (conceptual and theoretical) and their role in research. We will then discuss points to consider when critically analysing frameworks used in published research.

Earlier in this chapter, the importance of research studies being based upon what is already known – the existing body of knowledge – was discussed. Using the example of 'researching the garden', we suggested that ascertaining what is already known about a topic is work that should be undertaken very early on in the process of research.

Being able to clearly trace the researcher's thoughts, reasoning and decisions about all aspects of the research process throughout a research report conveys a sense of transparency to the work. Frames of reference can greatly enhance the ability of the researcher to share their thoughts and decision-making trails with the critical reader and hence facilitate transparency.

What is a frame of reference?

Burns and Grove (1993) suggest that frames of reference are abstract and logical structures of meaning, which guide the development of a study and, in time, enable researchers to link their findings to existing knowledge. Moody (1990) takes this further by suggesting that by helping to guide the researcher in decisions about data collection and the interpretation of data, the researcher is more able to weave the facts into an orderly system, which in turn facilitates understanding in the reader. Frames of reference are therefore necessarily derived from the existing body of knowledge.

Frames of reference can also be seen as mechanisms by which researchers attempt to share abstract conceptualizations with others (Burns & Grove 1993). This may entail the clarification and description of concepts to be investigated in the study, suggestions about how the researcher perceives a group of concepts relate together or both. All these attributes are important, as a theoretically sound, well-thought through and clearly presented frame of reference can act as a link between the researcher and the reader, affording a degree of insight into the thoughts, reasoning and conclusions of the researcher.

The conceptual framework presented in Figure 5.1, developed by Ellis (2001), demonstrates the functions indicated above and clarifies the various concepts, such as the barriers that inhibit access to continuing professional development (CPD) and barriers to subsequent changes to practice (Ellis 2001). Possible relationships between the various concepts are also indicated. As a result the reader is in a position to decide whether they concur with the lines of

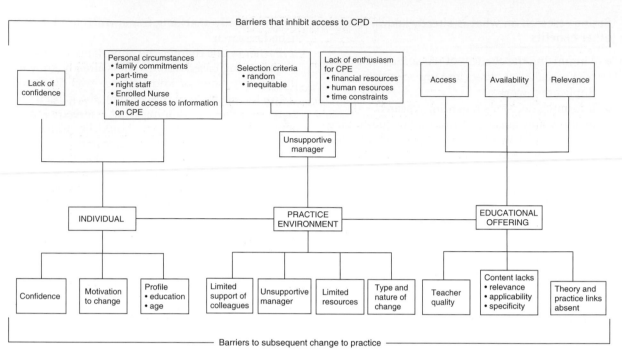

Figure 5.1   Conceptual framework to suggest the barriers that inhibit access to CPD and subsequent changes to practice (Ellis 2001).

Box 5.1 Example of a conceptual framework informing the development of a research instrument (Based on Thomson et al 1995)

In a study of the educational needs of community nurses in relation to their teaching role with students of nursing, Thomson et al (1995) drew on a theory known as Bradshaw's taxonomy of social need to provide a framework for the study. The researchers designed a questionnaire to reflect the four different types of need identified within the taxonomy. Bradshaw's definitions of each type of need are shown below, together with examples of questions from the questionnaire, designed to reflect the different types.

Normative need: need identified by a governing body or profession, e.g. *What qualifications or courses are you required by your employers to have attended in order to be allocated responsibility for supervising students?*

Comparative need: need identified by comparing individuals/organizations on the same attribute, e.g. *What arrangements for liaison exist between the educational centre from which the students come and the community placement areas?*

Felt need: need experienced/articulated by the individual, e.g. *What attributes/skills do you think community nurses and midwives need to help students to learn in community placements?* followed by: *In your opinion which of your own attributes/ skills require further development?*

Expressed need: 'felt' need expressed as a request or demand, e.g. *In the past three years have you identified any courses that you wished to undertake to assist you with your role in helping students to learn?*

---

argument that the researcher is putting forward, in this case what factors prevent the nurse from enrolling on a programme of study and which factors negate improvements in care, post CPD. Again, this can be seen as an example of transparency within a research process, as the researcher's thinking is laid open to scrutiny.

Frames of reference also guide researchers in the development of research methods and instruments, as exemplified in Box 5.1.

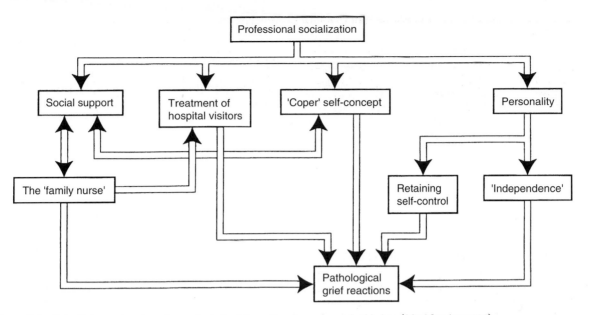

Figure 5.2   Potential causal routes of complicated grief reactions in nurses and midwives (After Crookes 1996).

Where do frames of reference come from?

In some cases a researcher may utilize an existing frame of reference, for example theories of nursing presented by Roper et al (1996) or Orem (1985). This can add credibility to a study as it should provide a firm theoretical basis to the work and facilitate comparison of findings with existing knowledge. However, this is only the case if the frame of reference chosen is clearly related to the study in hand. It is not unusual, for example, to find reports of studies examining adult learners such as nurses, using theory derived from work on how children learn.

Alternatively, a frame of reference may be generated by the researcher and may be quite original, though concepts within it may have been identified and refined by other researchers. An example of this is the conceptual framework of *potential causal routes of complicated grief reactions in nurses and midwives* (see Figure 5.2), which Patrick Crookes developed for his study on personal bereavement and Registered General Nurses (Crookes 1996). In the exploratory aspect of this work, previously clarified concepts such as 'social support' and 'coping' were utilized, along with less well-defined concepts such as 'the family nurse' role, to facilitate sharing of ideas about ways in which being a nurse may potentially complicate personal bereavement.

An interesting point to be made here is that conceptual frameworks reflect the thought processes and worldviews of those who develop them. While both Roper et al's and Orem's conceptual frameworks for nursing are based on the principle of promoting independence and 'self-care' in patients, the ways in which they articulate their ideas about how this can/should be applied to real life are very different. Theories (in this case in the form of conceptual frameworks) are only systematic versions of reality – not real life.

It is not uncommon to see a hybrid of the two approaches to the development of theory outlined above, with existing theory(ies) being incorporated within a new and perhaps wider application. An example of this is provided by McDonnell et al (1997) who utilized a number of theories related to health promotion and readiness to change (Prochaska & DiClemente 1986); and research utilization (Funk et al 1991) in their study of research utilization by practice nurses in the area of cardiovascular disease and stroke prevention.

How are frames of reference usually presented?

The way in which a frame of reference is shared with the reader varies. It may be in the form of descriptive text (e.g. Roper et al 1996), a diagram (as in Figures 5.1 and 5.2), or a combination of the two. Using both has the benefit of providing a visual summary along with written details of concepts and relationships considered in the study and can facilitate a greater understanding in the reader. This is obviously an important function of a framework, as others apart from those directly involved in a study need to be able to comprehend the theoretical bases on which a study is founded. Frameworks provide terms of reference within which the methods of enquiry used, the study findings, their interpretation and any conclusions or recommendations made, can be considered by the research consumer – therefore, a well thought-out and presented framework adds to the transparency of the work for the reader.

In summary, 'frames of reference' or 'frameworks' occupy a pivotal position within the process of research, acting variously as:

- A guide to the researcher and the critical reader to demonstrate that the work is pitched at a level which reflects what is already known about a research topic
- A means of clarifying concepts by offering 'visual' representations of abstract propositions about the topic being researched, to make them more accessible to the research consumer
- A bridge between what is 'known' and what is elicited by the current study
- An aid to both the researcher and the critical reader when examining the decision trails throughout a study
- An indication of the processes followed by the researcher in developing rigorous research methods and instruments.

Frames of reference should be considered where perceived relationships between concepts and decisions about method are discussed. However, overt discussion of the theoretical underpinnings of research projects is often lacking in published research papers. Frames of reference may also be offered or discussed in other areas (e.g. when findings and their implications are considered), depending very much upon the nature/level of the study, i.e. whether it is at the exploratory, descriptive or predictive level (Brink & Wood 1988).

RELATIONSHIPS BETWEEN LEVELS OF RESEARCH AND FRAMES OF REFERENCE

Frames of reference can be categorized as either conceptual or theoretical frameworks. A perusal of the research literature indicates that the terms are often used interchangeably, by both researchers and authors of research texts. Is it correct to do this? Are there any important differences between conceptual and theoretical frameworks?

Conceptual frameworks

Newman (1979) defines a conceptual framework as 'an organisation or matrix of concepts, that provides a focus for enquiry'. A conceptual framework is developed by linking concepts selected from theories, experience and/or other studies (Burns & Grove 1993) to form new and as yet untested propositions. They therefore reflect 'grand theories' (Moody 1990, p218) in that few of the concepts or relationships involved will have been formally tested. Their function is to act as a means by which hypotheses can be derived, which can then be submitted to testing at a later date (to generate middle-range theory). For those interested in a more detailed discussion of levels of theory, Moody's (1990) text is recommended.

In essence, conceptual frameworks are more correctly used in exploratory research studies. These are studies undertaken with the intention of exploring and clarifying concepts and possible relationships between them. Exploratory studies are appropriate when the existing body of knowledge is such that there is little or no empirical literature on either the topic or the population under examination (Brink & Wood 1988). In turn, such studies may act as 'groundwork' for further investigation at the descriptive or predictive level, where the identification of relationships between concepts indicated by the exploratory work provides the focus.

An example is provided by Crookes' (1996) study. As a result of this exploratory work, based around the conceptual framework in Figure 5.2, a theoretical framework was developed which proposes ways in which societal expectations of nurses and midwives *could* lead to complicated grief reactions in some individuals (see Figure 5.3). In other words, *possible* relationships between being a nurse and a predisposition to complicated grief reactions are put forward. It is intended that this will form the basis of further research aimed at testing such propositions.

Theoretical frameworks

Nieswiandomy (1993, p834) suggests that theoretical frameworks provide a framework for studies 'based on propositional statements from a theory or theories'; in other words, studies in which the concepts or variables involved have been truly substantiated by previous research and where the intention now is to test perceived relationships between them. At the descriptive level of research, this involves verification that relationships between

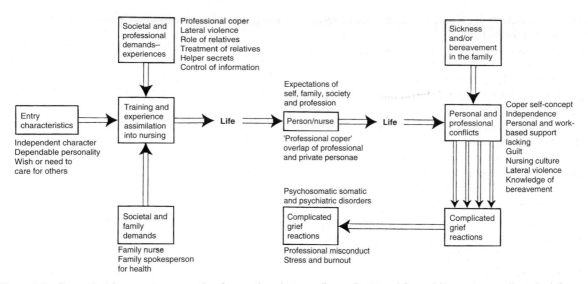

Figure 5.3 Theoretical framework representing factors thought to predispose Registered General Nurses to complicated grief reactions (Crookes 1996).

variables do exist. To return to the garden analogy, this would relate to the identification of a relationship between leguminous plants (such as Brussels sprouts and green beans) and high levels of nitrogen in the soil. The point to be made here is that while a relationship has been established between the two, cause and effect has not. That is, we cannot be sure without further research whether leguminous plants prosper in nitrogen-rich soil *or* that such plants cause the ground around them to become richer in nitrogen. Research at the predictive level, for example an experiment, involves the testing of possible explanations for observed phenomena and thus allows the identification of 'cause and effect' relationships. In this case, it is a fact that leguminous plants do have the ability to transfer nitrogen from the air into the soil around them – hence the centuries-old farming technique of growing such crops in rotation to allow fields to recover their nitrogen content and so become fertile again, without the need for artificial fertilizers. In this case, such research would *explain* why such practices have been successful over the years and might allow the translation of these principles to other settings.

The relationship between conceptual and theoretical frameworks

Whilst there are similarities between the two types of framework in that they both perform the functions listed on page 62, there are also fundamental differences. Using the terms interchangeably is not only confusing, particularly to those new to research, but also incorrect and imprecise.

The essential difference between conceptual and theoretical frameworks relates to:

- The level of knowledge which exists regarding the concepts examined within the study in question
- The direction and strength of the relationships thought to exist between those concepts
- The degree to which empirical testing of concepts and the relationships between them is valid.

The term conceptual framework refers to a fairly *informal* and relatively *untested* set of propositions regarding a number of concepts and the *possible* relationships between them. Such frameworks are most correctly used in exploratory research studies, where the intention is to gain more insight into concepts and their interrelatedness. A theoretical framework, on the other hand, is one which offers a more formal set of propositions and a well-developed mechanism for asserting relationships between concepts and thus forms the basis for descriptive and/or predictive research.

So there is a difference between conceptual and theoretical frameworks! That difference relates essentially to the absence or presence of clear statements about relationships between concepts included in the framework and thus should reflect what is already known about the topic under research.

WHERE ARE FRAMEWORKS FOUND?

In a detailed research report, a framework (conceptual or theoretical) will typically be found in a chapter of its own, often sandwiched between the literature review and the methods section. This is apt, as an effective framework acts as a bridge between what has gone before (theory and/or existing knowledge) and what is to come (the prospective study). It may be in the form of a diagram, a description and/or discussion of relevant concepts, or both. However, frameworks may also be found later in research reports, for example in discussion or conclusion sections, when a product of the research has been the refinement of a conceptual framework or the development of a theoretical framework. This demonstrates that frameworks can have relevance in various parts of research studies, as a linkage between the conceptual and empirical aspects of a study and also as an endpoint, to demonstrate perceived relationships between concepts. Their effectiveness therefore must be measured against the stated objectives of the work.

It is rare, however, for research consumers to have access to detailed reports. Usually they must rely on the brief overview papers published in professional journals. Historically, such papers have tended not to include overt discussion of – or even reference to – the conceptual underpinnings of the research (Polit & Hungler 1993), though this would appear to be changing within the 'quality' nursing journals. Absence may be as a result of the researcher not developing or using a frame of reference or they may have failed to articulate it adequately for the reader (perhaps even for themselves). Whilst this does not nullify the contribution of such work, its credibility and potential application to practice are inevitably brought into question. It may also mean that the report is much more difficult for the critical reader to 'appreciate', due to the effect on the transparency of the work.

Alternatively it may be the case that in brief reports, the theory underpinning the research is either presented under a specific heading, such as 'frame of reference', or clearly discussed in the literature review section. Examples of these include Graydon (1994), who utilized Lazarus and Folkman's (1984) theory of stress and coping to help explore the quality of life of women following mastectomy, and defined this under the heading 'theoretical framework'. Before undertaking a study exploring the abilities of cancer nurses to provide psychological care to patients in cancer care settings, Hanson (1994) explored three particular areas of the literature: stress theory and research; stress and its relationship with cancer; and psychological concepts pertaining to stress and persons with cancer. In this case the literature review structured around these areas presents pertinent theory to the reader and so clearly fulfils the remit of a framework discussed earlier, without overtly placing it under such a heading. It is the end and not the means that is therefore important when evaluating this aspect of a research report.

What to look for in the framework section of a study

Having discussed the function of frameworks and identified their importance in the research process, specific points to consider within research reports are offered here in brief:

- First and most obvious – is there a conceptual or theoretical framework? Is it made explicit?
- Has it been derived from – and with reference to – the existing body of knowledge?
- Is the framework appropriate for the study?
- Are the concepts clearly defined and understandable to the reader?
- Are relationships between the concepts clearly stated and understandable to the reader?
- Does the framework appear comprehensive?
- Is there an apparent linkage between 'theory', research methods and instrumentation, results and conclusions/recommendations?

If the answer to these questions is 'yes', then the frame of reference has done its job. Concepts and perceived relationships between them have clearly been articulated for the reader, having been derived from the existing body of knowledge and leading to the use of research methods which clearly focus on the research question(s). The framework will also have been effective because it is important that a critical reader is able to discern clear links between the research findings and the existing body of knowledge. It is surprising how often researchers fail to discuss their research findings adequately in the light of data from other studies.

If a theoretical framework has been put forward and so propositional statements are to be 'tested', then further questions can be asked:

- Are appropriate definitions provided for the concepts that will be tested?
- Is the propositional statement(s) which guides the research question or hypothesis clearly identifiable?
- Is the methodology chosen (questions/ hypotheses; instruments; analyses; findings; conclusions) consistent with the theory?
- Does the theory provide an adequate framework within which to describe, discuss and interpret the findings?

Summary

In research, correctly used conceptual frameworks are typically associated with exploratory studies where existing theory is inapplicable or insufficient. They allow the researcher to clarify concepts and *possible* relationships between them for the reader and thus provide a bridge between what is 'known' and what is intended to be elicited, by the study in hand, as discussed earlier. The point to remember is that if used correctly, the term 'conceptual framework' refers to a fairly *informal* and relatively *untested* set of propositions, regarding a number of concepts and the *possible* relationships between them.

The term 'theoretical framework', when correctly used, describes a rather more formal and well-developed mechanism for organizing phenomena to be examined than does a conceptual framework. The major difference is that a theoretical framework contains a set of propositions that assert relationships among the concepts. In descriptive research, such propositions can only indicate the existence of such relationships. On the other hand, predictive research seeks to substantiate cause and effect relationships and so verify or refute theory. Theoretical frameworks allow researchers to explain observations and make predictions about what is likely to happen in a given set of circumstances.

A theoretical framework may *sometimes* be a natural progression of a conceptual framework, as research based on a conceptual framework may

lead to substantiation and clarification of concepts and indicate relationships between a number of them (Crookes 1996). A theory of how concepts interrelate can then be developed, which is then articulated to the 'audience' as a theoretical framework.

The following exercise is designed to illustrate and reinforce points made in this text about frames of reference.

Exercise 5.1   Research questions

Consider each of the conceptual/theoretical frameworks in Box 5.2 together with the list of research questions below. Identify the framework(s) which could provide a useful basis for an exploration of each question.

- To what extent do hospital inpatients wish to be involved in planning their own care?
- What sort of interventions should practice nurses make in attempting to help people to stop smoking?
- How can nurses ensure that their work with older patients on a rehabilitation ward is optimally therapeutic?
- What factors affect compliance among young people with newly diagnosed diabetes?
- What nursing actions are most effective in meeting the needs of suddenly bereaved family members in the A&E department?

Exercise 5.2

Take time to think about your views on what knowledge is important and valid, and what is not.

Exercise 5.3

Find a number of research articles on a topic which interests you. In the light of points discussed in this chapter, identify the research paradigms which inform them. Having done that, decide whether the approaches chosen accurately reflect what the researcher(s) really wanted to know. Using the same articles, identify whether the research undertaken builds upon existing theory (what is known) or not. If it does, how is this link articulated for the reader?

Box 5.2 Conceptual and theoretical frameworks: an exercise

Health belief model (Becker 1978) Health-seeking behaviour is influenced by a person's perception of a threat posed by a health problem and the value associated with actions aimed at reducing the threat. The major components of the Health Belief Model include perceived susceptibility, perceived severity, perceived benefits and costs, motivation and enabling or modifying factors.

Learned helplessness theory (Seligman 1972) People tend to behave resignedly if their personal competency levels have been eroded and they feel that whatever behaviour they engage in, they cannot produce desired outcomes. Unless the environment is changed, apathy and depression are likely to result.

Readiness to change model (Prochaska & DiClemente 1986) When attempting to modify their own addictive behaviour, individuals move through a series of stages. The process begins with precontemplation (when the individual is not at all interested in changing their behaviour), through contemplation to preparing to change, making changes and finally maintaining change. Individuals who leap to action without adequate preparation or contemplation are at high risk for relapse.

Crisis theory (Aguilera & Messick 1980, Woolley 1990) Crisis is defined as an upset or disequilibrium in a steady state occurring when usual problem-solving strategies are ineffective. When an individual experiences an emotionally hazardous situation and is unable to use previously learned coping behaviours effectively or to reduce the stress using new problem-solving strategies, an emotional crisis may result. Immediately following a crisis event, prompt and skilful interventions are necessary to assist individuals towards maintaining or regaining emotional equilibrium.

Orem's theory of self-care (Orem 1985) Focuses upon each individual's ability to perform self-care. The need for nursing arises from self-care deficits, which occur when a person does not have the capacity for continuous self-care. Three categories of self-care requisites are proposed: universal requisites associated with physical life and the maintenance of human structure and functioning; developmental requisites associated with developmental processes at various stages of the life cycle; and health deviation requisites (arising as a result of an illness process or abnormality). The nurse's role may be wholly compensatory, partially compensatory or supportive–educative.

Maslow's theory of motivation (Maslow 1987) Individuals strive for holistic growth through a hierarchy of values and needs (which Maslow presented in pyramidal form). The base of the pyramid represents physiological and safety/security needs. These basic needs demand an individual's attention until satisfied. Only when these needs are met can attention be directed towards affiliation and self-esteem needs and eventually to self-actualization.

CONCLUSION

In this chapter we have explained and compared three research philosophies: the positivist, the naturalistic, and critical theory paradigms. We did this to highlight the fact that each has its strengths and weaknesses in terms of informing research processes. As such, we have attempted to undermine the traditional 'quantitative versus qualitative' debate and move you, the critical reader of research, to a position of judging the approach taken by a researcher on the basis of how well it asks the relevant questions, rather than how well it adheres to a particular worldview. Different research methods should not compete. What we need to understand is that they tell us different things.

We have also discussed 'theories', making the point that they are useful mechanisms for explaining and predicting phenomena – not merely abstractions with no real purpose. In research, theories are particularly useful because they offer a means of articulating just how the researcher believes a particular set of concepts or constructs are related together. We then presented arguments regarding the relationships which should exist between research and theory. The nature of theories and the processes of inductive and deductive reasoning were presented in support of these arguments, as was a classification of levels of knowledge ranging from exploration, through description, to explanation and prediction. The key point from this section is that research should stem from and build upon what is already known. It is up to the researcher to ensure that they do this and to demonstrate this clearly in the research report.

Finally we covered the issue of 'frames of reference' in research. This included explanations of what they are, their function within the research process, how they are generated and presented and what to look for in the framework section of a study. The fact that clear explication of the theoretical underpinnings of any research project facilitates 'transparency' for the reader, was a point repeatedly returned to within the chapter.

We hope that after reading this chapter, you will feel more confident about evaluating the theoretical aspects of research reports you read in the future. This should be so because you will be better prepared to evaluate the appropriateness of the research design and research methods; the suitability of the research questions; and the compatibility between the research methods, findings and conclusions.

References

Aguilera D and Messick J (1980) *Crisis Intervention: Theory and Methodology*. London: Mosby.

Becker M (1978) The Health Belief Model and sick role behaviour. *Nursing Digest* **6**: 35–40.

Benoliel JQ (1977) The interaction between theory and research. *Nursing Outlook* **25**: 108–113.

Brink P and Wood M (1988) *Planning Nursing Research: From Question to Proposal*. Boston, MA: Jones & Bartlett.

Burns N and Grove SK (1993) *The Practice of Nursing Research: Conduct, Critique and Utilisation*, 2nd edn. Philadelphia, PA: WB Saunders.

Carr W (1989) Action research: ten years on. *Curriculum Studies* **21**(1): 85–90.

Carper BA (1978) Fundamental patterns of knowing in nursing. *Advances in Nursing Science* **1**(3): 13–23.

Crookes PA (1996) *Personal bereavement in registered general nurses*. Unpublished PhD thesis, University of Hull, UK.

DePoy E and Gitlin LN (1994) *Introduction to Research: Multiple Strategies for Health and Human Services*. St Louis, MO: Mosby.

Elliott J (1991) *Action Research for Educational Change*. Milton Keynes: Open University Press.

Ellis LB (2001) *Continuing Professional Education for Nurses: an Illuminative Case Study*. Sheffield: Faculty of Medicine, University of Sheffield, unpublished PhD thesis.

Funk SG, Champagne MT, Wiese RT et al (1991) Barriers: the barriers to research utilisation scale. *Applied Nursing Research* **4**(1): 39–45.

Graydon J (1994) Women with breast cancer: their quality of life following a course of radiation therapy. *Journal of Advanced Nursing* **19**: 12–20.

Greenwood J (1984) Nursing research: a position paper. *Journal of Advanced Nursing* **9**: 77–82.

Hanson E (1994) An exploration of the taken for granted world of the cancer nurse in relation to stress and the person with cancer. *Journal of Advanced Nursing* **19**: 45–51.

Hart E (1995) Developing action research in nursing. *Nurse Researcher* **2**(3): 4–14.

Hunt M (1987) The process of translating research findings into nursing practice. *Journal of Advanced Nursing* **12**: 101–110.

Kerlinger FN (1973) *Foundations of Behavioral Research*, 2nd edn. New York: Holt, Rinehart & Winston.

Knowles (1984) *Androgogy in Action*. San Francisco, CA: Jossey Bass.

Lazarus RS and Folkmann S (1984) *Stress appraisal and coping*. New York: Springer.

Leininger MM (1985) *Qualitative Research Methods in Nursing*. Philadelphia: WB Saunders.

McDonnell A, Davies S, Brown J et al (1997) *A detailed investigation of the implementation of research-based knowledge by practice nurses in the prevention of cardiovascular disease and stroke prevention*. Report to the NHS Executive, Northern and Yorkshire Region.

Mackenzie AE (1992) Learning from experience in the community: an ethnographic study of district nurse students. *Journal of Advanced Nursing* **17**: 682–691.

McKay R (1969) Theories, models and systems for nursing. *Nursing Research* **18**: 393–399.

Maslow AH (1987) *Motivation and Personality*. London: Harper and Row.

Meerabeau L (1992) Tacit nursing knowledge: an untapped resource or a methodological headache? *Journal of Advanced Nursing* **17**: 108–112.

Moody LE (1990) *Advancing Nursing Science Through Research*, vol 1. Newbury Park, DC: Sage.

Newman M (1979) *Theory Development in Nursing*. Philadelphia: Davis.

Nieswiandomy RM (1993) *Foundations of Nursing Research*, 2nd edn. Norwalk, Connecticut: Appleton and Lange.

Orem DE (1985) *Concepts of Practice*, 3rd edn. New York: McGraw-Hill.

Polit DF and Hungler BP (1991) *Nursing Research: Principles and Methods*. Philadelphia, PA: Lippincott.

Polit DF and Hungler BP (1993) *Essentials of Nursing Research – Methods, Appraisal and Utilisation*. Philadelphia: Lippincott.

Prochaska JO and DiClemente CC (1986) *Towards a comprehensive model of change*. New York: Plenum.

Roper N, Logan WW and Tierney AJ (1996) *The Elements of Nursing: A Model For Nursing Based On a Model of Living*, 4th edn. Edinburgh: Churchill Livingstone.

Seligman MGP (1972) Learned helplessness. *Annual Review of Medicine* **23**: 407–412.

Seligman M (1975) *Helplessness*. San Francisco: WH Freeman.

Thomson A, Davies S, Shepherd B et al (1995) An investigation into the changing educational needs of community nurses, midwives and health visitors in relation to the teaching, supervising and assessing of pre- and postregistration students. Report to the English National Board for Nursing, Midwifery and Health Visiting, University of Manchester.

Titchen A (1995) Issues of validity in action research. *Nurse Researcher* **2**(3): 38–48.

Titchen A and Binnie A (1993) Action research as a research strategy: finding our way through a philosophical and methodological maze. *Changing Nursing Practice Through Action Research Report No. 6, National Institute for Nursing*, Oxford.

Wallace M (1987) A historical review of action research: some implications for the education of teachers in their managerial role. *Journal of Education for Teaching* **13**(2): 97–110.

Webb C (1990) Partners in research. *Nursing Times* **86**(32): 40–44.

Woolley N (1990) Crisis theory: a paradigm of effective intervention with families of critically ill people. *Journal of Advanced Nursing* **15**: 1402–1408.

Further reading

Bryman A (1993) Quantity and Quality in Social Research. Contemporary Social Research: 18 Series Editor: Martin Bulmer. London: Routledge.

Chalmers AF (1994) *What is This Thing Called Science?*, 2nd edn. Milton Keynes: Open University Press.

Ellis LB (1996) Evaluating the effects of continuing professional education on practice: Researching for impact. *Nursing Times Research* **1**(4): 296–306.

Kikuchi JF and Simmons H (1992) *Philosophic Inquiry in Nursing*. London: Sage Publications.

Leininger MM (1985) *Qualitative Research Methods in Nursing*. Philadelphia: WB Saunders.

Chapter **6**

The relationship between research question and research design

Jan Draper

INTRODUCTION

The whole emphasis of this book is to enable you to develop the skills needed to critically evaluate the research you read, so that this critical utilization of research might inform the development of your clinical practice. This chapter is concerned with the relationship between the question the research sets out to answer and the research design used to answer this question. This association between question and design is fundamental to the whole research process, because if an inappropriate design has been used to answer a research question, the quality of the research project will be fundamentally undermined. As the utility of any research depends on its quality and purpose (Closs & Cheater 1999), it is therefore important that a particular research question is matched with an appropriate design. So the 'fit' between research question and research design underpins the whole foundation of the research process and this chapter will explore the nature of this relationship.

The chapter is organized into two major sections. The first will explore what is meant by the term the 'research question' and will cover issues such as 'What do we mean by a research question?', 'What is the purpose of the research?', 'What is it that the researcher wants to know?', 'What is known already?', and 'What type of knowledge will be generated?'. The second section will examine what is meant by 'research design' and will provide an overview of the major different types of design, their strengths and limitations. The conclusion will bring these elements together and highlight the key issues you need to consider when reading research papers.

Key issues

- Types of research question
- Types of research design
- The relationship between research questions and research design
- The contribution of triangulation

Exercise 6.1

Take a few moments to consider the terms 'research question' and 'research design'. From your knowledge of research so far, brainstorm what you think these terms mean and note down your thoughts. We shall return to this activity later in the chapter.

THE RESEARCH QUESTION

In response to Exercise 6.1, you may have noted that, very simply, a research question is the essence of what the researcher wants to know or the question they want to answer. Parahoo (1997, p396) defines the research question as 'the broad question which is set at the start of a study'. The centrality of the research question to the whole research process is outlined by Rees (1997, p8) who suggests that 'research consists of extending knowledge and understanding through a carefully structured systematic process of collecting information which answers a specific question in a way that is as objective and accurate as possible'.

The overall purpose of the research is therefore to find an answer to the research question. An appropriate and well-executed research design ensures that this is done in the most rigorous way possible. So, at the outset of a study, the researcher outlines what it is they want to know. In the current climate of evidence-based practice, perhaps the researcher is interested in finding the most clinically and cost effective way of delivering care in a particular setting. In this instance, the research question should be tightly focussed; that is, it should be extremely clear exactly what aspect of practice the researcher is investigating and with which population of patients or clients. Or perhaps the researcher is interested in exploring the experience of a specific group of patients living with a particular chronic disease. In this kind of study the research question may well be somewhat broader, as the researcher is unsure exactly what type of answers they might uncover. These are examples of very different research questions which, as we shall see, require different research designs to answer them.

Exercise 6.2

Take a few moments to think about your clinical practice. No doubt there are areas of this practice that interest you and which you would like to explore in more detail. Perhaps you have already thought about some of these in detail, during your reading of the research literature or from discussion with colleagues. You might of course find answers to your queries by conducting a critical literature review. However, for the purpose of this activity, imagine that there is insufficient evidence available. How would you go about researching your topic? What might your research question be?

Developing a 'good' research question can be quite difficult, as perhaps Exercise 6.2 demonstrated. The question needs to be clear and well articulated so that there is no doubt about what it is the researcher wants to know. Cormack and Benton (1996) distinguish between two types of research question – interrogative and declarative. An interrogative research question is expressed as a question and alludes to a gap in health care knowledge. An example might be 'What is the experience of older people following discharge from hospital?'. A declarative research question is a statement that clearly defines the purpose of the study. For example, 'The purpose of this study is to examine the relationship between systematic discharge preparations and hospital readmission rates in a group of older people'.

Whatever style of research question adopted by a researcher, the question should be clearly expressed and, normally tightly focussed. A woolly or fuzzy question will lead to a woolly and fuzzy answer.

LEVELS OF KNOWLEDGE

The development of the research question is determined by the type of knowledge the researcher is intending to generate. Different types of research question will generate different types of knowledge, so the way in which the research question is expressed will be dependent upon whether the researcher is seeking to generate either descriptive, explanatory or predictive knowledge.

When little is known about a topic, research can be designed which provides a detailed description of the topic, generating descriptive knowledge. Research approaches which develop this type of knowledge can be either quantitative or qualitative but are more likely to be qualitative, as these methods more frequently, although not exclusively, allow detailed exploration of a particular topic. The question might also be interrogative in nature, for example 'What is women's experience of living with cervical cancer?'.

When a researcher is interested in explaining the relationship between different components of a specific topic, then explanatory knowledge will be generated. There is usually some knowledge already available on a number of aspects of this topic and so new research is designed to further explore relationships between the various components of this knowledge. Research questions are more likely to be declarative, for example 'The purpose of this study is to examine the relationship between surgical pre-assessment and post-operative pain' and research methods are most likely to be quantitative, such as surveys. Descriptive and inferential statistics are frequently used to explore the nature of the relationships between the variables identified in the research question.

When descriptive and explanatory knowledge about a topic is already available, a researcher may want to know whether some of these variables have a cause-and-effect relationship. In this instance, predictive knowledge is generated. Predictive knowledge is often regarded as the most powerful form of knowledge and is concerned with confirming or rejecting cause-and-effect relationships; in other words X will/will not have Y effect on Z. For example, does a preadmission home visit to women booked for planned hysterectomy lead to improved psychosocial functioning postoperatively? Experimental research is the methodology of choice here, as only a well-controlled experiment, such as a randomized controlled trial, will confidently establish such links.

WHAT IS KNOWN ALREADY?

The previous chapter suggested that research studies should build upon an existing body of knowledge. So, any new research study should develop what is already known, however limited this knowledge might be. For research intending to generate descriptive knowledge, it is likely that there will be less existing research available than for a study proposing to develop explanatory or predictive knowledge. However, irrespective of the amount of existing knowledge, prior to devising a research question,

the researcher must examine what evidence already exists with respect to their area of enquiry. Awareness of existing knowledge may well inform the way in which the researcher proposes to proceed with the research. (As we shall see later, grounded theory can be an exception to this approach.)

It is normal, therefore, that a literature review will be undertaken. Literature reviews fulfil a number of purposes including satisfying professional curiosity on a subject, locating evidence to inform practice development and finding solutions to immediate practice problems. In the context of this chapter, literature reviews are central to locating existing knowledge which might suggest directions for future research (Talbot 1995). There are, however, a number of limitations associated with literature reviews and awareness of these is important, as they may have a bearing on the development of the research question. Cullum (1994) suggests that the following can be common problems with literature reviews:

- Frequently reviews are insufficiently critical
- The process for selecting and including material in the review is often unclear
- There can be bias in favour of studies that demonstrate positive findings
- Insufficient information is provided about the review process in general.

In addition, implications for practice and for future research are sometimes inadequately explored.

As a result of these limitations the methodology of systematic reviews has developed over the last 10 to 15 years, to make the whole process of literature reviewing more rigorous. Systematic reviews differ from conventional critical literature reviews because they follow a 'strict scientific design in order to make them more comprehensive, to minimize the chance of bias and so ensure their reliability. Rather than reflecting the views of the authors or being based on only a (possibly biased) selection of the published literature, they contain a comprehensive summary of the available evidence' (CRD Report 4, 1996, pi). (For further information on literature reviews and systematic reviews, see Chapters 11 and 12).

Where it exists, then, reference to knowledge made available by the process of systematic reviewing is likely to indicate that a researcher has attempted to seek out the most rigorous knowledge available on the topic. However, despite their clear benefits to health care practice and their high profile in current research and development policy, systematic literature reviews have also received criticism. This is due in large part to their reliance on evidence generated via randomized controlled trials (see below) and their subsequent exclusion of evidence produced by other forms of research. I will return to this debate a little later in this chapter.

THE INFLUENCE OF THE RESEARCHER

It can be seen from the discussion so far, that development of the research question is informed by the response to a number of questions. What is the purpose of the research? What is it that the researcher wants to know? What type of knowledge is going to be generated? What is known already? So although framing of the research question is arguably the first hurdle to overcome, there are a series of preparatory stages the researcher must first negotiate.

It is important to acknowledge, therefore, that even this very first step in the research process is very much influenced by the researcher. Although the research question may appear 'objective' and 'scientific', particularly in the context of quantitative methods, it is important to remember that the question has not been conceived in a vacuum. Researchers do not 'arrive empty minded in the field' (James 1993, p67) but bring to the project their own beliefs and interests, which are influenced by their position in the world and their previous experience of research, including perhaps favoured ways of conducting research. Therefore, throughout the research process, including the development of the research question, the researcher is not a 'neutral spectator' (Denzin 1997, p35) who is abstracted and distanced from the research. Rather, their influence is woven throughout the project from inception to execution, analysis and presentation. Research design may attempt to remove traces of the researcher's existence, but their presence in and influence over the creation of the project (whether in the natural or social sciences) determines the framing of the research question, the methodological approach taken and ultimately the nature of the knowledge generated. So any investigation can never be devoid of the influence of the investigator (Koch & Harrington 1998). Carson and Fairbairn (2002, p25) argue that:

> Research questions are not grasped out of thin air but are the choice of the researchers in the field. Questions are developed from a particular theoretical perspective that a researcher chooses, and answers to these questions relate directly back to the research's theoretical perspective; the choice of research question will have a direct influence on the answers received.

Summary

It is particularly important when reading published research to be able to clearly identify the purpose of the study and what the researcher is attempting to find out. This is most often expressed as a research question or research aim/objective. For some studies using quantitative methods, the purpose of the research is expressed in terms of a hypothesis, which is 'a tentative statement, in one sentence, about the relationship, if any, between two or more variables' (Parahoo 1997, p126). Hypotheses should include reference not only to the variables and the relationship between them, but also the population involved in the study.

The researcher has a responsibility at the outset of a research report or paper to make this question clear. This may seem obvious and simple, but sometimes the research question is 'buried' away in the paper and is not obvious at all. As critical readers of research, we cannot make an accurate assessment of the methodology and methods used if we are unclear about the overall purpose of the research (Parahoo 1997). This makes our role as critical readers more difficult (Long 2002).

Exercise 6.3

Now that we have discussed the nature of the research question and some of the factors that determine its development in more detail, it is time to put this knowledge into action. Select a number of published papers reporting empirical research projects on topics that are of interest to you. Examine the research questions identified by the authors with reference to the following:

- *What is the purpose of the research?*
- *What is it that the researcher wants to know?*
- *What type of knowledge is going to be generated?*
- *What is known already?*
- *What is the influence of the researcher?*

Some examples of hypothetical research questions have been included below. We will return to these research questions in the section which follows, during our examination of some of the major research designs.

Research questions

1. What are men's experiences of the transition to contemporary fatherhood?

2. What are older women's experiences of becoming widows?
3. Is there a relationship between undertaking an in-house training programme on effective pain management and the quality of pain control on a hospital ward?
4. Is there a relationship between parental attendance in the anaesthetic room and subsequent length of hospital stay for the child following tonsillectomy?
5. Does restricted use of restraint lead to increased rates of falls in older people in a residential setting?

RESEARCH DESIGN

The research design is the overall plan of how the researcher intends to implement the project in practice. Parahoo (1997, p142) defines the research design as 'a plan that describes how, when and where data are to be collected and analysed'. The design also includes details 'for enhancing the internal and external validity of the study' (Polit & Hungler 1991, p653). It includes a description of how the sample is to be identified and recruited, ethical considerations, confidentiality, anonymity, access to the research site, how the data are to be collected and analysed and how the researcher intends to disseminate the findings of the study. So, in essence, the research design is concerned with the practical arrangements of getting an answer to the research question.

Research design is an umbrella term which encompasses the two concepts of 'research methodology' and 'research methods', terms which are frequently used interchangeably in the literature. Methodology is the overall research approach chosen by the researcher, for example whether experimental, survey, ethnography, phenomenology, grounded theory, action research or participatory research. Different research methodologies are influenced by different research perspectives or paradigms. Research method refers to the practical ways in which the researcher intends to collect and analyse data. In quantitative methods, these include structured questionnaires, rating scales and structured observation, and in qualitative methods, semi-structured or unstructured interviews, participant observation, narrative analysis and content analysis.

As we have already seen, research can generate different forms of knowledge (descriptive, explanatory or predictive) and it is the combination of a clear and focussed research question with the most appropriate research design, that is responsible for the level of knowledge generated. Some questions will be so specific that only one design will be appropriate, whilst other questions will be more ambiguous and may be informed by a number of different approaches.

It is extremely important that researchers select the most appropriate design for their study. In making their choice of the best approach to answer the research question, they must also take account of their own experience, any support or supervision they will need, any cost and other resource implications, the accessibility of the sample and whether there are any complex ethical considerations which may impede the progress of the research.

All of these factors influence the development of the overall research design. What is extremely important to this process is that there is congruence between the nature of the question posed by the researcher and the research design selected. In order to enable you to make decisions about the 'fit' between question and design, this section now provides a brief overview of quantitative and qualitative methods, prior to examining the different research methodologies in more detail.

OVERVIEW OF RESEARCH DESIGN

The relationship between philosophy and research is very influential in guiding (either consciously or not) a researcher's choice of research methodology.

You will recall from Chapter 5 that the paradigm of positivism is a world view which assumes that rules govern the social world in much the same way as rules and laws govern the natural world. Consequently positivism assumes that social reality exists in the same way as physical reality and that this reality can be captured and measured. In this process, the researcher is detached and 'objective', contributing unbiased and supposedly value-free knowledge. Emphasis within this paradigm is on testing theory and determining cause and effect, resulting in the generation of predictive knowledge. Consequently research within this paradigm uses predominantly quantitative research methods.

In contrast, the naturalistic paradigm assumes that there is no single and objective reality or truth because, as we are all different, a number of realities can simultaneously exist. This paradigm acknowledges therefore that different people will attach different meanings to the same phenomena. Research within this paradigm is concerned with understanding these different perceptions and meanings. The cultural context in which the research takes place and the position and influence of the researcher are not ignored in the research process but considered important. Emphasis in this paradigm is on generating theory and qualitative methods are predominantly used.

Over the last two decades there has been significant debate in the medical and health care literature about the relative merits of quantitative and qualitative research methods. Proponents of quantitative methods, for example, have suggested that all research should use such methods, as this is the only way to ensure the validity and reliability of research. Conversely, advocates of qualitative methods have suggested that it is only by using these methods that we can truly understand the experience of a patient or client.

Carson and Fairbairn (2002, p21) have been critical of researchers who appear entrenched in one paradigm and suggest that:

> One of the problems with some and perhaps many researchers in nursing and allied health areas is that they are so committed to a particular research paradigm, that they fail to notice whether it can deliver adequate answers to their research questions. Indeed, rather than looking for a method that is appropriate to the research questions that are raised, some will change those questions to allow them to make use of their favoured research method or methods.

In contrast to 'methodolatry' (Oakley 1990), other commentators argue that no one research methodology is fundamentally superior to another (Avis 1994). Arguments about which methods are the best are therefore fruitless (Begley 1996) and indeed, as we shall see later, different methodologies can be used complementarily (Poole & Jones 1996). Closs and Cheater (1999, p13) suggest that 'it is time to stop wasting energy on arguing whether qualitative or quantitative methods provide the "best" information for nursing. We need to choose whichever method is likely to answer clearly articulated questions of importance to the profession'.

So rather than framing a research question so that it can be answered using a researcher's favoured methodological approach, it is important that nursing and health care researchers first frame the question and then choose the most appropriate method to answer it. In other words, they should choose the correct tool to do the job rather than first choosing the tool and then asking 'Now, what job can I do?'.

Exercise 6.4

Go back to the research questions identified on pages 72–73. See whether you can identify which questions would be most amenable to examination via qualitative or quantitative methods.

QUANTITATIVE RESEARCH APPROACHES

When a research question is attempting to generate explanatory or predictive knowledge then quantitative methods are the methods of choice. This section examines two types of quantitative research methodologies, the randomized controlled trial and the survey.

Randomized controlled trial (RCT)

There are a number of experimental designs but the principal one used in health care research is the randomized controlled trial (RCT). The RCT rigorously and systematically studies cause-and-effect relationships between variables (Parahoo 1997) and aims to produce predictive knowledge. The methodology is characterized by three features – control, randomization and manipulation – which ensure as far as possible that the results obtained are a direct result of the effects of the intervention (Parahoo 1997). Most commonly, it is the uncertainty of a treatment effect that drives or is a prerequisite for an RCT (Oakley 1990) and in this circumstance, the RCT is considered the most appropriate research approach to use (Closs & Cheater 1999).

Within an RCT, subjects are drawn from a reference population using careful selection criteria and then randomly allocated to either a control or treatment group. These randomization procedures are carefully adhered to so that the features of the control and treatment groups are comparable. The intervention is then manipulated in that the treatment group receives the intervention whilst the control group does not. In this way, other variables which may have accounted for the difference between the treatment and control groups are controlled. The outcomes between the treatment and non-treatment groups are then measured and compared.

As a result of the RCT's ability to minimize the effect of bias 'the randomized controlled trial is commonly considered the "gold standard" by which other research designs are judged' (Evans & Pearson 2001, p597). However, although it is the major research methodology in medicine (Evans & Pearson

2001, Oakley 1990), there are only a small number of RCTs to evaluate nursing interventions (Cullum 1997, Magarey 2001, Parahoo 1997). One of the reasons for this is that it is difficult in nursing to maintain the degree of control required to undertake a RCT. Often, nursing practice is a highly complex affair where it is difficult to isolate and control variables. Patients and nursing are not static but dynamic and the emphasis on person-centred and individualized nursing care makes generalization difficult (Parahoo 1997).

So despite their clear role in generating predictive knowledge, RCTs have been criticized for being reductionist and for failing to take into account the real-life and 'messy' world of health care practice (Parahoo 1997). One of the limitations of RCTs is their sole reliance on the criterion of effectiveness (Evans & Pearson 2001) and one of the consequences of this is that 'nursing research is now being collected, sorted, appraised and summarized under a narrowly defined concept of what constitutes good evidence' (Evans & Pearson 2001, p594). Because the whole evidence-based-practice movement is defined almost exclusively in terms of the evidence generated via RCTs (Evans & Pearson 2001, French 1999), this results in a disregard of evidence generated in other traditions. So reliance on RCTs as the methodological 'gold standard' may serve to limit nursing's body of knowledge, as not all aspects of nursing practice are open to enquiry in this way. Evans & Pearson (2001, p595) argue that 'this is not to suggest that randomized controlled trials are not important to nursing, rather that they are not the only source of valid evidence that should inform and guide nursing practice'.

They suggest that in addition to effectiveness, there are two other components of evidence: feasibility and appropriateness. Appropriateness is concerned with 'the impact of the intervention from the perspective of the recipient' (Evans 2003, p81). So inclusion of this criterion into the design of RCTs and therefore systematic literature reviews, will allow for examination of the effect of the treatment on the patient. Feasibility is concerned with the context in which the intervention takes place and examines 'whether the intervention can and should be implemented' (Evans 2003, p81). So, for example, the findings of an RCT conducted in a hospital setting may not necessarily be relevant to patients in a primary care or intermediate care setting (Closs & Cheater 1999).

Evans (2003) argues therefore that the RCT provides only a partial picture and is unable to provide all the answers 'needed for a complete evaluation' (Evans 2003, p82). The implication of using a fuller range of criteria for establishing an evidence base for nursing and health care is that all valid and relevant evidence is brought together, not just that which pertains to effectiveness. Inclusion of appropriateness and feasibility would therefore permit examination of issues such as compliance. There is little point in carefully designing an RCT to examine the effectiveness of a particular intervention if the experimental group is going to encounter problems with compliance. For example, in a review of randomized and quasi-randomized controlled trials (i.e. a controlled trial that lacks the same degree of control as an RCT) that examined whether the use of hip protectors reduced the incidence of hip fractures among older people following a fall, Parker et al (2001) reported that there were significant variations in the rates of compliance across the studies reviewed, ranging from only 24% to 86%. If patients did not comply with wearing the hip protectors, perhaps because they were uncomfortable, this could have significantly affected the findings.

> Traditional quantitative approaches, such as the RCT, are an appropriate means of testing an intervention or treatment, but, and herein is the importance of qualitative approaches, beliefs and understanding must be explored to establish, for example, reasons why patients do not adhere to medication regimes. Without such insights clinical practice is unlikely to be either cost or clinically effective.
>
> (Colyer & Kamath 1999, p192)

In summary, it is clear that whilst RCTs cannot meet all our needs for research-based information (Black 1996), they remain important to the generation of nursing knowledge. Poole and Jones (1996, p108) argue that by 'ignoring the contribution of the experimental design, there is a risk of overlooking certain areas of potential nursing knowledge'. So what is called for is a recognition of complementarity between research methodologies and that what is important is that 'researchers should be united in their quest for scientific rigour in evaluation, regardless of the method used' (Black 1996, p1215).

Exercise 6.5

Go back to the hypothetical research questions on pages 72–73. Identify those you think are amenable to enquiry using a RCT.

Box 6.1 Example of an RCT

Robertson et al (2002) conducted an RCT to find out whether a home-based exercise programme for people over the age of 75 years was a cost-effective way of reducing the number of falls and injuries related to falls. Two hundred and forty people over the age of 75 (mean 81 years) took part: 121 were allocated to the exercise programme run by a district nurse and 119 received usual care. The outcome measures were the number of falls and injuries due to falls, the cost of implementing the programme and the falls-related hospital costs. Participants in the exercise group had significantly fewer falls than those in the no-treatment group and the programme resulted in cost savings.

You may have concluded that perhaps questions 3, 4 and 5 could be explored using a RCT. For example, the relationship between restricted use of physical restraint practices and the rates of falls in older people in a residential setting could be explored using a carefully designed RCT. Patients could be randomly allocated to either a control group (that receives standard physical restraint practices) or a treatment group (that receives restricted physical restraint practices). The incidence of falls in both groups could then be measured.

Survey

Surveys are a frequently used methodology in nursing and health care research as they are a relatively cost-effective way of gathering information from a large number of people. They enable us to achieve a 'snapshot' of a situation and ask questions such as 'What is going on?' or 'What do people think?'. They are also used widely in other arenas, for example in market research and general population surveys such as the General Household Survey or the Population Census.

Surveys can be described as either descriptive or analytical. Descriptive surveys attempt to identify descriptive statements about the population under study, whereas analytical or explanatory surveys attempt to suggest relationships or associations between a number of different variables under study (Atkinson 1996).

The most commonly used methods of data collection in survey research are questionnaires and structured interviews. Questionnaire and interview

schedule design is therefore important as the quality of these will determine the quality of the data collected. These data are usually quantitative and are analysed using descriptive and inferential statistics. The knowledge generated is therefore predominantly descriptive (for descriptive surveys) and explanatory (for analytical or explanatory surveys).

However, although familiarity, relative cost-effectiveness and the ability to reach a large audience are advantages of surveys, there are a number of limitations to this research approach. As the usual aim of survey research is to make generalizations from the survey sample to the wider population, it is important that the survey sample is indeed typical and therefore representative of that total population. Clear descriptions of the sampling decisions taken are therefore important. Related to the concept of generalization is the issue of response rates. Frequently, surveys rely on respondents self-completing a questionnaire. So even if the survey sample is representative of the population at large, the utility of the data can be undermined if there is a low response rate. If there is a poor response rate, for example under 50%, researchers must take care in making generalizations to the wider population, as the survey respondents may be systematically different to non-responders.

Linked to the nature of the sample and response rates, is the issue of validity in survey research. The validity of survey data can be compromised because of the self-report nature of the data collection procedure. Although attempts can be made in the design of the questionnaire to minimize threats to validity, validity is always vulnerable in survey research. We have already described how surveys are a very efficient way of capturing a lot of data from a relatively large sample. However, if the questionnaire has not been designed carefully, the amount of data generated can be overwhelming, making analysis difficult. Consequently it may be possible to paint a picture of *what* is happening without understanding *why*. In this instance, the survey is a missed opportunity as only superficial data may have been collected. A further limitation of survey research is that the questions used may reflect the researcher's ideas and theoretical insights. Researchers can therefore be criticized for influencing the nature of the responses given.

Exercise 6.6

Go back to the hypothetical research questions on pages 72–73. Which of these questions could be answered using survey research?

Box 6.2 Example of survey design

Griffiths (2002) conducted a survey to examine multidisciplinary care and discharge planning processes on a number of wards and on a nurse-led intermediate care inpatient unit (NLIU) in one NHS trust in England. The survey was conducted in parallel with an RCT and so the research design is an example of methodological triangulation (see page 81). Questionnaires were sent to 18 wards that had referred patients to the NLIU within the last 18 months, and also to the NLIU itself. The questionnaire was based on an already validated questionnaire designed to examine multidisciplinary discharge planning practice. Sixteen questionnaires were returned. The findings show the NLIU appeared similar to the wards in terms of how care was organized and that overall input from professions other than nursing was not substantially lower on the NLIU.

Perhaps you concluded that only the first two questions are open to investigation using surveys. So, for example, a survey could be used to examine older women's experiences of widowhood. Using a carefully constructed questionnaire, informed by the available literature, a representative sample of older women could be surveyed and their responses analysed using descriptive and inferential statistics.

QUALITATIVE RESEARCH APPROACHES

When a research question is attempting to generate exploratory or descriptive knowledge then qualitative research methods, influenced by the naturalistic paradigm, are most appropriate. Closs and Cheater (1999, p15) describe the usefulness of qualitative methods:

> *Evidence from qualitative studies provides the essential groundwork from which many clinical problems are identified and understood, and hypotheses are generated and tested. A great strength of qualitative research is its attention to detail and context. Qualitative methods are particularly appropriate when little is known about a topic.*

In this section we will examine three research methodologies that generate qualitative data: ethnography, phenomenology and grounded theory.

Ethnography

Essentially ethnography is concerned with describing people in their cultural context. It is both a process (a methodology) and an end-product (an ethnography). Ethnography has its roots in social anthropology and, traditionally, it is focussed on small scale communities, in 'other' or 'exotic' cultures. However, contemporary ethnography no longer just focuses on 'other' but also settings 'at home', in what has come to be described as 'anthropology at home' (Jackson 1987, Rapport 2000). The challenge of anthropology at home is to 'make strange the familiar' (Draper 2000). It is therefore a research approach that helps us to literally 'describe culture'.

Anthropology and the tool of ethnography seek to understand the culture under study, through a process of thick description, which is detailed and concerned with the nitty-gritty ins and outs of every-day life. So ethnography enables the capture of multiple and different voices in their everyday context. The researcher uses known methods of data collection such as semi-structured or open interviews, observation, diaries and historical documents, and then analyses these in the context of the culture under study. During this process of data collection the researcher becomes part of the culture under study and is therefore exposed to the nuances of every day life in that culture. Ethnography has the potential therefore to be highly reflexive, because the researcher acknowledges how their particular cultural location, who they are and their values and beliefs, shape the conduct of the study and the interpretation of the data.

Box 6.3 Example of ethnographic research

Holland (1999) explored the transition from student nurse to qualified nurse using an ethnographic approach. She undertook participant observation and interviews in the practice setting, along with an open-ended questionnaire. Her sample was four groups of adult branch student nurses in a college of nursing in England. Using thematic data analysis 8 key themes were identified. Drawing on ritual transition theory, her findings indicated 'an ill-defined transition' for the students which was perpetuated by their dual role as both student and worker.

> ## Box 6.4 Example of Husserlian phenomenology
>
> King and Turner (2000) undertook a Husserlian phenomenological study to explore the experiences of registered nurses caring for adolescent girls with anorexia, in Victoria, Australia. Five female registered nurses were interviewed in order to explore their experiences of caring for these anorexic girls. The researcher used a number of bracketing strategies as a way of suspending their prior beliefs and these included not doing the literature review until after data collection was complete and 'undertaking an audio-taped exegesis of own understandings prior to commencement of the study' (p141). Data were analysed and 6 themes emerged: personal core values of nurses; core values challenged; emotional turmoil; frustration; turning points; and resolution. King and Turner describe these themes as accounting for the journey nurses take when caring for adolescent anorexic females and call for preparation and continued support for registered nurses.

> ## Box 6.5 Example of Heideggarian phenomenology
>
> Hodges et al (2001) conducted a study to explore the perceptions of nurses, students and older people about living with chronic illness. Sixty-five participants were involved in 7 focus group interviews, which were transcribed and analysed thematically. A key aspect of the focus group interviews was that participants were shown 5 slides of art masterpieces and then questions in the focus group included 'If this painting were the cover of a book about chronic illness, what would be the story?', 'Does the painting remind you of a feeling you might have had related to health?'. Themes that were developed from the data were: social isolation, role changes, and movement and inertia.

Phenomenology

Based on Husserlian philosophy, phenomenology, in contrast to ethnography, is concerned with understanding the individual experience. So a researcher adopting a phenomenological research approach seeks to understand an individual's (lived) experience of a phenomenon as expressed by the individual. It is an approach 'that emphasizes the complexity of human experience and the need to study that experience as it is actually lived' (Polit & Hungler 1991, p651). The aim is to develop descriptions and insights that provide a clear picture of the phenomenon from the perspective of those involved. Qualitative data collection methods are commonly used, such as open or semi-structured interviews, stories and diaries.

Husserlian phenomenology stresses the notion that only those who experience the particular phenomenon are capable of communicating their experiences to the outside world (Parahoo 1997). The researcher attempts to put aside their own preconceptions about the phenomenon through the process of 'bracketing'. This technique is intended to exclude personal bias from the study in order to ensure that the description of the participant's experience is as impartial and accurate as possible. It involves researchers examining their own assumptions, values and prejudices and attempting to set them on one side, or bracket them, whilst conducting the research. This process of bracketing is in stark contrast to the reflexivity inherent in ethnography.

A development of Husserlian phenomenology is Heideggarian phenomenology. This approach emphasizes the 'experience of understanding' (Parahoo 1997, p44) rather than just the experience itself. So it is concerned with how people make sense of what is happening to them. Heidegger rejects Husserl's concept of bracketing, as he argues that it is impossible for the researcher not to come to the research setting influenced and informed by their own beliefs and values.

Grounded Theory

Grounded theory has its roots in symbolic interactionism, which is an 'approach to the interpretation of social action and the formation of identity' (Billington et al 1998, p259). It is an inductive approach to generating knowledge, where theories or hypotheses emerge from or are 'grounded' in the data. So grounded theory attempts to develop

Box 6.6 Example of grounded theory

Levy (1999) conducted a grounded theory study to investigate the processes by which midwives facilitate women to make informed choices over their pregnancy and delivery. Interactions between midwives and women were observed and interviews were also conducted with the midwives. Data were analysed using grounded theory approaches to analysis and the main category that emerged was what Levy called 'protective steering', 'whereby midwives were concerned to protect the women in their care, as well as themselves, when choices were made' (Levy 1999, p104). Other categories that emerged were orienting, protective gate-keeping and raising awareness.

explanatory theory from the data that have been collected.

A key difference from other qualitative methods is that researchers start their data collection and from these initial data begin to formulate a theory, which is then subsequently developed and confirmed (or not) through further data collection. The grounded theory approach attempts therefore to build theory inductively through an iterative process of data collection and analysis. In order to ensure that it is the data leading the development of theory, researchers using grounded theory will not usually examine the relevant literature concerning the topic, prior to the data collection process. Strauss and Corbin (1990 cited in Parahoo 1997, p45), who were early pioneers of this approach, describe how 'data collection, analysis and theory stand in reciprocal relationship with each other. One does not begin with a theory, then prove it. Rather, one begins with an area of study and what is relevant to that area is allowed to emerge'.

So these three different approaches to the generation of qualitative data, share some similarities and yet are also distinctive. Sometimes, however it is difficult to distinguish between the three approaches, and Parahoo (1997, p46) summarizes it thus:

Phenomenology collects data on individuals' experiences as its focus is on individuals. In ethnography, individuals are studied as part of their environment and the focus is on individuals not in isolation, but in relation to their institutions,

organizations, communities, customs or policies. Both these approaches seek mainly to describe phenomena rather than to explain them. In grounded theory, the focus is on the generation of theories from data and it therefore matters little if individuals are studied in isolation or as part of their cultural and social environment.

However, despite their advantages in producing 'thick description', it is important to identify that qualitative research methods are commonly criticized on a number of counts. First, the influence of the researcher on qualitative methods is considered to be more 'subjective' and therefore a threat to the rigour of the study. Second, purposeful rather than random sampling techniques are frequently used, making it impossible to generalize the findings to a wider population. However, it is important to remember that these criteria for judging research – objectivity, random sampling/randomization and generalization – are drawn from an alternative research paradigm and are therefore inappropriate for qualitative research methods. As we have already seen, qualitative research seeks to do different things to quantitative research so it is inappropriate to use evaluation criteria designed for quantitative studies. What is important is that researchers using qualitative methods describe their approach to ensuring rigour and credibility.

Exercise 6.7

Go back to the research questions identified on pages 72–73. Think carefully about which would be amenable to examination using ethnography, phenomenology or grounded theory. How might you need to modify the research questions in order to 'fit' with these different approaches?

You will have perhaps concluded that only the first two research questions could be answered using these approaches. So, for example, ethnography could be used to explore a group of middle-class men's experiences of their transition to contemporary Western fatherhood. Alternatively, phenomenology could be used to explore women's lived experiences of their widowhood.

NEW PARADIGM RESEARCH

In the final part of this section, we examine two research approaches associated with the critical theory paradigm, action research and participatory research, which have been described as 'new paradigm' research (Henderson 1995).

Action research

Action research has its home in the critical theory paradigm, as its overriding purpose is to achieve change and move practice on. Originally used in education, it is now becoming more popular in health care settings. Waterman et al (2001, p11) define action research as 'a period of enquiry that describes, interprets and explains social situations while executing a change intervention aimed at improvement and involvement. It is problem-focused, context-specific and future oriented'. This definition is particularly helpful in that it identifies the key distinguishing elements of action research:

- It is frequently undertaken over time
- It attempts to explain why things are happening
- It is concerned with introducing change
- It emphasizes involvement
- It is concerned with improvement in practice.

In its truest form action research embraces the notion of doing research *with* rather than *on* people. It is participatory and involves research 'participants' rather than 'subjects' or 'respondents'. It is therefore more democratic as participants are involved as key stakeholders in 'defining problems, implementing solutions and evaluating them' (Williamson & Prosser 2002, p587). Furthermore, it is located in the 'real life' context of clinical practice. So in contrast to how the messy real world of nursing can challenge an RCT, this messy world becomes a crucial feature of action research.

In doing research and solving a problem at the same time (Webb 1996), action research involves establishing the research question, identifying the most appropriate research design, implementing the desired change, and collecting and analysing data. Its stages mirror those of the nursing process: assessment of the problem, identification of the research question/action, planning the appropriate change and then evaluating this change.

The strengths of action research are that it can really help to develop practice and because it directly involves those for whom the change is very relevant, it is more likely to succeed. So, action research places emphasis on the process as well as the outcome. However, its limitations are that because of its context specificity, generalizability to other settings is difficult. Also, just as one of its strengths evolves from the involvement of those around, conversely it *depends* on their involvement. Furthermore, Williamson and Prosser (2002) suggest that although action research has great potential for changing health care practice due to its collaborative nature, it can raise political issues (such as the questionning of organizational structure and process) and ethical challenges (safeguarding anonymity, informed consent, confidentiality and protection from harm) for researchers.

Exercise 6.8

Go back to the research questions identified on pages 72–73. Which would most suit an action research approach?

It is possible that the third research question could be explored using action research. Involving the multidisciplinary team, the impact of the introduction of the in-house training programme could be evaluated by assessing the quality of pain management on the ward, as measured by possible changes in pain assessment scores.

Participatory research

This is a relatively new and developing research approach in health care and shares some of the principles of action research, for example reciprocity, participation and change. It cannot be described as a single method or design as the methods used will vary from project to project (Northway 2000). However, the essence of participatory research is that it emphasizes working in partnership with users, in order to hear their voices and test out different approaches to delivery (Tetley & Hanson 2000). It is 'carried out by local people rather than on them' (Cornwall & Jewkes 1995) and can involve prolonged contact with collaborators (Aranda & Street 2001). Although familiar research methods might be used (such as interviews and questionnaires), the crucial difference between participatory research and other conventional research methodologies is the relocation of power in the research process (Cornwall & Jewkes 1995).

Tetley and Hanson (2000, p69–88) describe how participatory research provides 'new ways of giving people a voice in the research process' and they contrast other more 'traditional' forms of either scientific or social research which espouse knowledge generation, control and power, with the more egalitarian principles of participatory research. So the emphasis is on collaboration, participants setting the research agenda, advising on data collection and analysis procedures and dissemination of results (Henderson 1995). Participatory research therefore involves a complete shift in the power dynamics of the research relationship where control and power is held by the participants and not the researchers.

Northway identifies a number of features of participatory research:

- It relies on active participation throughout all stages of the research project
- It examines power relations within the research
- It is an educational process in which researchers and participants learn together
- It has the capacity to generate different types of knowledge
- It enables action and 'rather than imposing solutions it recognizes that people have the capacity to develop and implement their own solutions' (Northway 2000, p45)
- It examines personal and professional values.

So when examining participatory research, or in fact any research which claims to have involved users, we need to explore the extent of this participation and examine the degree to which the researchers have been true to their word or whether they have merely paid lip service to the concept of participation.

TRIANGULATION

From this brief description of some of the key research designs, it can be seen that lots of different research designs can be used to answer the very many different types of research questions asked within the health care community. We have also already noted that rather than perpetuating the qualitative versus quantitative debate, we should acknowledge the relative merits of these different methods, as they are all needed to build a research base for nursing (Close & Cheater 1999). As each of these methods has its own strengths and limitations (Black 1996), it is possible to combine different methods within a single research study, in order to maximize the strengths of each and provide a fuller picture of the phenomenon under study. This is called triangulation and offers an alternative to what can be regarded as the bipolar qualitative versus quantitative debate (Cowman 1993), thereby contributing to a more balanced approach to the generation of research evidence.

Begley (1996) distinguishes between five types of triangulation:

- *Data triangulation* – which is the use of multiple data sources, at different time intervals, at multiple sites, from different people
- *Investigator triangulation* – when more than one experienced researcher examines the data
- *Theoretical triangulation* – when data are exposed to all possible theoretical interpretations
- *Methodological triangulation* – when two or more methods are used in the same study. This can be across-method (from different research traditions) or within-method (from the same research tradition)
- *Analytical triangulation* – when two or more approaches to the analysis of the same data are taken.

An example of across-method methodological triangulation might be the use of a RCT to determine the effectiveness of an intervention and a phenomenological exploration of the impact of this intervention on the client's lived experience. In this instance it may be possible that data generated from one 'arm' of the study may contradict that generated in another and the researcher's task is then to explore the possible reasons for this.

Triangulation is therefore not just about confirmation of research data but also about ensuring completeness of data (Begley 1996), capturing as much as possible about a particular phenomenon. So triangulation 'must be chosen deliberately, for the correct reasons and an adequate description of the rationale, planning and implementation of the method should be given' (Begley 1996, p127).

CONCLUSION

In this chapter we have explored the nature of the relationship between research question and research design. We first examined what is meant by the research question and how different research questions result in the generation of different types of knowledge. We then explored some of the major research designs involving both quantitative and qualitative research methods and discussed some of their strengths and weaknesses. Using hypothetical research questions and real examples of research, we have illustrated the ways in which different questions demand different methods. Our aim in doing this is to demonstrate the key issue in the relationship between question and design – that research design should be driven by the research question, not the other way around. When critically appraising research reports it is therefore crucially important that you are able to establish an appropriate fit between the question asked by the researcher and the methodology proposed. So what are the key issues to look for in a published paper that provide clues about the fit between question and design? It might be helpful to bear in mind the following questions when considering this issue. A carefully written research report should include reference to most of the following questions.

What is the purpose of the research?
Is its purpose to describe, explain or predict? Are the aims of the research clearly stated?

Is this expressed as a clear research question?
Is the question interrogative or declarative (see page 70)?

Does the proposed research design reflect existing knowledge of the subject?
Does the researcher make reference to what is currently known about the topic? Remember you would not expect to see this in grounded theory.

What is the researcher's previous experience of research?
Is the researcher experienced across a range of methodologies?

Does the framing of the research question enable the use of the researcher's favoured approach?
Is the research question leading?

Are the methods of data collection and analysis appropriate for the design?
For example, direct measurement in RCTs and interviews, observation and historical documents in ethnographic research.

Does the researcher appropriately discuss mechanisms to ensure the rigour and quality of the research?
Is there a discussion of reliability and validity in quantitative methods and credibility, trustworthiness and authenticity in qualitative methods (see Chapter 7)?

Does the sample size reflect the research design?
You would expect a large sample for a RCT, for example, and smaller samples for qualitative methods (see Chapter 9).

Is the role of the researcher in the research process discussed?
You would expect quantitative methods to discuss this in terms of minimizing bias and extraneous variables; qualitative methods to discuss this in terms of reflexivity; and action research and participatory research to discuss this in terms of their action/role in the project.

Is the position of those researched made clear?
In quantitative methods, the researched are likely to be known as 'subjects', in qualitative methods as 'respondents' or 'informants', and in participatory research as 'participants'.

What implications for practice are made?
The results of a large RCT may have significant implications for practice, whereas making large claims to change practice on the basis of a small ethnographic study are inappropriate.

Are there any misfits?
For example, this could be a research study which collects qualitative data that are then analysed quantitatively.

References

Aranda S and Street A (2001) From individual to group: use of narratives in a participatory research process. *Journal of Advanced Nursing* 33(6): 791–797.

Atkinson FI (1996) Survey design and sampling. In: Cormack DFS (ed) *The Research Process in Nursing*, 3rd edn, Oxford: Blackwell Science, pp202–213.

Avis M (1994) Reading research critically. I. An introduction to appraisal: designs and objectives. *Journal of Clinical Nursing* 3: 227–234.

Begley CM (1996) Using triangulation in nursing research. *Journal of Advanced Nursing* 21: 122–128.

Billington R, Hockey J and Strawbridge S (1998) *Exploring Self and Society*. Basingstoke: Macmillan Press.

Black N (1996) Why we need observational studies to evaluate the effectiveness of health care. *British Medical Journal* 312: 1215–1218.

Carson AM and Fairbairn GJ (2002) The whole story: towards an ethical research methodology. *Nurse Researcher* 10(1): 15–29.

Closs SJ and Cheater FM (1999) Evidence for nursing practice: a clarification of the issues. *Journal of Advanced Nursing* 30(1): 10–17.

Colyer H and Kamath P (1999) Evidence-based practice. A philosophical and political analysis: some matters for consideration by professional practitioners. *Journal of Advanced Nursing* **29**(1): 188–193.

Cormack DFS and Benton DC (1996) The research process. In: Cormack DFS (ed) *The Research Process in Nursing*, 3rd edn. Oxford: Blackwell Science, pp53–63.

Cornwall A and Jewkes R (1995) What is participatory research? *Social Science and Medicine* **41**(12): 1667–1676.

Cowman S (1993) Triangulation: a means of reconciliation in nursing research. *Journal of Advanced Nursing* **18**: 788–792.

CRD (Centre for Reviews and Dissemination) (1996) Undertaking systematic reviews of research on effectiveness: CRD guidelines for those carrying out or commissioning reviews. York: NHS Centre for Reviews and Dissemination.

Cullum N (1994) Critical reviews of the literature. In: Hardey M and Mulhall A (eds) *Nursing research: theory and practice*. London: Chapman and Hall, pp43–57.

Cullum N (1997) Identification and analysis of randomised controlled trials in nursing. *Quality in Health Care* **6**: 2–6.

Denzin NK (1997) *Interpretive Ethnography: Ethnographic Practices for the 21st Century*. Thousand Oaks: Sage Publications.

Draper J (2000) Fathers in the making: men, bodies and babies. Unpublished PhD Dissertation (Social Policy). Hull: University of Hull.

Evans D (2003) Hierarchy of evidence: a framework for ranking evidence evaluating healthcare interventions. *Journal of Clinical Nursing* **12**: 77–84.

Evans D and Pearson A (2001) Systematic reviews: gatekeepers of nursing knowledge. *Journal of Clinical Nursing* **10**: 593–599.

French P (1999) The development of evidence-based nursing. *Journal of Advanced Nursing* **29**(1): 72–78.

Griffiths P (2002) Nursing-led in-patient units for intermediate care: a survey of multidisciplinary discharge planning. *Journal of Clinical Nursing* **11**: 322–330.

Henderson DJ (1995) Consciousness raising in participatory research: Method and methodology for emancipatory nursing inquiry. *Advances in Nursing Science* **17**(3): 58–69.

Hodges HF, Keeley AC and Grier EC (2001) Masterworks of art and chronic illness experiences in the elderly. *Journal of Advanced Nursing* **36**(3): 389–398.

Holland K (1999) A journey to becoming: the student nurse transition. *Journal of Advanced Nursing* **29**(1): 229–236.

Jackson A (ed) (1987) *Anthropology at Home*. London: Tavistock Publications.

James A (1993) *Childhood: Identities, Self and Social Relationships in the Experience of the Child*. Edinburgh: Edinburgh University Press.

King SJ, Turner de S (2000) Caring for adolescent females with anorexia nervosa: registered nurses' perspective. *Journal of Advanced Nursing* **31**(1): 139–147.

Koch T and Harrington A (1998) Reconceptualising rigour: the case for reflexivity. *Journal of Advanced Nursing* **28**(4): 882–890.

Levy V (1999) Protective steering: a grounded theory study of the processes by which midwives facilitate informed choices during pregnancy. *Journal of Advanced Nursing* **29**(1): 104–112.

Long AF (2002) Critically appraising research studies. In: McSherry R, Simmons M and Abbott P (eds) *Evidence-informed Nursing: a Guide for Clinical Nurses*. London: Routledge, pp41–64.

Magarey JM (2001) Elements of a systematic review. *International Journal of Nursing Practice* **7**: 376–382.

Northway R (2000) The relevance of participatory research in developing nursing research and practice. *Nurse Researcher* **7**(4): 40–52.

Oakley A (1990) Who's afraid of the randomised controlled trial? Some dilemmas of the scientific method and 'good' research practice. In: Roberts H (ed) *Women's Health Counts*. London: Routledge, pp167–194.

McSherry R, Simmons M and Abbott P (eds) (2002) Evidence-informed nursing: a Guide for Clinical Nurses. London: Routledge, pp41–64.

Parahoo K (1997) *Nursing Research: Principles, Process and Issues*. Basingstoke: Macmillan.

Parker MJ, Gillespie LD and Gillespie WJ (2001) Review: hip protectors reduce hip fractures after falls in elderly people living in institutions or supported home environments. *Evidence Based Nursing* **5**: 23.

Polit DF and Hungler BP (1991) *Nursing Research Principles and Methods*, 4th edn. Philadelphia: Lippincott.

Poole K and Jones A (1996) A re-examination of the experimental design for nursing research. *Journal of Advanced Nursing* **24**: 108–114.

Rapport N (2000) 'Best of British': The new anthropology of Britain. *Anthropology Today* **16**(2): 20–22.

Rees C (1997) *An introduction to research for midwives*. Cheshire: Books for Midwives.

Robertson MC, Devlin N and Gardner MM et al (2001) Effectiveness and economic evaluation of a nurse delivered home exercise programme to prevent falls. 1: randomised controlled trial. *British Medical Journal* **322**: 697–701.

Talbot LA (1995) *Principles and Practice of Nursing Research*. St. Louis: Mosby.

Tetley J and Hanson L (2000) Participatory research. *Nurse Researcher* **8**(1): 69–88.

Waterman H, Tillen D, Dickson R et al (2001) Action research: a systematic review and guidance for assessment. *Health Technology Assessment* **5**(23). www.hta./nhs.uk/fullmono/mon523.pdf

Webb C (1996) Action research. In: Cormack DFS (ed) *The Research Process in Nursing*, 3rd edn. Oxford: Blackwell Science, pp155–165.

Williamson GR and Prosser S (2002) Action research: politics, ethics and participation. *Journal of Advanced Nursing* **40**(5): 587–593.

Further reading

Evans D (2003) Hierarchy of evidence: a framework for ranking evidence evaluating healthcare interventions. *Journal of Clinical Nursing* **12**: 77–84.

In this very recent paper, Evans draws on some of his earlier work. He argues that the sole criterion of effectiveness, upon which RCTs and the evidence-based practice movement are based, is inappropriate because it only provides a partial picture as to the impact of an intervention on a patient or client. In this paper he fleshes out an alternative hierarchy of evidence, which he suggests should include the other criteria of feasibility and appropriateness.

French P (2002) What is the evidence on evidence-based nursing? An epistemological concern. *Journal of Advanced Nursing* **37**(3): 250–257.

In this paper, French examines the meaning of the term 'evidence-based nursing' and argues that its meaning is unclear. He suggests that the term is frequently used as a euphemism for other terms such as 'research-based practice', 'professional practice development', 'clinical judgement/problem solving' and 'managed care'. He concludes that there is little evidence that EBP is a stable construct.

McSherry R, Simmons M and Abbott P (eds) (2002) *Evidence-informed Nursing: a Guide for Clinical Nurses*. London: Routledge.

This is a useful and compact book which explores the key issues that contribute to the development of evidence-based nursing practice.

Parahoo K (1997) *Nursing Research: Principles, Process and Issues*. Basingstoke: Macmillan.

This is a classic contribution to the nursing research literature and explores in detail the different research designs.

- Used together, qualitative and quantitative methods can support theory to a greater degree than the use of either method alone.

SAMPLING (See also Chapter 9)

A further issue for the critical reader is that of sampling in qualitative research. When collecting qualitative data from a particular group, it is often impractical and indeed may be inappropriate to use a probability (random or representative) sample not only because such data collection methods require a list of the total population, but because they also take longer and hence are more expensive on resources. It is also inappropriate to use a random sample when the objective of the research is to understand and give meaning to a social process, since the intention is not to apply statistical tests and generalize the findings to a wider population. Rather, the intention is often to explore, describe and interpret a range of experiences and views. For this reason, qualitative data are often collected using a *purposive non-probability* sample. This is different from a convenience sample since its purpose is to identify specific groups of people who exhibit the characteristics of the social process or phenomenon which is being investigated. The researcher can then include all sorts of people who have different perspectives as well as particular knowledge of the topic under investigation.

If a researcher wishes to develop a social theory, a *theoretical sampling* technique may be used. The idea here is that the researcher selects the subjects and collects and analyses data to produce an initial theory which is then used to guide further sampling and data collection from which further *theory* is developed (*iteration*).

QUALITATIVE DATA COLLECTION METHODS

To ensure rigour in qualitative research it is important that researchers not only make explicit their data collection method but also apply them in a consistent and systematic way. The methods of data collection used in qualitative research include:

- Observational methods
- Interviews
- Focus groups
- Consensus methods
- Analysis of documents.

OBSERVATIONAL METHODS

Observational methods generally use the researcher as the research instrument to collect the data. Although observational methods of collecting data may involve questioning or analysis of documentary evidence, they are primarily based on observation per se, either as complete participant (covert observation), participant as observer (overt observation) or observer as participant (Mays & Pope 1995b). Patterson (1995), for example, collected qualitative data during participant observation in a nursing home over a period of 12 months, with the objective of examining the process of social support, in particular how residents adjusted to life in a nursing home. All observations were recorded daily in computerized field notes using a strategy developed by Schatzman and Strauss (1973) which included observational, theoretical and methodological notes.

In reviewing the findings, Patterson quotes examples from the observational data for illustrative purposes. She was able to conclude that emotional support and practical assistance are primary supportive behaviours from others. Although she does not use the terms credibility, dependability, transferability and confirmability (see above), some of these concepts are embodied within the research. For example, in addition to observation she also conducts informal and semi-structured interviews to increase the confirmability of her study. She also states the precise parameters of her research (including details of the interview guide, for example) to improve the study's credibility. She suggests some supportive interventions for others and her confidence that her findings are transferable is based on the rigour of her data collection methodology. Good qualitative researchers are cautious about the generalizability of their findings and often can only *suggest* that interventions *may* be appropriate in other settings.

The details of how *field notes* are recorded can be very helpful when appraising a published qualitative research study. In an excellent paper on the field experience of a white researcher 'getting in' a poor black community, Kauffman gives a good example of how a field note can be used to illustrate one of the central themes of a piece of research when she describes how an 'outsider' can appear non-judgemental: '… yep, everybody like you cos you like everybody!' (Kauffman 1994). This is a highly appropriate use of field notes within a publication which enables the critical reader to make some assessment of the rigour with which the data have been collected.

INTERVIEWS

A great deal of the qualitative data in published literature are collected by interviews. White (1995) undertook an in-depth series of interviews amongst a small group of older, Caucasian women in Auckland, New Zealand, to determine how perceptions of cervical cancer and cervical screening services might be affecting health-seeking behaviour. She gives a good description of her interview schedule in sufficient detail to enable the critical reader to assess this part of her methodology.

Smith (1999) illustrated the importance of reflections on the research process and using these reflections as a valuable source of data and as a means of enhancing ethical and methodological rigour. He conducted six in-depth interviews with problem drinkers to explore the 'lived experience' of their suffering and reports excerpts from his reflective journal in his paper. This provides previously hidden contextual information which increases the understanding of the suffering experienced by problem drinkers. This use of a reflexive journal in conjunction with in-depth interviews can increase the credibility of the data provided by transcripts and field notes.

It is clearly important to see at least some detail of how an interview has been conducted when appraising the rigour of a piece of qualitative research. To conduct a good in-depth interview, or indeed any interview, interviewers need to be trained and not rely solely on their existing clinical skills. This training includes familiarizing a researcher with the skills of, for example, reflective questioning, summarizing and 'controlling' an interview. Whyte (1982), for example, gives a 'directiveness scale' for analysing interview technique. Authors who report data from interviews should normally also give details of the training which interviewers received or the skills which they used.

Details of how the data were recorded are also import- ant in the evaluation of qualitative research. For example, field notes written at the time of an interview may interfere with the data collection but field notes written afterwards may miss out on some of the details! For most situations, audio-taping is an appropriate method for recording data, although transcription is an immensely time-consuming and expensive (in time and resources) activity. Interviews may be classified as shown in Box 7.1.

Box 7.1 Types of interview

- Structured – questionnaire-based
- Semi-structured – open-ended questions
- Depth – reflective questioning, covering a few issues in great detail

---

FOCUS GROUPS

The idea of using focus groups is to collect qualitative data by encouraging group interaction and recording that interaction, rather than a researcher asking individuals questions individually (Kitzinger 1995). Such groups can encourage participation from reluctant interviewees or those who feel they have nothing to say, as well as monitoring changes in the group's opinions or attitudes. As with individual interviews, this method does not discriminate against those who cannot read or write.

In their study of barriers to managing the chronic pain of older adults with arthritis, Davis et al (2002) used focus groups to collect data with 57 older adult participants who had self-reported arthritis. The focus groups were conducted with participants who resided independently in their own homes or congregated in residential settings. Objectives for the research were as follows:

- To explore the pain management barriers experienced
- To identify themes and their properties by conceptually grouping these barriers
- To develop a theoretical model of the relationships among the themes.

Nine themes were identified to describe barriers to chronic pain management experienced by the older people and the resulting model showed the importance of personal decision making in the use of pain management methods. This paper is a good example of how a focus group can be part of a systematic qualitative methodology.

CONSENSUS METHODS

These methods of data collection include the:

- Delphi technique
- Nominal group technique
- Consensus development conferences.

The Delphi technique is not new and has developed into an accepted method of achieving consensus between experts. However, concern has been expressed about the subjectivity associated with its use and perhaps the major deficiency in studies using the Delphi technique is the question of what is meant by 'consensus' (Duffield 1993). Mobily et al (1993) report a validation study of cognitive behavioural techniques to reduce pain. Using a Delphi survey, nurses selected for their expertise in pain management were asked to validate definitions and activities considered important in the implementation of three non-pharmacological pain management interventions. Considerable care was taken in the selection of subjects to provide expert opinion and 42 out of 97 completed a first round of the Delphi survey. As the authors correctly pointed out, the actual response rate is not critical in this type of study where the most important factor is range of expertise rather than representation.

Space does not permit detailed examination of nominal group techniques and consensus development conferences which are similar in principle to the Delphi technique. The interested reader is referred to Mays and Pope (1995c).

A NOTE ON CASE STUDIES

Case studies can be considered to be a qualitative research methodology and are discussed in more detail elsewhere. They usually focus on one or a limited number of settings and are used to explore specific social processes, especially where complex, interrelated issues are involved. Kearney et al (1995), for example, developed a grounded theory methodology to describe how pregnant crack cocaine users perceived and responded to their problems. They collected their data using in-depth interviews with 60 pregnant or post-partum women (cases) who used crack cocaine on average, at least once per week during pregnancy. Their sample was derived from a larger study of pregnant drug users and all participants were screened for eligibility, including confirmation of pregnancy or post-partum status. This was particularly important, not only for reasons of credibility, but also because the sources of referrals (which resulted in interviews) were paid. This paper is an excellent example of the detail that is necessary for the critical reader to evaluate the rigour with which a qualitative methodology such as this has been used.

A further example of a case study involving the collection of qualitative data is described in a paper by Thomas and De Santis (1995) on the feeding and weaning practices of Cuban and Haitian immigrant mothers in south Florida. Once again, the inclusion criteria are detailed enough to enable evaluation of the credibility of the data collection. Conclusions drawn from publications which omit such criteria should be treated with caution by the critical reader.

Although case studies in themselves are not really a distinctive method of qualitative research, they are increasingly used in the study of health care systems. For example, in a hypothetical study of the impact of general management in the UK National Health Service, an investigator, when confronted by different accounts from stakeholders, would either probe or return to interviews to try and account for discrepancies with the theoretical framework. Case studies in particular should try to get an accurate picture by means of triangulation so that degrees of convergence and divergence in the data can be carefully considered and included within the framework. Critical readers should also evaluate published case studies with this in mind.

Summary

A range of methods are used to collect data within qualitative research studies, including interviews, observation and focus groups. Since these methods invariably involve the researcher directly, there is potential for the researcher to influence the data collected. It is important, therefore, that qualitative researchers reflect on – and acknowledge within papers – the effect which their presence or their own views and experiences may have had on the data. In addition, qualitative data collection methodologies should be explicit and applied in a consistent, systematic and self-conscious way.

QUALITATIVE DATA ANALYSIS

In very basic terms, qualitative methodologies use *words* rather than numbers to express the information gathered to answer a particular question, and in evaluating the rigour with which a piece of research has been conducted, it is important to be clear about what a qualitative study is not. A paper reporting a small number of subjects is not a qualitative study simply because the sample size is too small for statistical analysis; nor is it qualitative because it is based on questionnaire responses to subjective material or data collected by interview.

published literature is necessary for both qualitative and quantitative research. In evaluating qualitative research, not only is it essential to be familiar with the scientific principles described in this chapter, but it is also essential that when reporting the results of our own work, we present findings which are readily accessible to the diverse audiences for whom they are intended, including researchers, practitioners and users of health and social services.

Sandelowski and Barroso (2002) describe the challenges of 'finding the findings' in qualitative studies. They analysed 99 reports of qualitative studies on women with HIV infection and describe varied reporting styles, misrepresentation of data and analytic procedures as findings, misuse of quotes and theories and a general lack of clarity concerning pattern and theme. Theses and dissertations in particular presented special challenges because they often contained several of these problems.

In addition, Schulmeister (1998) reviewed a random sample of 60 references from each of three nursing research journals for citation and quotation accuracy. Errors were classified as major or minor and of the 180 references reviewed, 58 (32%) had citation errors, with 43 of the 58 errors classified as major which made retrieval of the cited work difficult; even worse, 12 of the 180 articles contained a major quotation error, including four instances where the content of the original article contradicted or was unrelated to the author's contention. This rate of citation and quotation errors in the three sample nursing journals is comparable to rates previously published for other medical and nursing journals. However, errors of citation and quotation clearly diminish the value of published papers. We should ensure, therefore, that when we evaluate the published work of others it is not a case of the 'kettle calling the pot black!'

In conclusion, Hegyvary (1999) has emphasized the importance of moving beyond the advocacy of the inherent superiority of any particular theory, method or procedure when conducting nursing research. The methods used must be worthy and appropriate tools to address a particular research question, just as the question must be worth asking. She calls for nursing researchers to expend their professional energies in asking salient questions, in applying any and all reasonable methods that promise and ultimately produce advancement of professional knowledge, in using and writing clear language to communicate our findings and in applying and further testing that knowledge in nursing and health care practice. We would add a plea that *all* nurses and health care practitioners become critical readers of the resulting research papers.

Exercise 7.1

Read the following published article and answer the questions below:

Holmberg LI and Wahlberg RN (2000) The process of decision-making on abortion: A grounded theory study of young men in Sweden. *Journal of Adolescent Health,* **26**: 230–234.

Questions

1. What is the objective/research question of this paper?
2. How was 'grounded theory' used to analyse the data?
3. Which themes emerged from the interviews?
4. How were these categorized?
5. To what extent are the nursing implications of the study supported by the data analysis?
6. In the reader's judgement, have the researchers used a systematic and self-conscious methodology?

References

Britten N and Fisher B (1993) Qualitative research and general practice (editorial). *British Journal of General Practice* **43**: 270–271.

Carr LT (1994) The strengths and weaknesses of quantitative and qualitative research: what method for nursing? *Journal of Advanced Nursing* **20**: 716–721.

Davis GC, Hiemenz ML and White TL (2002) Barriers to managing chronic pain of older adults with arthritis. *Journal of Nursing Scholarship* **34**(2): 121–126.

Donovan J (1995) The process of analysis during a grounded theory study of men during their partners' pregnancies. *Journal of Advanced Nursing* **21**: 708–715.

Duffield C (1993) The Delphi technique: a comparison of results obtained using two expert panels. *International Journal of Nursing Studies* **30**(3): 227–237.

Glaser BG and Strauss AL (1965) Temporal aspects of dying as a non-scheduled status passage. *American Journal of Sociology* **71**: 48–59.

Hegyvary ST (1999) Editorial image. *Journal of Nursing Scholarship* **31**(3): 203.

Kauffman KS (1994) The insider outsider dilemma: Field experience of a white researcher 'Getting in' a poor black community. *Nursing Research* **43**(3): 179–183.

Kearney MH, Murphy S, Irwin K et al (1995) Salvaging self: a grounded theory of pregnancy on crack cocaine. *Nursing Research* **44**(4): 208–213.

Kitzinger J (1995) Introducing focus groups. *British Medical Journal* **311**: 299–302.

Lincoln YS and Guba EG (1985) *Naturalistic Enquiry*. Thousand Oaks, CA: Sage.

Mays N and Pope C (1995a). Rigour and qualitative research. *British Medical Journal* **311**: 109–112.

Mays N and Pope C (1995b) Observational methods in health care settings. *British Medical Journal* **311**: 182–184.

Mays N and Pope C (1995c) Qualitative interviews in medical research. *British Medical Journal* **311**: 251–253.

Mobily PR, Herr KA and Kelley LS (1993). Cognitive-behavioural techniques to reduce pain: a validation study. *International Journal of Nursing Studies* **30**(6): 537–548.

Nolan M and Behi R (1995) Triangulation: the best of all worlds? *British Journal of Nursing* **4**(14): 829–832.

Patterson BJ (1995) The process of social support: adjusting to life in a nursing home. *Journal of Advanced Nursing* **21**: 682–689.

Risjourd MW, Dunbar SB and Moloney MF (2002) A new foundation for methodological triangulation. *Journal of Nursing Scholarship* **34**(3): 270–275.

Sandelowski M and Barroso J (2002) Finding the findings in qualitative studies. *Journal of Nursing Scholarship* **34**(3): 213–219.

Schatzman L and Strauss AL (1973) *Field Research: Strategies for a Natural Sociology*. Englewood Cliffs and NJ: Prentice-Hall.

Schulmeister L (1998) Quotation and reference accuracy of three nursing journals. Image: *Journal of Nursing Scholarship* **30**(2): 143–146.

Smith BA (1999) Ethical and methodological benefits of using a reflexive journal in hermeneutic-phenomenologic research. *Image: Journal of Nursing Scholarship* **31**(4): 359–363.

Stake RE (1995) *The Art of Case Study Research*. Thousand Oaks: Sage.

Strauss A and Corbin J (1990) Basics of Qualitative Research. Thousand Oaks, CA: Sage.

Thomas JT and DeSantis L (1995) Feeding weaning practices of Cuban and Haitian immigrant mothers. *Journal of Transcultural Nursing* **6**(2): 34–41.

Yin RK (1994) *Case Study Research: Design and Methods*, 2nd edn. Newbury Park: Sage.

White GE (1995) Older women's attitudes to cervical screening and cervical cancer: a New Zealand experience. *Journal of Advanced Nursing* **21**: 659–666.

Whyte WF (1982) Interviewing in field research. In: Burgess RG (ed) *Field Research: a Sourcebook and Field Manual*. London: George Allen and Unwin pp111–122.

Further reading

The main topics outlined in this chapter are covered in greater depth in these texts. Denzin and Lincoln (2000) is a comprehensive review of qualitative research methodology.

Baker C, Wuest C and Stern PN (1992) Method slurring: the grounded theory/phenomenology example. *Journal of Advanced Nursing* **11**: 1355–1360.

Carr LT (1994) The strengths and weaknesses of quantitative and qualitative research: what method for nursing? *Journal of Advanced Nursing* **20**: 716–721.

Denzin NK and Lincoln YS (eds) (2000) *A Handbook of Qualitative Research*. Thousand Oaks, CA: Sage.

Horsburgh D (2003) Evaluation of qualitative research. *Journal of Clinical Nursing* **12**(2): 307–312.

Morse JM (ed) (1991) *Qualitative Nursing Research: A Contemporary Dialogue*. Newbury Park, CA: Sage.

Pretzlik U (1994) Observational methods and strategies. *Nurse Researcher* **2**(2): 13–29.

Russell C and Gregory D (2003) Evaluation of qualitative research studies. *Evidence-Based Nursing* **6**(2): 36–40.

Webb C (1989). Action research: philosophy, methods and personal experiences. *Journal of Advanced Nursing* **14**: 403–410.

Chapter 8

Evaluating quantitative research

Nigel Mathers, Yu Chu Huang

INTRODUCTION

When evaluating quantitative research the critical reader should not only review the appropriateness of the design used for a study (discussed in Chapter 6) but also the rigour with which the *methodologies* of data collection and analysis have been applied. Without appropriate data collection methods and rigorous analysis of data, the conclusions which have been drawn by the authors may not be supported.

In the broadest sense of the term, methods of analysis are the way researchers interpret the data they have collected to support their claim. If, for example, it is claimed that y is caused by (or associated with) x the critical reader should be asking themselves the sort of questions which are outlined below:

- Have appropriate methods been used to collect and analyse the data?
- How valid is the link claimed between x and y?
- In statistical terms, how robust is the statistical test that has been used?

The objectives of this chapter are to discuss these issues of quantitative data collection and analysis and enable the reader to critically evaluate the rigour with which a study has been conducted.

Key issues

- Rigour in quantitative research
- Quantitative data collection methods
- Sampling in quantitative research
- Methods for analysing quantitative data

EVALUATING QUANTITATIVE RESEARCH

Crucial to the process of evaluating quantitative research are the concepts of *validity* and *reliability*. Without a clear understanding of these central concepts, the critical reader will find it difficult to assess the rigour with which a quantitative study has been conducted.

The concepts of validity and reliability have become increasingly well defined and more complex to assess during the past 40 years. However, it is not unusual for published literature to gloss over these important issues even though they are crucial in evaluating a quantitative study.

VALIDITY

In its broadest sense, validity is the extent to which a study using a particular instrument measures what it sets out to measure. Reliability is an important precondition for validity – if an instrument is unreliable, it lacks adequate validity. However, a reliable instrument is not necessarily valid since it may be measuring something other than what it is supposed to measure. This relationship between validity and reliability is outlined in Figure 8.1.

It may be seen from this figure that the ideal situation is when there is high reliability and high validity and measurements are clustered around the true

RELIABILITY

	HIGH	LOW
HIGH **VALIDITY**	CELL 1 XX X XX X X XXX X ● X XX XX XX XX XX XXX	CELL 3 ●

LOW	CELL 2
	
	XXXXX
	XXXX
	XXX
	
	●
		CELL 4
		
		    X X X
		X X X
		    X ● X X
		    X X X
		X X

Note: It is not actually possible to have high validity without reliability (**Cell 3**)

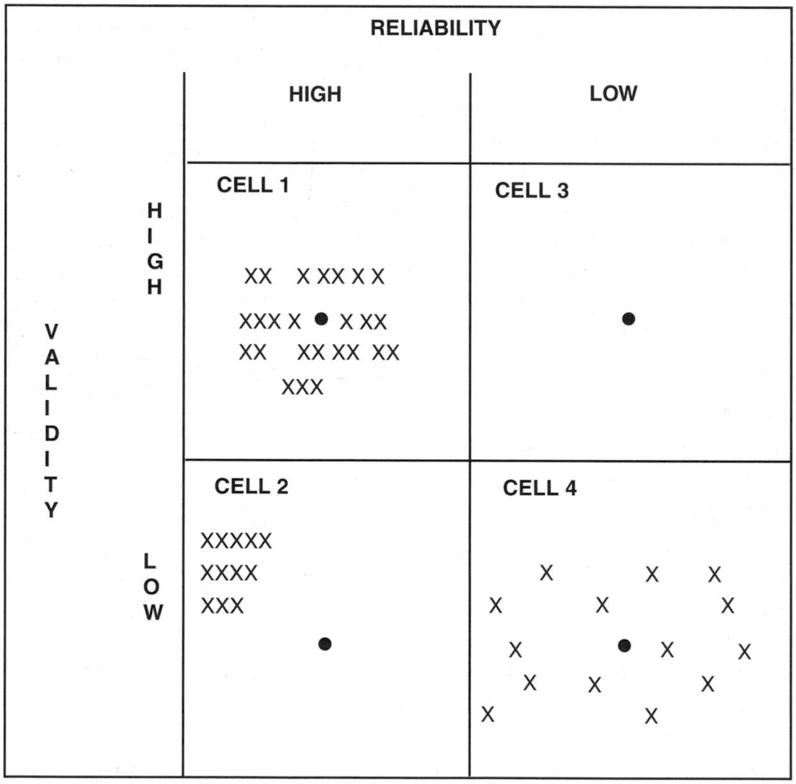

● is the 'true' result
X represents attempts to measure the 'true' result

Cell 1 High reliability/high validity. This is the 'ideal' situation where measurements are clustered around the true result.

Cell 2 High reliability/low validity. In this situation the measure produces a consistent result but this is not close to the true result.

Cell 4 Low reliability/low validity. This is the worst of all worlds where the measure not only fails to give a consistent result but there may also be evidence of systematic bias in that the target or 'true' result is missed completely.

Figure 8.1   Validity and reliability in quantitative research.

result (Cell 1). By contrast, the situation of low reliability and low validity is the 'worst of all worlds' where the measure not only fails to give a consistent result but there may also be evidence of systematic bias in that the target or 'true' result is missed (Cell 4).

In the situation of high reliability but low validity the measure produces a consistent result but this is not close to the true result (Cell 2). It is, however, not possible to have a situation of low reliability but high validity since if a particular measure hits the target (true result) occasionally but not consistently, the validity of such a measure is likely to be inadequate (Cell 3).

Types of validity

Face or content validity   This relates to whether, 'on the face of it', the instrument or study measures what it is supposed to measure. For example, Yamashita (1995) used a well-established questionnaire for measuring the occupational satisfaction of hospital nurses. The face or content validity of this questionnaire used in her particular setting was established by submitting an appropriately modified version to a panel of experts for content analysis. Since the assessment of face validity is essentially subjective, a panel of experts should be used for this process rather than an individual researcher.

Criterion or convergent validity   This assesses a measure against another measure of the same phenomenon. This is usually an already existing and well-accepted measure. For example, the General Health Questionnaire (GHQ), a mental health screening instrument, was developed by independent comparison of the score on the questionnaire with the mental state examination by an experienced psychiatrist (Goldberg & Williams 1991). This process established the *concurrent convergent* or *criterion validity* of the instrument. *Predictive convergent validity* assesses the degree to which a measure can predict future events. For example, risk scales are often used to predict the probability of ischaemic heart disease and the agreement of the scales with subsequent cardiac events gives a measure of their predictive convergent validity.

Construct or hypothesis validity   This is the most important and highest level of validity in quantitative research. It expresses the confidence we can have that a particular construct or hypothesis is valid. It can be used to find out, for example, how

closely an instrument correlates with another variable to support a hypothesis. For example, if a hypothesis that wheezy children had unhappy parents was correct, then a questionnaire to measure degrees of unhappiness in parents which was able to distinguish between the parents of wheezy and non-wheezy children would give the hypothesis construct validity. The more ways in which the construct validity of a hypothesis has been tested, the more confidence the critical reader can have in the conclusions drawn by particular authors in relation to their hypotheses.

RELIABILITY

Test/retest reliability

Within quantitative research studies, reliability is the extent to which a test or an instrument such as a questionnaire gives consistent results. For example, a questionnaire can be given to the same person on two separate occasions and the consistency of their responses examined. A good correlation between the results would suggest that the test/retest reliability of the questionnaire was good. However, if the correlation coefficient (a measure of the degree of association between two sets of responses) is low (e.g. <0.5), one should question any conclusions the author has drawn from the data collected using such a questionnaire. It is important to remember that the time between administrations of the questionnaire is key – if it is too long, what is being measured may have changed; if it is too short, then the second set of results will be affected by the individual's memory of the previous administration of the questionnaire.

INTEROBSERVER (BETWEEN OBSERVERS) RELIABILITY

If two different people administer the same questionnaire to the same person, to what extent is there agreement between the results obtained? This agreement or otherwise is usually reported in the literature as a *Cohen's Kappa* (or *K coefficient*). This expresses the level of agreement that is greater than that expected by chance alone. In reviewing the literature, a K coefficient of 1 is perfect agreement.

Such a statistical analysis can also be used to assess the *intraobserver* (within observer) reliability of an instrument such as a questionnaire. The *Pearson correlation coefficient* may also be used for this purpose.

'INTERNAL' OR 'SPLIT-HALF' RELIABILITY

This is a measure of how much a respondent gives similar answers to similar questions. For example, a respondent may be asked in a questionnaire whether he or she agrees with the statement that the government should regulate chemical additives in food. Towards the end of the questionnaire, the subject is asked if he or she agrees with the statement that the government should not regulate chemical additives in food. Agreement by the subject with the first statement but disagreement with the second gives an indication of the internal reliability or consistency of the questionnaire. This would typically be expressed as *Cronbach's alpha*, with a result greater than 0.5 indicating an acceptable level of consistency between responses. The same process can be used to look at a series of questions or a subscale to assess the extent to which a questionnaire reliably reflects an attitude, for example.

Phillips and Wilbur (1995) evaluated adherence to breast cancer screening guidelines among African-American women of differing employment status. Data were collected using the Breast Cancer Screening Questionnaire (BCSQ). This was developed using published instruments and a review of the literature. The reliability of the published instruments was quoted as previously established, and although the individual components of test/retest or intra/inter-observer reliability were not specified, they were expressed as a Cronbach's alpha coefficient. For example, the alpha coefficients for Champion's Health Belief Model Scale ranged from 0.72 to 0.88 in the study and this was judged acceptable. However, the Knowledge Scales of Dickson's Breast Cancer Screening Inventory produced alpha coefficients of 0.22, 0.30 and 0.29 and as a result these measures were dropped from further analysis. The paper is a good example of the care which is necessary in choosing and applying a questionnaire. When appraising a piece of literature, such efforts give added credibility to the conclusions drawn from a particular piece of research. Such detailed consideration of reliability gives the critical reader an indication of the rigour with which the authors have conducted their study.

Summary

Validity and reliability are crucial concepts in evaluating research studies that have used quantitative methods. Validity is concerned with whether the study has accurately identified the concepts of interest and examined the relationships between them and reliability is concerned with the consistency (or replicability) of research processes. In order to be valid, a study must also be reliable.

QUANTITATIVE DATA COLLECTION METHODS

QUESTIONNAIRES

All too often when reading a published paper, the critical reader finds that only a single sentence has been used to refer to the design or piloting of a questionnaire – giving the impression that all that is needed to construct a questionnaire is common sense and enthusiasm. However, constructing a reliable and valid questionnaire to collect high-quality data is a subtle and sophisticated art. Poorly designed questionnaires collect poor quality data. Lydeard (1991) describes a number of steps necessary for developing a questionnaire to use as a research tool:

● Define the area of investigation
● Formulate the questions
● Choose the sample and maximize the response rate
● Pilot and test for validity and reliability
● Recognize sources of error.

However, there is little to be gained in trying to reinvent the wheel! There are many 'off the peg' questionnaires which can be used for particular purposes whose authors have already established their reliability and validity. When reading a published study which has used a well-established questionnaire to collect data, it is more important to make a judgement as to whether it has been used appropriately rather than assess how it has been developed. This information is readily available from the texts referenced at the end of this chapter (for example, McDowell & Newell 1987).

Some studies, however, are concerned primarily with the development and psychometric testing of a questionnaire rather than its use. Hagerty and Patusky (1995), for example, in a careful and well-written paper, describe the process of developing a questionnaire to measure a 'sense of belonging'

(SOB). They used the following steps:

- The area of investigation was defined by reviewing the relevant literature.
- The questions were formulated from a number of sources, including the literature review, clinical experiences and statements by people who had participated in earlier focus group interviews.
- The process of sampling and piloting took place amongst community college students and clients diagnosed with major depression in hospital. A third group of Roman Catholic nuns was subsequently sampled. Details of how response rates were maximized – such as paying respondents $5 for completed questionnaires – are also given.
- A good description of how the validity and reliability testing of the questionnaire was established is also included. For example, content validity was assessed by a panel of experts and retest reliability was examined through the studies with the three subject groups.
- Finally, some consideration was also given to the possible sources of error in the whole process of developing the instrument.

This detailed description of how a particular questionnaire was developed gives the critical reader confidence in the rigour of the study. In a study which has used a self-developed instrument for data collection, sufficient detail should be given to allow for an appraisal of how it was developed before application.

Timms and Ford's paper on nurses' perceptions of the need for continuing education in gerontology (Timms & Ford 1995) is a further example of a research report which gives sufficient detail about the development of a questionnaire to allow an assessment by the critical reader. For example, the questionnaire was pilot tested by a convenience sample of 30 nurses for clarity, completeness, readability and for test/retest reliability. The use of a convenience sample may be criticized on the grounds of representativeness but the important point is that the reader can find out from the paper how the instrument was piloted and evaluate this process.

The alert reader will, at this point, recognize that whether or not a questionnaire is an appropriate data collection method depends on the research question which has been asked. A good example of the use of well-validated questionnaires can be seen in the paper by Blixen and Kippes (1999). The purpose of their study was to develop an understanding of the quality of life of older adults with osteoarthritis,

with varying levels of depression and social support as a basis for nursing interventions. Using a convenience sample of 50 adults in a cross-sectional survey, they administered the Arthritis Impact Scales, the Centre for Epidemiological Studies Depression Scale, the Social Support Questionnaire and the Quality of Life Survey to measure the severity of osteoarthritis, depression, informal social support and quality of life. The details of the questionnaires used are given in a very comprehensive methodology section of the paper which enables the reader to evaluate the rigour with which they have conducted their research. In this study, because of the specific nature of the research question being asked and the fact that a well-defined hypothesis was being tested, it is entirely appropriate that these specific questionnaires were used to collect the data.

The pilot study

Hanson et al (1995) conducted a pilot study of the psychological support role of night nursing staff on an acute care oncology unit. This impressive paper used observation field techniques to explore the nature of the nurse-patient relationship. The study revealed eleven main categories leading to indicators distinctive to night nursing which need to be explored through further research. Such a pilot study is usually the preliminary to a main study and as such should follow the design of the main study as closely as possible. In addition, the sample used should consist of subjects who resemble as closely as possible those who will be used in the main study.

Another criterion a pilot study should meet is the extent to which the areas covered or the questions asked by interview or questionnaire measure what they are supposed to measure. In Hanson et al's excellent paper, considerable attention is paid to this criterion and it may be considered a 'benchmark' by which any published pilot study can be appraised by the critical reader.

Summary

Careful questionnaire design is essential in quantitative research for the collection of good quality data and critical readers should look for evidence that research methods have been piloted and modified accordingly.

SAMPLING

SAMPLE SIZE AND QUANTITATIVE METHODS

The question of sample size is inextricably linked to the subject of statistical power which is discussed in some detail in the following sections.

Axton and Smith (1995), for example, in their comparison of brachial and calf blood pressures in infants, used a convenience sample of 79 infants. They reported no statistically significant differences in their measurements when assessed by a paired t-test (see Figure 8.2). Although less than 100 subjects, this sample size allowed for adequate power for this particular statistical test when both effect size and level of significance were taken into account. (This is discussed later in this chapter.)

However, in many studies, not only are inappropriate sampling methods used but also the size of the sample is inadequate to demonstrate the effect of one variable on another (Sherman and Polit 1990). In other words, the confidence one can have that there is a link between a cause (the *independent* variable) and an effect (the *dependent* variable) must be tempered by the knowledge that the sampling method used, and the size of the sample, are both crucial in establishing this relationship and its generalizability.

TYPES OF SAMPLING

Convenience (opportunistic) sampling

Snowdon and Kane (1995) obtained a convenience sample from the paediatric ward of a large, acute care hospital in Canada to identify the needs of parents following the discharge of a child from hospital. This was a descriptive study of sixteen families. The authors, quite rightly in our view, are cautious about the conclusions which can be drawn from such a small convenience sample and describe the study as preliminary. A convenience or opportunistic sample is just that – resources may only allow for a sample to be drawn from a convenient population and any conclusions which are drawn must, of necessity, be cautious. Even when evaluating a study with a much larger convenience (opportunistic or non-probability) sample, such as that by Stein (1995) who recruited a sample of 149 children into an investigation of pain, the critical reader needs to have considerable reservations about the generalizability

of the results, since whatever makes the sample 'convenient' may also be related to the variables of interest. This could introduce bias into a study.

Random sampling and randomization

It is important to distinguish between random sampling and randomization. *Random samples* are chosen to obtain a representative sample of the population. By ensuring that the method of choosing the sample is purely random, any statistics calculated from the sample will be an unbiased estimate of the relevant population parameter. For a *simple random sample*, every member of the population has an equal chance of being selected, and choosing one individual does not affect whether any other individuals are chosen.

Randomization, on the other hand, is a method of allocating treatments to subjects completely at random. There are two reasons for randomization. First, it can be shown that in the long run patients will be balanced in both known and unknown prognostic factors. Second, before a patient is recruited to a trial, there should be no way of predicting which treatment they are likely to receive. Bitter experience has shown that trials that have not used random allocation methods can be biased in unexpected directions (see also Chapter 6).

Random sampling techniques are discussed in more detail in Chapter 9. They can be split into *simple* random sampling and *systematic* random sampling. If selections are made purely by chance this is known as *simple* random sampling. For example, numbers could be drawn out of a hat having first given a number to every member of the population. However, this is a very laborious way of carrying out sampling and *systematic* random sampling is a more commonly employed method. After numbers have been allocated to everybody in the sampling frame (population), the first individual is picked using a random number table and then subsequent subjects are selected using a *fixed sampling interval*, i.e. every nth person.

Random sampling technique   Stratified random sampling is a way of ensuring that particular strata or categories of individuals are represented in the sampling process. For example, if approximately 4% of the patients in our practice is made up of particular ethnic minority groups then, with a simple random selection, there will be a chance that there are no people from ethnic minorities in the sample. If the study requires a sample which is representative of the population frame, then a stratified sampling method would have to be used:

- The population would be split into different strata, in this case separating out those individuals with the relevant ethnic background (minority group).
- Random sampling techniques would then be used to sample each of the two (majority and minority) ethnic groups separately using the same sampling interval in each group.
- This will ensure that the final sampling frame is representative of the minority group in a pro rata basis to the actual population.

However, if the aim of the research was to compare the results of the minority group with the larger group, a *disproportionate sampling method* would have to be used. This is because the numbers achieved in the minority group, although pro rata to those of the population, would not be large enough to demonstrate statistical differences. With disproportionate sampling the strata are not selected pro rata to their size in the wider population. For instance, if a comparison of iron status was being made between a particular minority group and a larger majority group, then it would be necessary to oversample the smaller group (include more members of this group) in order to achieve statistical power, i.e. in order to be able to demonstrate statistically significant differences between groups.

HOW BIG SHOULD A SAMPLE BE?

This is a bit like asking 'how long is a piece of string?' Most nursing studies continue to rely on relatively small convenience or opportunistic samples. Brown et al (1984) looked at four journals between 1952 and 1980 and reported a median sample size of 84 in 1952 and 80 in 1980. Clearly, it is the nature of nursing research to ask research questions whose answers are both complex and difficult to measure. However, for a quantitative study to have enough *statistical power* to give the critical reader confidence that a relationship exists between two variables, larger sample sizes are required than are currently used in much nursing research.

Sherman and Polit (1990) looked at 62 articles in nursing research published in 1989 and concluded that 'a substantial number of nurse studies ... have insufficient (statistical) power to detect real effects primarily because the samples used are too small'. They calculated that for two-thirds of the articles

reviewed which had sample sizes less than 100, to demonstrate sufficient power, an average sample size of 218 subjects per group was required rather than the actual average of 83. Does this mean 'the larger the better'? For some quantitative research questions this may only be the case up to a point since a study can be 'overpowered'! However, the confidence one can have in a reported association between two variables in a quantitative study also depends on the data collection methods, the design of the study and the use of valid and reliable measuring instruments. A detailed discussion of statistical power can be found towards the end of this chapter.

QUANTITATIVE DATA ANALYSIS

When reading a published study which has collected quantitative data, the critical reader should ask themselves which sort of data has been collected. Different methods of statistical analysis are used for different types of data. In deciding if an appropriate test has been used, it is necessary to be clear about the type of data that has been collected. The different methods of statistical analysis for quantitative data may be broadly classified into *parametric statistics*, which assume the data have a normal distribution and which are used to manipulate *interval* or *ratio* data, and *nonparametric statistics* which make no assumptions about distribution and are used to analyse *ordinal* or *nominal* data.

INTERVAL AND RATIO DATA

An *interval* or *ratio* scale is one in which data are recorded on a measurement scale where the gaps between the numbers are the same wherever the researcher is on the scale. For example, in measuring the level of iron in the blood, data are recorded in milligrams. Wherever the researcher is on the scale, 'a milligram (mg) is a milligram', i.e. the difference between 3 mg and 4 mg is the same as between 11 mg and 12 mg. This is an interval or ratio scale. A ratio scale specifically is one which has an absolute zero (i.e. there is a meaningful zero point on the scale such as nil volume) which allows the researcher to make meaningful ratio comparisons such as 100 ml is twice as much as 50 ml. This distinction between interval and ratio data is less important as far as the critical reader is concerned, since interval and ratio data may be analysed statistically in the same way.

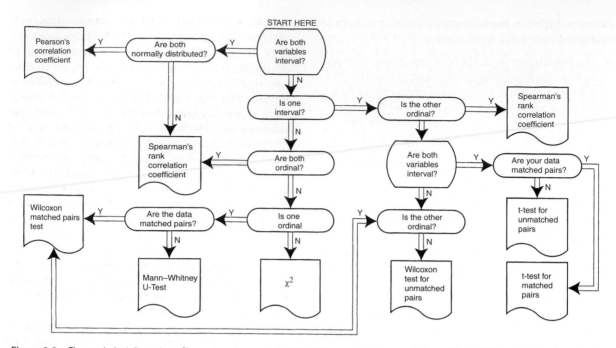

Figure 8.2   The statistical flow chart (From Armstrong et al 1990: 158, reprinted by permission of Oxford University Press).

ORDINAL DATA

Here, data are collected on a scale which has *an order* but there is no mathematical relationship between different points on the scale. For example, the classification of Social Class stretches from Social Class V to I. However, although the measurement has an order, in no sense can Social Class II be regarded as twice Social Class I.

NOMINAL DATA

When nominal data are collected, there is *no mathematical relationship* at all between the different categories. For example, in the Registrar General's classification of occupation, although one may wish to categorize and number the different occupations for analysis, there is no sense of a mathematical relationship between the categories – a refuse collector is not twice a teacher!

WHICH STATISTICAL TEST FOR WHICH TYPE OF DATA? (Fig. 8.2)

When comparing two samples to see if there is any statistically significant difference between them (i.e. differences which are highly unlikely to have

occurred by chance), appropriate statistical tests for interval or ratio data are the *t-tests* for matched or unmatched pairs. Matched pairs of samples are used, for example, to assess the effect of an intervention before and after in the same subjects. If more than two samples are being compared, then an ANOVA test (**An**alysis **of Va**riance) should be used to analyse the data.

Janke (1994) in her development of a breastfeeding attrition prediction tool, reported a one-tail (see following section) t-test of mean instrument scores of women with and without prior breastfeeding experience. Statistically significant (p = 0.001) group differences were found in two components of the instrument; the negative breastfeeding sentiment and the breastfeeding control contrast. Although the scales of her instrument are chosen to measure the attitudes of women (nominal data), she has treated these data as interval in her analysis. This is because it is possible – although controversial – to sum the items of a subscale in a questionnaire to create an index which, although it is derived from nominal data, may be treated as interval data for analysis.

In her study of job satisfaction in Japanese nurses, Yamashita (1995) used a one-way ANOVA to look for differences among medical (*n* = 175), surgical (*n* = 199) and ICU (*n* = 240) nurses. She was able to demonstrate statistically significant differences among the three practice areas of nurses in terms of their job satisfaction. A *one-way* ANOVA is used when there are sets of data from three separate groups of subjects and we want to know whether there is a difference between the three groups. A *two-way* ANOVA is used when there are two (or more) independent (cause) variables and we wish to test a hypothesis that they affect a dependent (effect) variable; similarly, a *three-way* ANOVA may be used to test for the statistical significance of increasing numbers of independent variables. The interested reader is referred to Campbell and Machin (1997) for a more detailed discussion of these issues.

Berg et al (1994) performed a two-way ANOVA to analyse the differences in nurses' creativity, tedium and burnout between a ward for severely demented patients and a similar ward which acted as a control. The comparisons over time within each sample showed that the creativity and innovative climate of an intervention group (consisting of systematic clinical supervision and individualized planned care) increased during the year of the study. In this example, two independent variables (the intervention and time) are examined for their effect on the dependent variables of creativity, tedium and burnout. Their results are tabulated very clearly in the original paper and this is a good example of the necessary transparency for the critical reader to evaluate the rigour with which the authors have approached the analysis of their quantitative data.

A more recent example of the use of ANOVA comes from a study which examined the disparities in cardiovascular health between southern rural, African American and white women to determine if their cardiovascular risk index differed by race, education or income levels and if differences persisted when controlling for body mass index (BMI) (Appel et al 2002). Using a three way ANOVA test, which included race, income and education, education and race were significant predictors of the cardiovascular risk index but when adjusted for BMI, race was no longer a statistically significant predictor; the only significant predictors were BMI and educational level. Using this statistical analysis, the authors were able to conclude that women with the least education had the highest cardiovascular risk index regardless of race.

ONE- AND TWO-TAILED HYPOTHESES

If the aim of a particular study is to test a hypothesis (H_1) that there is a difference between the scores of two groups of subjects, then the corresponding *null hypothesis* (H_0) (see later) is that no such difference exists. The original hypothesis (H_1) therefore merely states that there is a difference. It does *not* say, for example, that group 2 will score higher or lower than group 1, only that group 1 and 2 will differ. This is called a *two-tailed hypothesis*: group 2 could score less than or more than group 1. If, however, the original hypothesis was that group 1 would score less than group 2 (i.e. if the direction of the difference between the two groups is predicted) then this would be a *one-tailed hypothesis*. Similarly, if H_1 was that group 1 would score more than group 2, this would also be a one-tailed hypothesis since the direction of the difference would still be predicted. This distinction may seem arcane to the uninitiated but it is important when applying significance tests. Statistical printouts usually show the two-tailed probability of a calculated statistic. One-tailed probabilities are the two-tailed probabilities divided by two.

The appropriate statistical tests for comparison of ordinal data sets are the *Wilcoxon test* for paired or related samples and the *Mann–Whitney* test for unpaired or independent samples. For example, a researcher wishes to find out if there is an improvement in the quality of life for hypertensive patients following the introduction of new clinical guidelines. Ordinal data are collected to assess the impact of the intervention and the scores of the patients are compared before and after the intervention. In this situation the Wilcoxon test for paired or related samples should be used. The point here is that the Wilcoxon test is used when the subjects are the same.

However, if a researcher wished to compare the performance of two groups of nurses, one of whom used the new clinical guidelines and the other who did not, then, assuming once again that ordinal data have been collected, the Mann–Whitney test should be used to make comparisons between the groups since they contain *different* subjects.

The Claybury community psychiatric nurse stress study (Fagin et al 1995) asked the question: is it more stressful to work in hospital or the community? The authors collected data on the stress levels of 250 community-based and 323 ward-based psychiatric nurses. The Mann–Whitney test was used to compare the mean scores for each group for job satisfaction and 'occupational burnout'. By means of this analysis, the authors were able to conclude that the ward-based psychiatric nurses were achieving less personal fulfilment from their work and that 'stress was reaping its toll on mental health nurses'. This is a well-written paper which gives the critical reader plenty of information to evaluate the methods of data analysis which the authors have used.

The statistical test used for comparing groups when nominal data have been collected is generally χ^2 (chi-square). A good example of the use of χ^2 may be found in Dealey's paper (1994) on monitoring pressure sore problems in a teaching hospital. Using the χ^2 test, each grade of pressure sore was assessed for any differences between two surveys done in 1989 and 1993. There was no statistically significant difference in the grades of pressure sores although the survey did show an improvement in the management of established pressure sores. The paper itself is well written and sufficient detail is given for the critical reader to evaluate the appropriateness of the statistical tests used.

ANALYSING DIFFERENT TYPES OF DATA

The critical reader will find that some authors use nonparametric tests (e.g. Mann–Whitney U-test) for interval data and that this is often accepted by the editors of journals. The difficulty is, however, that if a nonparametric test is used for interval data, then the calculated *p-value (significance level)* will always be greater than that obtained using, for example, the t-test (a p-value of <0.05 is generally accepted as statistically significant). This means that a researcher is less likely to find a significant result with a nonparametric test using the same data, so such tests are less powerful. Nonparametric tests are also much less flexible when used to analyse interval data. For example, multiple regression and analysis of covariance are not possible with such tests.

Sometimes it is necessary for a researcher to compare interval with ordinal data rather than the same type of data (i.e. interval). More detailed discussion of the statistical manipulations which then become necessary is unfortunately beyond the scope of this text. However, a statistical flow chart is shown in Figure 8.2 which is an easy guide for the novice through the sometimes bewildering world of statistics.

CONFIDENCE INTERVALS

The published literature often reports confidence intervals for populations. These are the range of values within which a researcher can be confident that the population value falls. Confidence intervals can be set at different levels. A 95% confidence

interval (CI 95) means that one can be 95% confident that the population value falls within a certain range. These values should not be too wide if the critical reader is to believe that the sample represents the attributes of the rest of the population.

A study might report, for example, that 40% of a sample of 1000 people were smokers and that the calculated 95% confidence interval was plus or minus 3% of this value. The critical reader could then be 95% confident that the frequency of smoking in the population was between 37% and 43%.

However, sample sizes have a crucial influence on confidence intervals. If the sample size was only 100 and the percentage of smokers was still 40%, the corresponding 95% confidence interval might be 12% either side, a range of between 28% to 52% for the population. Unfortunately, much of the published literature does not include confidence intervals and it is often difficult to evaluate this aspect of data analysis in a study. The interested reader is referred to Gardner and Altman (1989).

Summary

A number of factors determine the appropriate statistical test for the analysis of quantitative data in a given set of circumstances. These include the level of measurement of the data (ratio, interval, ordinal or nominal), the question to be answered (i.e. is a description of the data required or an indication of the relationship between variables?) and the number of groups in the study. Although decisions about the use of different methods of analysis often require advanced statistical knowledge, it is usually possible for the critical reader to assess whether a researcher has provided sufficient justification for the approach they have used. However, if in doubt, ask a statistician for advice!

INDEPENDENT AND DEPENDENT VARIABLES

In addition to describing population parameters, the aim of quantitative data analysis is often to establish an association between two variables: the independent variable (cause) and the dependent variable (effect). The strength of the association is determined partly by the 'robustness' of the statistical test used.

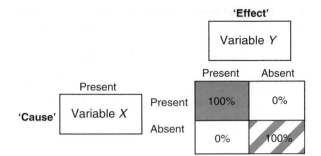

'Effect'

Variable *Y*

		Present	Absent
'Cause' Variable *X*	Present	100%	0%
	Absent	0%	100%

Legend:

  when *X* is present, *Y* is always present

  when *X* is absent, *Y* is also always absent

Figure 8.3   'Perfect' relationship between *X* and *Y*.

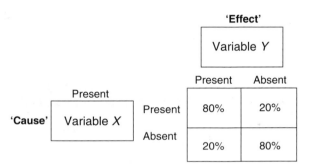

'Effect'

Variable *Y*

		Present	Absent
'Cause' Variable *X*	Present	80%	20%
	Absent	20%	80%

Figure 8.4   Relationship between variables in the 'real' world.

Deaths from lung cancer

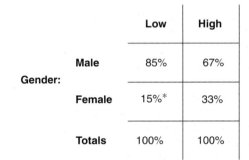

Gender:	Low	High	Totals
Male	85%	15%	100%
Female	67%*	33%	100%

[*Note: This means that 67% of females had low death rates from lung cancer]

Figure 8.5   Gender and death from lung cancer.

Death rates from lung cancer

Gender:	Low	High
Male	85%	67%
Female	15%*	33%
Totals	100%	100%

[*Note: This means that 15% of low death rates from lung cancer were observed in females]

Figure 8.6   Deaths from lung cancer and gender.

In a 'perfect' world, variable *X* may cause effect *Y* as shown in Figure 8.3.

However, when data are analysed in the real world, such 'perfect' relationships are rarely found! This is illustrated in Figure 8.4 where variable *X* is sometimes present when *Y* is absent and *Y* is sometimes present when *X* is absent. These sorts of data imply that 'something else' is disturbing the relationship between *X* and *Y*. This 'something else' may be another variable often referred to as the 'confounding variable'. The influence of a confounding variable on a relationship between an independent and dependent variable is known as 'Simpson's paradox' and the process of taking it into account when inferring a cause-and-effect relationship is known as *specification* or *elaboration*. The interested reader is referred to Campbell and Machin (1997) for a far more detailed discussion of this topic. Such an analysis of three variables (dependent, independent and confounding) is admirably presented in Lauver and Tak's paper (1995) on optimism and coping with a breast cancer symptom.

The distinction between the independent and the dependent variables is important. A further example may make this clearer. A hypothesis might be: *Men have a higher death rate from lung cancer than women.* Prevalence data are collected and tabulated as shown in Figure 8.5, in which the gender was totalled to 100% of the observations. In Figure 8.6 it is the death rate from lung cancer which is totalled to 100% of the observations.

Exercise 8.1

Which hypothesis is being tested by each table? (Clue: the independent variable must total 100%.) What is the likely confounding variable?

Summary

When reading reports of research investigating the relationship between one or more variables, it is important to identify which is the independent variable (or presumed cause) and which the dependent variable(s) (or presumed effect). It is also important to be aware of the effects of confounding influences which mean that, in the real world, 'perfect' relationships between variables are rarely observed. An important function of quantitative analysis is to determine the probability or 'likelihood' that a relationship between variables observed in the context of a research study could have occurred simply by chance.

THE NULL HYPOTHESIS, STATISTICAL SIGNIFICANCE AND STATISTICAL POWER

When quantitative data are analysed for relationships between variables a *null hypothesis* is tested. The null hypothesis (H_0) states that there is no difference between the two groups which are being compared. If the null hypothesis can be rejected on the basis of analysis using appropriate statistical tests (see above) then one can infer that there *is* an association between two variables which *may* be cause and effect. The strength of such an association depends on the statistical test used and the statistical power of the study.

Fox and Mathers (1997) analysed 1422 statistical tests in 85 quantitative original papers for statistical power in the *British Journal of General Practice*. The median power of tests analysed was 0.71, representing a slightly greater than two-thirds likelihood of rejecting false null hypotheses. Thirty-seven (44%) of the 85 studies achieved a power of 0.8 or more. Ten studies had power of >0.99 suggesting 'overpowering'. Twenty-one of the papers, however, had a likelihood of gaining significant results poorer than that obtained by tossing a coin when a null hypothesis is false.

What is statistical power and why is it important?

Statistical power is at the heart of quantitative research and may best be understood in conjunction with the null hypothesis. There are four situations which can arise when the data from a particular study have been analysed. These are illustrated in Figure 8.7. Each cell is discussed in turn below. The possible combinations of study and 'real world' results with the null hypothesis are as follows:

Cell 1. One possibility is that the results from a study support the null hypothesis and this is, in fact, the situation in the 'real' world. Again there are no problems with this since the results reflect 'reality' and there is *no* association between the variables demonstrated either by the study or in the 'real' world.

Cell 2. If, however, the null hypothesis is supported by the results of the study (i.e. found to be true), but in the 'real' world, the null hypothesis is in fact incorrect this is known as a *type II error (beta)*. The concept of statistical power is used to try and minimize the likelihood of this type II error. The lower the power of the study, the more likely it is that any lack of association which has been found

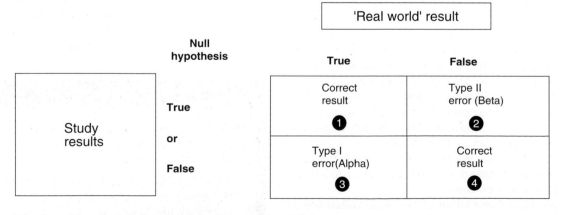

Figure 8.7 The null hypothesis (H_0), statistical significance and statistical power.

between two variables is due to chance. Clearly, sample size is crucial here in determining the power of a study and the smaller the sample, the greater the likelihood of the negative results being due to chance. Conventionally, a value of 0.80 is acceptable as a measure of sufficient statistical power to minimize the chances of such a type II error.

Cell 3. However, the situation may also arise that the study results show the null hypothesis to be false (i.e. it shows that there is an association between two variables) but in 'reality' the null hypothesis is true (i.e. there is *no* association between the variables). This is known as a *type I error (alpha)*. Again, sample size is crucial here, in determining the likelihood of a statistically significant result and whether such results might have arisen by chance. This is usually expressed in the published literature as a *p-value*. The higher the p-value, the more likely it is that such results have occurred by chance and there is no 'real' association between the variables. Conventionally, a value of <0.05 is acceptable as a measure of sufficient statistical significance to demonstrate a 'real' association between two variables (i.e. a statistically significant difference between two groups).

Cell 4. The null hypothesis is not supported by the results of the study (i.e. found to be false) and this is also the situation in the 'real' world. There are no problems with this and there *is* an association between the variables.

Apart from sample size, two other factors affect the statistical power of a study. The first is the *significance level* or *alpha* (above). Power increases with higher type I errors. However, if the significance level which is required is less than the conventional 0.05 (i.e. the risk of a type I error is required to be lower than is conventionally acceptable, e.g. 0.01) then the statistical power would also decrease.

The second factor affecting statistical power is effect size. The effect size is merely a measure of how 'wrong' the null hypothesis is, i.e. it measures the strength of the association between the independent and the dependent variable. There is a reciprocal relationship between effect size and sample size: the larger the effect size, the smaller the sample size needs to be and the greater the power. Of course, in non-experimental (or non-intervention) research, the researcher does not manipulate or control the independent variable but nevertheless its value can be estimated.

As outlined above, much of the published literature of nursing research is based on relatively small sample sizes. This means that unless effect sizes are large, many of these studies are underpowered and have a high probability of committing a type II error (showing no association between two variables, when 'in reality' there is an association). Some assessment of statistical power by the critical reader is particularly important when non-significant results are reported and the study inconclusive. In addition, many research studies in nursing are concerned with small effect sizes and consequently are likely to be underpowered. When a study is designed, a statistical power of about 0.80 should be aimed for which means that only one in five times would a false null hypothesis be accepted. Lower values, for example 0.66, would mean that the chance of accepting a false null hypothesis would be one in three.

The calculations of statistical power are complex but tables are available (e.g. Cohen 1977) to identify the necessary sample size to achieve a statistical power of 0.80 for each of the different statistical tests. Some estimate of effect size is also necessary and as a 'rule of thumb', a medium effect size is visible to the naked eye: anything less clear should be counted as a small effect. In other words, a medium effect can be discerned from everyday experience without recourse to formal measurement. For example, the difference between male and female adult heights in the UK would be counted as medium effect size. Most effects encountered in biomedical and social research should therefore be assumed to be small unless there is a good reason to claim a medium effect, while a 'large' effect size would probably need to be defined as one which is so large that it hardly seems necessary to undertake research into something so well established. Cohen (1977) offers the example of the difference between the heights of 13 and 18-year-old girls as a large effect. For a fuller discussion of these issues the reader is also referred to Fox and Mathers (1997).

Summary

The further questions which a critical reader needs to ask about quantitative data analysis in a published paper are as follows:

- Has an appropriate statistical test been used by the authors for the particular type of data which have been collected?

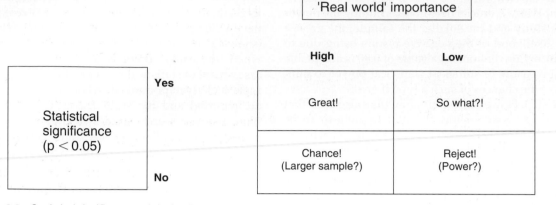

Figure 8.8   Statistical significance and the 'real' world.

- Have justifiable statistical inferences been made about a relationship between different variables?
- In other words, are the authors justified in their claim that an intervention (variable *X*) has resulted in a particular effect (variable *Y*)?
- What is the level of statistical significance which has been chosen by the authors?
- Is there sufficient statistical power in the study to support any claimed association between an intervention and a result?
- Has 'real world' (or clinical) significance been considered as well as statistical significance?

The last question is particularly relevant for the weary critical reader of the academic literature. If the results of a study have statistical significance but not 'real world' (or clinical) significance, then so what?! (See Figure 8.8)

CRITICAL APPRAISAL OF QUANTITATIVE RESEARCH

In its broadest sense, critical appraisal is defined as the systematic application of rules of evidence to a piece of published literature to determine its validity and applicability. However, with the increasing availability of specialist journals in which to publish and changes to the current funding systems of Universities to reward research, the volume of scientific literature is expanding exponentially. In 1985, for example, there were over 20 000 active biomedical journals and the number has increased very

substantially since then. Unless researchers have some systematic way of appraising what is published, filtering it and incorporating it within their own canon of literature then quite simply they will be overwhelmed!

THE RESEARCH PROCESS

Before starting to evaluate a quantitative research paper the researcher needs to decide whether it is worth reading in the first place. Starting with the abstract, the researcher should ask the following questions:

- Why did the authors do their study?
- What did the authors do?
- What were the findings?
- What do the findings mean?

If the answers to these questions are not readily apparent on reading the abstract and skimming through the paper, then it may not be worthwhile reading it. However, if the results of the researcher's first filtering are good then read on.

RESEARCH QUESTION/AIMS AND OBJECTIVES

The first question a critical reader needs to ask when reading a paper is: have the authors defined a clear and important research question? Or alternatively have they formulated a clear aim or specified objectives for their study? In some cases a hypothesis will be stated which the authors wish to test. If this is not clear from an initial review then it is unlikely that the effort involved in reading, appraising and making notes on this particular paper is worthwhile.

Unfortunately many authors remain confused about the difference between aims and objectives. (An aim is the purpose of a study. The objectives are the steps necessary to achieve that purpose.)

In summary, the researcher should ask:

- What is the major aim (objective) of the study?
- Is it unambiguously defined?
- Is it a question worth asking?
- Are objectives clearly stated?

METHODOLOGY

Subsumed under this heading are both design and methods. The most important initial question to ask about the methodology is:

- Is the chosen design appropriate for the research question?

Unfortunately, many authors do not state their design explicitly and it may be necessary to tease this out from the paper. The sorts of question a critical reader needs to ask if a questionnaire has been used to collect data, for example, are as follows:

- Has an 'off the peg' questionnaire been used appropriately by the researchers?
- If a questionnaire has been developed by the authors, has the process been described in sufficient detail for an assessment of its reliability and validity?
- Has the questionnaire been piloted?
- What response rate has been obtained? (Most biases disappear at response rates of >70%.)

Sampling is another important aspect of evaluating quantitative research. There are a number of different random sampling methods which include simple, systematic and stratified. The key questions to ask are:

- Is the sampling frame representative or could it be biased?
- Has an appropriate sampling method been chosen?
- Is the sample large enough? (i.e. is the power of the study sufficient to detect a 'real' difference?)

In addition to this, the critical reader should be aware of both the subject and setting in which the research was carried out and, if there has been a comparison of a treatment and control group, then to what extent did matching occur. Similarly, if the response rate in a particular study was low it is particularly important for authors to have collected data on non-responders or non-participants so that some assessment of the representativeness or otherwise of the control group may be made.

OUTCOME MEASURES

There are a number of issues to consider:

- The study should state the criteria used for the outcome measures. How were they developed?
- If it is a clinical study which is being reported then to what extent were the outcomes clinically relevant?
- Were they accurate and reproducible?
- Would all clinicians accept the particular end-point of the authors?
- How has the problem of observer bias been dealt with?
- If the process of care has been studied, then do the described outcomes depend on that process?
- Have all relevant outcomes been reported?

RESULTS

Clearly, data must be displayed explicitly to enable judgements to be made. There should be good use of graphs, tables and bar charts, and numbers should be used in addition to percentages. Remember that logarithmic scales amplify small differences in results. Unfortunately, it is sometimes the data that are not published, which are the very data that would enable a critical reader to assess the validity of the results.

Judgements will also need to be made as to whether an appropriate statistical test has been used by the authors for the particular type of data which have been collected. For example, have tests designed for interval data been used on nominal data? In addition, have justifiable statistical inferences been made about a relationship between different variables? In other words, to what extent are the authors justified in their claim that an intervention (independent variable), for example, has resulted in a particular result (dependent variable)?

Response rates are also important as mentioned above and some data on non-responders to a questionnaire should be reported, since a poor response rate of <70% can introduce bias. For example, only those with a good response to a particular treatment might have bothered to return the questionnaire.

Specific questions to ask are:

- Have any non-responders been followed up to see if they differ in significant ways from the responders?
- Have the data been reweighted to compensate for the non-response and to make the findings more representative?
- Have any confounding variables been considered which might influence the results?

Having made some judgements about the validity of the results which have been presented, critical readers should start to consider their applicability to their own research or practice. In a sense applicability is dependent on validity. If the results presented are not valid, either because an inappropriate design has been chosen or the methods of analysis are faulty, then clearly the applicability of a particular study is in doubt.

CONCLUSIONS/RECOMMENDATIONS

In summary, the important questions to ask before applying research results to either our own or others' studies or practice are as follows:

- Do the conclusions and recommendations follow from the results?
- Have any conclusions been drawn that are not supported by the data presented?
- Indeed, are any results left out and if so, is there any explanation of why these results have not been discussed?
- Has there been any reflection on the limitations of the study or methodology and how significant are the conclusions in a practical and statistical sense?

Answers to these questions will enable the critical reader to decide whether a piece of published work is both valid and applicable. Applying these criteria to issues of the *British Medical Journal* published in 1980, Sackett et al (1985) rejected 53% of published

articles. *The British Medical Journal*, however, did well compared with the *New England Journal of Medicine* which had 82% of its content rejected for failing to satisfy the requirements for scientific proof or clinical significance.

CONCLUSION

Evaluation of quantitative research is a sophisticated art and we can only hope to give the researcher a flavour of some of the skills and knowledge required in the course of this chapter. Like all skills they are, of course, best learnt by practice. We hope that on completing these two chapters, the diligent reader will have the necessary understanding, confidence and skills to evaluate the rigour with which studies using both quantitative and qualitative research methodologies have been conducted.

Exercise 8.2

Read the following published article and answer the questions below.

Gullicks JN and Crase SJ (1993). Sibling behaviour with a newborn: parents' expectations and observations. *Journal of Obstetric, Gynaecological and Neonatal Nursing* 22: 438–444.

Questions

1. What is the research question/objective of this paper?
2. How was the data collection method chosen and developed?
3. How was the 'internal' or 'split-half' reliability of the questionnaire determined?
4. Which sort of data have been collected?
5. How have these data been analysed?
6. Which statistical test has been used to compare the parents' expectations and observations?
7. How confident is the researcher that parents expect more negative behaviour than they actually observe?

References

Appel SJ, Harrell JS and Deng S (2002) Racial and socioeconomic differences in risk factors for cardiovascular disease among southern rural women. *Nursing Research* 51(3): 140–147.

Armstrong D, Calnan M and Grace J (1990) *Research Methods for General Practitioners*. Oxford: Oxford University Press.

Axton SE and Smith LF (1995) Comparison of brachial and calf blood pressures in infants. *Paediatric Nursing* 21(4): 323–326.

Blixen CE and Kippes C (1999) Depression, social support, and quality of life in older adults with osteoarthritis. *Image: Journal of Nursing Scholarship* 31(3): 221–226.

Brown JS, Tanner CA and Padrick KP (1984) Nursing's search for scientific knowledge. *Nursing Research* **33**(1): 26–34.

Campbell MJ and Machin D (1997) *Medical Statistics: A Commonsense Approach*, 3rd edn. Chichester: John Wiley.

Cohen J (1997) *Statistical Power Analysis for the Behavioural Sciences*. New York: Academic Press.

Dealey C (1994) Monitoring the pressure sore problem in a teaching hospital. *Journal of Advanced Nursing* **20**: 652–659.

Fagin L, Brown D, Bartlett H et al (1995) The Claybury community psychiatric nurse stress study: is it more stressful to work in hospital or the community? *Journal of Advanced Nursing* **22**: 347–358.

Fox N and Mathers N (1997) Empowering research: statistical power in general practice research. *Family Practice* **14**(4): 324–329.

Gardner MJ and Altman DG (1989) *Statistics with Confidence, Confidence Intervals and Statistical Guidelines*. London: BMJ Books.

Goldberg D and Williams P (1991) *A Users Guide to the General Health Questionnaire*. Windsor: Nfer-Nelson.

Hagerty BMK and Patusky K (1995) Developing a measure of sense of belonging. *Nursing Research* **44**(1): 9–13.

Hanson EJ, McClement S and Kristjanson LJ (1995) Psychological support role of night nursing staff on an acute care oncology unit. *Cancer Nursing* **18**(3): 237–246.

Janke JR (1994) Development of the breastfeeding attrition prediction tool. *Nursing Research* **43**(2): 100–110.

Lauver D and Tak Y (1995) Optimism and coping with a breast cancer symptom. *Nursing Research* **44**(4): 202–207.

Lydeard S (1991) The questionnaire as a research tool. *Family Practice* **8**(1): 26–33.

McDowell I and Newell C (1987) *Measuring Health: a Guide to Rating Scales and Questionnaires*. Oxford: Oxford University Press.

Phillips JM and Wilbur J (1995) Adherence to breast cancer screening guidelines among African-American women of differing employment status. *Cancer Nursing* **18**(4): 258–269.

Sackett DL, Haynes RB and Tugwell P (1985) *Clinical Epidemiology. A Basic Science for Clinical Medicine*. Boston: Little, Brown.

Sherman RE and Polit DF (1990) Statistical power in nursing research. *Nursing Research* **39**(6): 365–369.

Snowdon AW and Kane DJ (1995) Parental needs following the discharge of a hospitalised child. *Paediatric Nursing* **21**(5): 425–428.

Stein PR (1995) Indices of pain intensity: construct validity among pre-schoolers. *Paediatric Nursing* **21**(2): 119–123.

Timms J and Ford P (1995) Registered nurses' perceptions of gerontological continuing education needs in the United Kingdom and in the USA. *Journal of Advanced Nursing* **22**: 300–307.

Yamashita M (1995) Job satisfaction in Japanese nurses. *Journal of Advanced Nursing* **22**: 158–164.

Further reading

The main topics outlined in this chapter are covered in greater depth in these texts.

McDowell and Newell (1987) contains a large number of questionnaires particularly suitable for the collection of data in nursing research.

Gibbon B (1995) Validity and reliability of assessment tools. *Nurse Researcher* **2**(4): 48–55.

Howe T (1995) Measurement scales in health care settings. *Nurse Researcher* **2**(4): 30–37.

Lynn MR (1988) Should you believe what you read? Reliability and validity in published paediatric nursing research. *Journal of Paediatric Nursing* **3**(3): 197–199.

McDowell I and Newell C (1987) *Measuring Health: A Guide to Rating Scales and Questionnaires*. Oxford: Oxford University Press.

Oldham J (1995) Biophysiologic measures in nursing practice and research. *Nurse Researcher* **2**(4): 38–47.

Wilkin D, Hallam L and Doggett M (1992) *Measures of Need and Outcome for Primary Health Care*. Oxford: Oxford University Press.

Chapter **9**

Populations and samples: identifying the boundaries of research

Christine Ingleton

INTRODUCTION

Sampling considerations encompass all aspects of the research enquiry. Yet in many health care research studies the sampling design is the weakest part of the study. The correct match of the sampling procedures to the research aims and methods is an important consideration in assessing the trustworthiness or rigour of research findings and implications. Consequently an appreciation of the process of sampling and the rationale underpinning sampling decisions are essential for both researchers and consumers of research. Moreover, an understanding of how sampling decisions may affect findings will help in making more informed decisions about their applicability to clinical practice.

In this chapter I will first discuss why researchers base their work on samples. I will then examine ways in which researchers set boundaries in quantitative designs and then consider how boundaries are constructed in qualitative studies. It will become clear that qualitative and quantitative approaches address boundary setting differently and therefore judgements about the appropriateness and rigour of the sampling strategy in published research should be made with this in mind.

Key issues

- Populations and samples
- Sampling within quantitative designs
- Sampling within qualitative designs
- Evaluating a sampling strategy

Box 9.1 Reasons for taking a sample

Including the whole population may be:

- **Too expensive** – the use of sampling saves time and money
- **Impractical** – because the population may be vast and/or information on each member of the population may not be available
- **Inappropriate** – a more detailed investigation of a smaller number of subjects may be preferable to a more superficial consideration of the whole population
- **Unnecessary or unethical** – if correctly undertaken, sampling will ensure that the sample chosen and the findings elicited from that sample will reflect the wider population

WHY DO RESEARCHERS NEED TO IDENTIFY SAMPLES?

Research in health care settings usually involves the collection of data on a sample of people, rather than on the entire population of cases in which the researcher is interested (known as a census). Often, because of the number of people involved, the researcher does not have the resources to study the whole population. There are other reasons (see Box 9.1) why researchers may choose not to measure the whole population.

TYPES OF SAMPLE

The methodological literature on sampling generally makes a distinction between *probability sampling* (where each person in the population has an equal and non-zero chance of being included) and *non-probability sampling* (where each person's chance of being included in the sample is not known and may be zero). The purpose of most quantitative research is to examine the distribution of previously identified phenomena (or variables) within a population and/or exploring and testing relationships between variables (Bryman 2001, May 1997). Given the purpose of quantitative projects, it is appropriate that probability sampling should be used whenever possible in order to permit an estimate of sampling error and a calculation of the degree of confidence with which findings may be generalized to a wider

population. In the next section of this chapter I will discuss some of these terms and consider how probability or random sampling as it is sometimes referred to, works in practice.

REASONS FOR TAKING A SAMPLE

There are a number of reasons why researchers do not operate censuses but instead choose to investigate a sample of the population of interest. From Box 9.1 we can see that some of these reasons are pragmatic (that is, the researcher has no real choice) while others have a more theoretical basis (that is, there is no requirement that the views of a whole population are canvassed). Sampling decisions affect the value or credibility of research findings, particularly when the researcher attempts to extrapolate findings to a wider population than the one studied. The process of sampling and the rationale underpinning sampling decisions are therefore important issues to consider when critically analysing published research with a view to its applicability to clinical practice.

BOUNDARY SETTING IN QUANTITATIVE RESEARCH

DePoy and Gitlin (1994) describe boundary setting in the quantitative domain as *deductive*. That is, the researcher begins with a notion of the kinds of people they wish to study, and clearly defines the characteristics or attributes of that group. This is referred to as the *population*. The population for a study is typically reported as being composed of two groups – the *target population* and the *accessible population*. The target population is the entire set of cases about which the researcher would like to make generalizations. A *target population* might include *all* undergraduate nursing students enrolled on a degree programme in the UK. It is often not feasible, because of time, money and personnel, to obtain this sample so an *accessible population* may be used as an alternative. An accessible population is one that meets the population criteria and is *available*. For example, *an accessible population* may include all full-time undergraduate students enrolled on a degree in one region of the UK.

The sample is drawn from the population so the sample is a subset of the defined population. Table 9.1 shows examples of populations and samples.

Table 9.1   Examples of populations and samples

Population	Possible sample selection
All district nurses working in one region in the UK	100 district nurses selected for a study of job satisfaction
All deaths occurring in one city in the UK between 1995–1996	300 case notes selected by researcher to establish place of death
The pulse rate of a patient during a 24 hour period	Hourly measurements of patient's pulse rate recorded by staff
Nurse/patient interactions in a care of the elderly setting	6 patients observed and video recorded during interactions with trained nurses at meal times, over 3 days

Probability sampling refers to techniques that are based on probability theory (see Kumar 1999, Bland 1995 for an in-depth discussion). The two central features of probability theory as applied to sampling are that:

- the researcher has access to every member of the population;
- every member or element of the population has an equal and non-zero chance of being selected for the sample (i.e. they must not have 'no chance' of being selected).

The important point to remember is that the probability of each member or element being included in the sample is known and is greater than zero. By knowing the size of the population and the degree of chance that each element may be selected, a researcher can calculate the sampling error. Sampling error refers to the estimated difference between data obtained from a random sample and the data that would be obtained if the entire population were measured. Importantly, it indicates how representative the sample is likely to be of the population – an important criterion given that the main purpose of quantitative research is to generalize to a wider population. However, it is important to bear in mind that every study will contain a degree of sampling error to the extent that results are never 100% representative of the population; every sample will be slightly dissimilar from a subsequent sample drawn from the same population. Put simply, there is no such thing as the 'perfect sample'. There are a number of different ways of obtaining a probability sample. Four of the most common ways are discussed in this chapter:

- Simple random sampling
- Systematic sampling
- Stratified random sampling
- Cluster sampling.

An overview of these approaches and their advantages and disadvantages is shown in Table 9.2. It should be noted that sampling techniques discussed under the headings of quantitative and qualitative sampling issues are concerned with the identification of respondents for studies. Later in the chapter we will consider other indications for sampling.

SIMPLE RANDOM SAMPLING

This method of probability sampling attempts to ensure that every person or every element in the population has an equal chance of being included in the study. Hence, the sample is deemed to be 'representative' and the findings generalizable to a wider identified population. This method involves the selection, at random, of the required number of individuals for the sample from a list of the population (*sampling frame*). Once the sampling frame is obtained, individuals are assigned numbers consecutively. Then a random selection of the required number is made. Random numbers may be generated by using a lottery method (such as numbers being drawn out of a hat), random number tables or a computer. Many text books on statistics contain random number tables (see Kumar 1999). It is important to bear in mind that a researcher cannot select a simple random sample without a full and up-to-date list of the population. Bjorkstrom and Hamrin (2001) used a random sample of Swedish nurses in order to study attitudes towards research and development in nursing (see Box 9.2). The implications of this approach were that the findings could be generalized to the population of Swedish nurses working in a variety of areas of the profession. However, it is worth noting that the sample size and not just 'randomness' is important before assertions can be made about whether findings can be generalized to the wider population so confidently.

Table 9.2   Probability sampling – description, advantages and disadvantages

Type of sample	Description	Advantages	Disadvantages
Simple random	Obtain sampling frame Number members consecutively Select sample through table of random numbers	Little knowledge of population required Most unbiased of probability methods	Complete sampling frame essential Time consuming Expensive
Stratified	Divide into strata Ascertain number of cases for each stratum Randomly sample each sub group	Assures certain characteristics of the population are represented Increases probability of sample being representative by lowering sampling error	Requires complete sampling frame Costly and time consuming to stratify lists Statistics more complex
• Proportionate	Sample is drawn so that each stratum is equal to its proportion		
• Disproportionate	Oversample a disproportionately small stratum to ensure they are represented and allow comparisons		
Systematic	Obtain sampling frame Decide on sample size Agree sampling interval Select every (n)th element	Easy to select sample Economical Time saving and efficient	Bias in the form of non-randomness After the first case is selected, population members do not have equal chance of selection
Cluster	Groups or 'clusters' are selected from population Successive selections are made (region, district, hospital) Random sampling from cluster	Economical Useful when sampling frame unavailable. Characteristics of clusters can be estimated	Subjects may not accurately reflect characteristics of population and therefore generalization should be limited to the population of the clustering variable Larger sampling error than other probability samples Statistics are complex

SYSTEMATIC SAMPLING

Simple random sampling can often be time consuming and laborious. Systematic sampling offers a simpler method to randomly select a sample. It involves the selection of every 'nth' case drawn from a sampling frame at fixed intervals, for example, every 'nth' patient on a waiting list for orthopaedic surgery or every 'nth' qualified nurse on the ward 'off duty' list. However, for systematic sampling to fulfil the requirements of a probability sample, the population must be listed in a random order. To return to the example of ward off duty as a means of selecting a sample of nurses, if the population was

listed in order of seniority starting with the sister, every 'nth' nurse selected would clearly not be random. Because of the non-random order of the 'off-duty' list, bias would be introduced and this in turn would affect the external validity (generalizability) of the study. It is also important that the first element or member of the sample must be selected randomly. To do this, the researcher first divides the population (N) by the size of the desired sample (n) to obtain the sample interval width (k). In short, the sampling interval is the distance between the elements selected for the sample. Supposing a researcher wishes to study a group of 50 practice nurses and knows from the sampling frame that

Box 9.2 Example using simple random sampling (from Bjorkstrom & Hamrin 2001, with permission)

Title: *Swedish nurses attitudes towards research and development within nursing*

The aim of this study was to test an assessment instrument in order to study attitudes towards research and development within nursing. A **random sample** of 407 registered nurses were selected nationally by the Swedish Nurses Association of Health (**sampling frame**). The sample was drawn from all categories and areas of the profession, and at least 100 nurses from each of four groups of nurses from decennial examination years were selected. The number of completed questionnaires was 289, giving an overall **response rate** of 71%. There was no follow up of **non-responders**.

there is a population of 500, the sampling interval would be as follows:

$$k = 500/50 = 10$$

Therefore, every tenth name on the list of practice nurses would be sampled. After the sampling interval has been set, the researcher would use a table of random numbers to obtain a starting point for the selection of the 50 subjects. As the population size in this case is 500 and a sample size of 50 is required, a number between 1 and 500 is randomly selected. If, for example, the number selected is 54, the practice nurses assigned numbers 54, 64, 74, and so forth would be included in the sample until 50 cases had been chosen.

STRATIFIED RANDOM SAMPLING

In stratified random sampling, the population is divided into smaller homogenous sub groups called strata, where members of the group share a particular characteristic (e.g. stratum A may be males and stratum B may be females). These characteristics are chosen for stratification based on the assumption that they will have an effect on the variables under study. The researcher then randomly samples within the strata. There are two ways of achieving this. The

researcher may sample proportionately (in relation to the relative size of the stratum) or disproportionately. For example, if a patient population in a GP practice consisted of 10% Asian, 5% Afro-Caribbean, and 85% white people, then a proportional stratified sample of 100 patients, with ethnic background as the stratifying variable, would consist of 10, 5 and 85 patients from the respective sub populations. Clearly it would be inappropriate to draw conclusions about the characteristics of Afro-Caribbean people based on only 5 cases. If comparisons are sought between strata of unequal membership size, such as in this example, a disproportional sampling design would be appropriate. The sampling portions may be altered to ensure there is some representation of minority groups, even to the extent of including all members.

Teasdale et al (2001) employed proportional stratified random sampling to assess the effects of clinical supervision and informal support on qualified nurses (see Box 9.3). Interestingly, Teasdale and colleagues used a combination of sampling strategies within their study, illustrating that simple sampling designs are not always feasible or appropriate and that on occasion (and depending on the complexity of the research question) more multi-facetted design solutions are required (Marsland & Murrell 2000). For example, the study setting may change from that envisaged at the outset and this will have ramifications for the sampling design.

A study by Payne et al (2002) which sought to identify service providers' and commissioners' understanding of specialist palliative care in one area of South London, faced a number of unanticipated changes which could not have been predicted at the beginning of the study. These included a 30% reduction in beds (from 18–12), a cost saving exercise that required a reduction in costs by £350 000 in the short term, and a consequent reduction in staff. These sorts of major changes often occur in health care settings and this means that researchers need to be flexible and open minded when searching for sampling solutions to complex health care problems.

CLUSTER SAMPLING

This involves dividing the population into a number of units, or clusters, each of which contains individuals having a range of characteristics. The clusters themselves are chosen on a random basis. To illustrate what is in involved in cluster sampling, imagine

> **Box 9.3** Example using stratified sampling, combined with opportunistic sampling (from Teasdale et al 2001, with permission)
>
> **Title:** *Clinical supervision and support for nurses: an evaluation study*
>
> The aim of this study was to assess the effects of clinical supervision and informal support on qualified nurses. The **population** from which the sample was drawn comprised all qualified nurses working in general medical, general surgical and community adult nursing in the Trent regional health authority. The NHS Trusts in the region were stratified into 3 groups comprising: i) hospital trusts with 500 or more beds; ii) hospital trusts with fewer than 500 beds and iii) community trusts. A **random sample** of 3 larger hospitals, 4 smaller hospitals and 4 community hospitals was invited to participate. Co-coordinators in each trust then distributed questionnaires to an **opportunistic sample** of qualified nurses. A power analysis was conducted using Cohen's (1977) table for the chi-square test to estimate the number of questionnaire returns required to detect differences. Cohen's table indicated a requirement of a minimum of 196 returns to give an 80% chance of detecting differences. A 40% **response rate** was predicted, which meant 510 questionnaires had to be issued.

approach is sometimes known as multistage or area sampling. Marsland and Murrell (2000) used a multistage sampling technique to select study sites for in-depth case studies in a longitudinal study of the careers of nurses qualifying in the UK from the pre-registration Project 2000 diploma course.

Exercise 9.1

Read the article by Marsland and Murrells (2000) and answer the following questions:

- Which sort of sampling methods did they use and why?
- What factors complicated their sampling strategy?
- What were the key factors which determined the size and composition of the sample?
- What implications did the sampling strategy have for subsequent data analysis?
- What are the key learning points from this paper in terms of selecting a sample?

QUOTA SAMPLING

Although quota sampling is *not* a probability sample, it shares some of the characteristics of stratified random sampling in that the first phase entails dividing the population into homogenous strata and selecting elements from each. The crucial difference lies in the procedure by which potential subjects from each stratum are secured. Whereas stratified random sampling involves a random sampling method of obtaining sample members, quota sampling obtains respondents through convenience samples.

Age, sex, designation or grade, religion, ethnicity, medical diagnosis, educational attainment and socio-economic status are examples that are likely to be relevant stratifying variables in health care research. For example, if the researcher is interested in exploring whether the experience of managing an ileostomy is different for people depending on age and sex and a sample of 100 is desired, a quota of 25% older males, 25% older females, 25% young females and 25% young males may be set. This sampling strategy is considered inherently inferior in quantitative research as a way of guaranteeing a sample representative of the population (Schofield 1997) because it is not possible to calculate sampling error. Equally, within a qualitative framework this

that a researcher wishes to interview 100 nurse lecturers in the UK. If the 100 names were chosen through a simple random sampling procedure, it is likely that the researcher would be confronted with the prospect of travelling around a vast geographically scattered sample in order to conduct the interviews. Clearly, this would not only be expensive and time consuming, it may also prove difficult or impossible to obtain a full list of the population (sampling frame). In cluster sampling, large groups or clusters make up the sampling units. If we imagine there are 100 departments of nursing in the UK, lecturers within each site would form a cluster. Ten sites or 'clusters' could be randomly selected and a random selection of ten lecturers within each cluster could be taken. Because the sample is selected from clusters in two or more separate stages and involves sampling different geographical areas, this sampling strategy is treated with caution since it selects a sample on the basis of predetermined criteria and hence reduces the inductive analytical power of naturalistic inquiry (Polit & Hungler 1999). However, in the absence of a full list of the population, a quota sample at least ensures that various sub-groups within the population are represented.

Summary

A 'sample' is the term given to any subset of a wider population under scrutiny. In quantitative studies the researcher will typically attempt to utilize a probability sample of some kind, so as to allow at least tentative generalization to a wider population. There are a number of ways in which probability samples can be drawn, each of which has its own particular strengths and weaknesses (see Table 9.2). Information regarding how a sample is identified is therefore of particular importance to the critical reader of quantitative research papers, as a failure to do this correctly can negate any claims to 'generalizability' to any other population than the one under scrutiny.

SAMPLING IN THE QUALITATIVE DOMAIN

As described in previous chapters of this book, qualitative research seeks to explore and understand phenomena. Since the most appropriate and fruitful research subjects (or informants) may not be equally dispersed within a population, it is logical for researchers to make use of sampling techniques which allow them to identify those with the specific information they require. Also, since the basic purpose of qualitative enquiry is exploration and understanding, the researcher often does not know the boundaries of the research population at the outset. Accordingly, researchers often find that the most appropriate boundaries for the sample emerge during the process of data collection and analysis rather than being predetermined at the start.

Grbich (1999) describes the process of sampling within the qualitative domain as inductive. The researcher often starts broadly and frequently samples all events and individuals within the sphere of interest. As fieldwork and interviewing progress, the broad ideas, concepts and questions become more clearly defined and focused. Throughout this process the researcher is making decisions about who to interview and who and/or what to observe. The chosen sampling techniques need to be appropriate to the purpose of the study. The three main types (convenience, purposive [including theoretical] and snowball sampling) are now considered.

CONVENIENCE SAMPLING

As the name implies, convenience sampling invites the most readily available people who meet the inclusion criteria to act as subjects in a study. The process of selecting participants is continued until the required sample size has been attained. This approach is also sometimes referred to as volunteer, opportunistic or accidental sampling. Researchers may perhaps rely on respondents already known to them or identify respondents via their membership of a group. For instance, a researcher interested in studying the experiences of women combining a nursing career with motherhood might begin by interviewing friends in this situation. He/she might also contact a self-help organization such as the Working Mothers Association or advertise in the nursing press for respondents to contact them. Although there are limitations with this approach in terms of its ability to generalize to a wider population, it is sometimes the only feasible way of obtaining a sample. For example, it is not always possible (or indeed necessary) to identify the total population and problems may exist with respondent accessibility, time and money. Alternatively, there may be ethical constraints. Kenney (2000) encountered some of these problems in a qualitative study of stressors, personality traits and health problems among women by age group (see Box 9.4). It is useful to note that many studies undertaken by health professionals utilize convenience samples, even when the study is quantitative in orientation. This is particularly the case when research has been carried out in the pursuit of an academic qualification and so time and money have been at a premium. In this context sample designs are frequently a compromise between the ideal and limitations imposed by both the nature of the study and the resources available. This does not necessarily negate the results of such studies. It does, however, place some doubt on their generalizability and so this is a possibility of which the critical reader should be aware.

For example, recruiting participants as they attend an outpatient clinic on a particular day of the week

Box 9.4 Example using convenience sampling (from Kenney 2000, with permission)

Title: *Women's 'inner-balance': a comparison of stressors, personality traits and health problems by age groups*

The main purpose of this descriptive study was to identify differences in women's stressors, personality mediating traits and symptoms of health problems by age groups. No **sampling frame** was available and a **convenience sample** of 299 women representing 4 ethnic groups was recruited through notices in a university newsletter, and by invitation of the investigator. Women between 18 and 65 years old, who could read English, and resided in the south western United States were recruited. **Volunteers** were given a cover letter explaining the nature and purpose of the study and a questionnaire. To attract minority women, a small remuneration of $5 was offered as an incentive for completing the questionnaire.

to a research study focussing on satisfaction with the quality of care received in the clinic will mean that respondents are convenient and accessible to the researcher but they will not be representative of the population attending outpatient clinics.

PURPOSIVE SAMPLING

Purposive sampling is also referred to as judgemental sampling and involves the 'hand-picking' of individuals by the researcher based on certain pre-defined criteria. As the name suggests, the researcher purposively chooses informants who are seen as able to add to, support or refute the developing theory in relation to the topic under investigation and thus provide the most relevant information in relation to the aims of the study. Initially the researcher may select a range of informants whose experience is broadly typical. Then as the study progresses, informants with more particular knowledge and experience are intentionally sought. For instance, if a researcher wished to conduct a study on experiences of pain in labour, they might begin by interviewing a cross section of women and then conduct more in-depth interviews with women who had experienced either a 'good' or 'bad' experience of pain relief during labour.

In a grounded theory approach to research (see Chapter 6), this type of sampling is known as *theoretical sampling* (Coyne 1997, McCann & Baker 2001). Theoretical sampling is the process of data collection for generating theory whereby the researcher jointly collects, codes and analyses data and decides what data to collect and who to collect it from, in order to develop his/her theory as it emerges. This type of sampling is based on the underlying assumption that the researcher has sufficient knowledge about the population of interest to choose specific subjects for the study.

Mays and Pope (1995) provide an example of how theoretical sampling might work in relation to a study to explore how and why team work in primary health care is more or less successful in different GP practices. In this study theoretical sampling is proposed as the strategy of choice because some of the theoretically relevant characteristics of general practice affecting variations in team work, such as the frequency of opportunities for communication among team members and the local organization of services, are relevant to the research question. Though not statistically representative of general practices, such a sample is theoretically informed and relevant to the aim of the research, that is to understand social processes. Purposive sampling is commonly used in nursing studies, and many examples exist in current published research. For example, McCann and Baker (2001) used a combined strategy of both purposive and theoretical sampling to elucidate how community mental health nurses develop interpersonal relationships with young adult consumers who have an early episode of psychotic illness (see Box 9.5). In the research literature there is often much confusion surrounding the difference between purposive and theoretical sampling. Both sampling approaches are concerned with selecting *information rich cases* and thus both approaches are *purposeful*. For example, McCann and Baker (2001) used theoretical sampling for their grounded theory study (see Chapter 6) as a way of sampling on the basis of concepts that were proven theoretically relevant to their evolving theory. For a detailed discussion of how theoretical sampling can be applied in practice, see Strauss and Corbin (1990).

The main limitation of both purposive and theoretical sampling is that, since these strategies rely on the researcher's knowledge of the population, bias may enter the selection process.

Box 9.5 Example using combined purposive and theoretical sampling (from McCann & Baker 2001, with permission)

Title: *Mutual relating: developing interpersonal relationships in the community*

This study aimed to elucidate how community mental health nurses develop interpersonal relationships with young adult consumers who have an early episode of psychotic illness. The study took place in the community, in rural and regional New South Wales, Australia and involved consumers ($n = 9$), significant others such as parents and partners ($n = 8$) and community mental health nurses. **Purposive sampling** or sampling using certain pre-determined criteria was used initially to guide data collection. Thereafter, sampling of the potential participants and the setting for data collection were determined by **theoretical sampling,** where decisions about sampling participants, setting and type of data collected were based on the emerging theory. **Theoretical saturation** of the main concepts identified in the data collected determined the actual number of participants and time spent in the field.

Exercise 9.2

Read the article by McCann and Baker (2001) and answer the following questions:

- What predetermined criteria were used to guide sampling and data collection? Were they appropriate?
- In what ways was theoretical sampling based on their evolving theory?
- How did the authors decide on the sample size? Was this an appropriate strategy?

SNOWBALL OR NETWORK SAMPLING

Another method of obtaining a convenience sample is through snowball or network sampling. This method is also referred to as nominated sampling. The researcher makes contact with one or two people 'in the field' and once trust and rapport have been established, asks the first respondent to nominate or introduce them to another person to interview. In this way the sampling frame is built around social networks. This technique is particularly useful when the researcher is regarded with suspicion by the population of interest. It is also a useful approach when there is difficulty in identifying members of the population, for example when this is a clandestine group. As an illustration, a researcher interested in studying the health needs of prostitutes or intravenous drug users might find it impossible to access respondents other than through the use of a snowball sample.

Summary

In qualitative research, the identification of a sample as representative as possible of the parent population is considered less of an imperative than a sample which provides the information required by the researcher. As a result, the qualitative researcher may not identify the total population at the outset, not least because they may not know what it is. Within such a system there is obviously a concern regarding bias introduced by not necessarily using a sample that might provide a range of opinion. Three recognized methods for sampling in the qualitative domain have been discussed in this section. The critical reader of qualitative research must therefore make some decisions regarding whether an unreasonable degree of bias has been introduced due to the requirement for the most relevant data to answer the research question. If the researcher has provided details of their sampling processes, this should not be difficult. Furthermore, knowledge of how sampling impacts upon the quality and range of the data collected, as well as the appropriateness of generalizing from that data, is important when seeking to evaluate the rigour of a research study.

SAMPLING FOR OTHER REASONS

The different sampling techniques detailed so far have been concerned with identifying respondents or 'informants' for study. However, there are other aspects of sampling which are more concerned with ensuring that the researcher gains a 'truthful' or valid understanding of the phenomena being studied. These include:

- Time sampling
- Event sampling
- Setting sampling.

To some degree, these processes have relevance to research carried out in both the quantitative and qualitative domains.

TIME SAMPLING

Within any social organization, activities and events may alter and vary with time. Hence, researchers have to consider the time dimensions in all field situations (Creswell 1998, Silverman 2001). Often it is necessary to sample activities and events that occur over a period of time, as well as activities or established routines that occur at particular hours in the day. Similarly it might be appropriate to observe the research setting at different days of the week or even at different times of the year. Supposing a researcher was interested in exploring the experience of triage in an accident and emergency department, it would be likely that they would discover very different patterns of activity at different times of the week; for example, at weekends when patients do not have easy access to a GP. In time sampling, some rationale is used to select the time intervals during which data gathering takes place.

EVENT SAMPLING

Within any research setting, the researcher typically has to make decisions about which events to observe. In order to obtain a comprehensive picture, it may be necessary to sample discrete sets of events. These events have been delineated as the *routine*, the *special* and the *untoward*. For example, a study of liaison between community nurses and GPs may need to focus upon 'routine' mechanisms for communication exchange (such as the weekly primary health care team meeting); 'special' events when opportunistic liaison may take place (such as a one-off staff seminar); and the 'untoward' or unplanned (such as informal communications in car journeys when visiting patients). Payne et al (2000) used event sampling as a strategy to explore the role of nursing interactions within the context of 'handovers' (see Box 9.6).

Exercise 9.3

Read the article by Payne et al (2000) and answer the following questions:

- Was the sampling strategy appropriate given the research aims?

> **Box 9.6 Example using event sampling (from Payne et al 2000, with permission)**
>
> **Title:** *Interactions between nurses during handovers in elderly care*
>
> This study sought to explore the role of nursing interactions within the context of 'handovers'. The **study setting** was five wards in an acute elderly care unit in a district general hospital in the south of England. **Event sampling** was employed by two research assistants who undertook **non–participant observation** on each ward sequentially. They observed both formal information exchanges (handovers) and informal exchanges. Observations were made from 06.50–00.30 Monday to Friday to cover all nursing shifts. Periods of observation ranged from 1 to 5.5 hours (mean 3.5 hours).

- How was the sampling of 'events' determined? Was this appropriate?
- What are the advantages and disadvantages of observing:
  - 'formal exchanges'
  - 'informal exchanges'?

Both time sampling and event sampling can be random or non random depending on the study aims and are often used in observational studies.

SAMPLING BY SETTING

It is important for researchers to select an appropriate setting for data collection as the situation has an effect upon the phenomena under study and the kind of data that can be gathered. For example, if a researcher was attempting to describe relatives' involvement in patient care, it might be necessary to sample wards with different layouts and designs since the degree of privacy might be a factor influencing their decision to become involved in the care. Whether the researcher chooses to select one location (as in a single in-depth case study) or a number of locations (as in multiple case designs), decisions should be determined by the research aims and methodological framework underpinning the design (see Gomm et al 2000, Grbich 1999, Schwandt 1997).

Qualitative studies are more likely to stress the setting and site of the research study. For example, ethnographic studies typically describe the informants, setting and context in great detail. The reason for this is that qualitative research is usually conducted in a naturalistic setting; thus the study context in which the phenomenon of interest takes place is considered to be a part of the phenomenon itself (Ingleton et al 1998). Seymour's (2001) study of nursing patients who were dying in an intensive care unit provides an example of the importance of understanding contextual factors in order to understand phenomena.

Summary

To gain greater understanding of any phenomenon or concept involving human behaviour, it is often necessary to collect data from subjects at different times (time sampling), doing a range of different things (event sampling), in a range of settings. Evidence of these sampling processes is important if the results are to be considered valid and trustworthy.

WHAT SIZE OF SAMPLE?

We have so far concentrated on the reasons for selecting a sample and some of the ways in which that selection is made. After deciding upon the approach, the next step is to decide on the sample size. Regardless of the research approach, the issue of sample size is an important consideration particularly as the optimum number of cases that should be included in the sample is one of the less well understood aspects of sampling.

One of the most common views held by people new to research is that *the* most important thing is to have a large sample. So does sample size matter? And if it does, how do we decide whether a sample is big enough? There are no simple rules for determining the most appropriate sample size. While a number of formulae are to be found in the literature (Faithfull 2001), they do not produce conclusive answers. These formulae take into account factors such as the level of confidence that needs to be attained in the findings, the size of the population and the variability of the measures when they are applied to the study population (Bland 1995). Whilst

decisions regarding sample size are often determined with scientific principles in mind, they have to be achieved within the pragmatics of the real world. Broadly speaking, most researchers working within a positivist framework would agree that larger samples are more representative of the population than smaller samples. This is because the sampling error will decrease as the sample size increases. Whilst this is so, it must be remembered that a large sample cannot correct or compensate for a faulty sampling design or loosely formulated rationale. Equally, the suggestion that a larger sample is always better does not apply in studies where the type of sample is purposive or theoretical – quite the contrary, as too many informants could cloud the issues and overcomplicate the complex process of analysis (Schwandt 1997). For this reason, the number of informants is usually smaller than in quantitative studies. When deciding on a sample size a number of factors, both scientific and practical, need to be borne in mind:

1. Homogeneity of population
2. Orientation of the study
3. Type of analysis
4. Practical considerations.

HOMOGENEITY OF POPULATION

If individual subjects are very much alike with regard to all variables other than the one being measured, a small sample may be sufficient. In other words, the more variability there is in the population, the larger the sample size needs to be. If the researcher needs to be very precise in generalizing to the population based on sample data, a larger sample may be required to accurately represent the variability within the population and so add weight to their claims to generalizability.

ORIENTATION OF THE STUDY

The orientation of the study also has implications for the required sample size. If the research is qualitative in nature, then the sample size is guided by different principles than for quantitative studies. When using a grounded theory approach, for example, the researcher continues asking questions until they are persuaded that a conceptual framework has emerged that is integrated, that explains the phenomena of interest, and that no new phenomena are emerging. In such studies the number of informants is not determined in advance as the researcher continues to collect data until no new information is forthcoming. This means that it is not possible to predict the required sample size at the outset. However, when presenting the final report, the researcher should describe and justify the final sample size. The critical reader will be observing that this is indeed so.

When probability sampling is used, it is possible to calculate the precise number of subjects needed by using a statistical procedure called *power analysis* (see Chapter 8). Kumar (1999) gives an introduction to the topic, which is recommended if you wish to acquaint yourself with the theory and practice of this procedure. However, it is a complex activity that usually requires the assistance of a statistician. It is not discussed further here.

TYPE OF ANALYSIS

The type of analysis planned has a bearing on sample size, as does the number of strata or categories into which the data may be subdivided. If the intention is to tabulate information, respondents will need to be divided into different categories, for example, male and female. Figure 9.1 shows how the division of a relatively large sample of 84 people by only two variables (sex and team in which individuals work)

can substantially reduce the sample size within each cell of a table. This has implications for analysis since a number of common statistical tests, such as the chi-squared test demand certain minimum cell frequencies.

Because qualitative data are more cumbersome and time consuming to manipulate and analyse, most qualitative studies are confined to a small sample. This does not mean that descriptions of the sampling strategy are any less important. Providing a clear and systematic account of the sampling strategy will allow readers to judge how trustworthy or rigorous the study is. Adequate sample size is generally determined through saturation (Glaser & Strauss 1967, McCann & Baker 2001) and recurrent patterning, whereby the researcher discovers that further participants give similar rather than dissimilar information.

PRACTICAL CONSIDERATIONS

Practical considerations such as the length of time available to complete the study, the availability of respondents, and financial and human resources at the researcher's disposal will invariably influence the size of the sample. Because of these constraints many nursing research studies are confined to small, convenience samples. Even though these studies

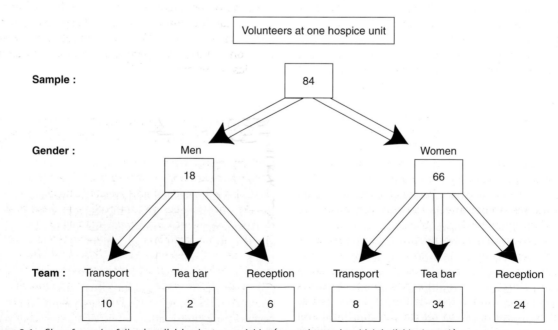

Figure 9.1 Size of samples following division by two variables (sex and team in which individuals work).

may be limited in terms of their ability to generalize to a wider population, they can generate valuable information if they are well planned and conclusions are consistent with the level of existing nursing knowledge.

Summary

It is clear that determining the sample size is an integral and complex part of any research study. The rationale used to determine an adequate size for the sample is linked to the homogeneity of the population, the purpose and design of the study, the type of analysis planned as well as the practicalities of conducting research in the 'real world' of health care. Even if meticulous attention is given to the sampling plan, the **risk** of sample bias is always present and the reasons for this will now be discussed.

SOURCES OF SAMPLING BIAS

Whereas sampling error may occur by chance, sampling bias is systematic, and although the terms are sometimes used interchangeably in the literature, these two concepts should be considered separately. Sampling bias is caused by the researcher and occurs when samples are not planned sufficiently carefully. A degree of bias will be present in all sampling strategies, either from procedural or personal reactivity. Procedural reactivity occurs if the procedures used distort or bias the data. This may result from factors such as the time of day or year of data collection; the place the data were gathered; the language used; and the social circumstances of the subjects. Another source of procedural bias may be the sampling frame. Either it may prove impossible to obtain a list of the population or such a list may be out of date or otherwise incorrect. Personal reactivity occurs when the researcher affects the way responses are given, thereby distorting or biasing the data.

Non-response may also be a problem. For instance, if questionnaires were sent to a carefully selected random sample of nurses to examine their knowledge of primary nursing, it is possible that nurses who possessed more knowledge of these issues would be more likely to return the questionnaire than nurses with little knowledge of this subject.

The basic issue here is that those who do not participate may differ from those who do. For this reason anything other than a relatively high response rate (over 65%) may cast doubts on the representativeness of the sample achieved. When faced with this problem, the question of how people who have not responded differ from those who have needs to be addressed. May (1997) suggests some ways in which researchers can tackle this crucial question. For example, in a postal survey it is possible to compare late returners of questionnaires with earlier ones or those responding after one or two reminders with those responding without prompting. If the researcher knows some of the characteristics of the population it may be possible to check to see whether the sample obtained is reasonably typical of the population. In any survey where there is differential responding between categories (for example, a low response rate from GPs working in rural areas), comparison can be made between their responses and those from other categories. However, there are no absolute solutions, only palliatives (Robson 1993).

Within a qualitative framework, the 'reluctant informant' can be likened to the non-responder in quantitative research. Some lack of response is inevitable but nevertheless, a clear description of those declining to participate in the study is important to the credibility of the research (Polit & Hungler 1999). Equally relevant is the use of the 'volunteer' as a potential research subject. Regardless of the type of sampling strategy, the ethics of health care research demand that subjects agree to participate in research voluntarily. Not all selected subjects will consent to participate and therefore a potential for bias is present.

Summary

Sampling bias occurs when a researcher fails to plan their sampling processes adequately. Having knowledge of how sampling **should** take place provides some protection for the critical reader of research. The important thing to remember is that bias will be present to some degree, in any research project. The critical reader needs to be able to make a decision as to whether or not that bias can reasonably be seen to contradict the conclusions and generalizations asserted from the findings.

CRITIQUING THE SAMPLE

It is worth noting that in many nursing investigations, the sampling plan is the weakest aspect of the study. You will usually find a section of the research report that describes the study sample, setting or site, population, or some combination of these terms, in varying degrees of depth. These research concepts are an integral component of the study and should be carefully and systematically made explicit by the researcher, regardless of the design or orientation of the research. Sampling is judged to be one important facet of the methodology and as such, is generally presented in the 'methods' section of the report, although there may be a separate section on the sample. There are many examples of published guidelines for critiquing the sampling section of a research report (see, for example, Burns & Grove 1997, Lo-Biondo Wood & Haber 2000, Polit & Hungler 1999). These guidelines are generally comprehensive but some list up to sixteen criteria for critiquing the sampling plan, rendering them impractical and unwieldy to apply in everyday practice. Five key criteria by which to critique the sampling plan are presented here (see Box 9.7). The following discussion will focus upon these criteria.

Initially the parameters or characteristics of the study population and/or setting should be specified. This should include a description of the population and how it was identified and should state both the inclusion and exclusion criteria for the study.

Next, the sampling plan's appropriateness to the research design should be evaluated. When critiquing qualitative research designs, you should apply criteria related to sampling strategies that are relevant for the particular type of qualitative study. As we have seen, these are generally inductive and purposive. Equally, when critiquing quantitative research designs, you should apply criteria related to sampling strategies that are consistent with the type of design. These, as we have observed above, are commonly deductive. Lack of adherence to the principles of random selection in the case of quantitative designs jeopardizes the representativeness of the sample and thus the external validity of the study.

You will then be seeking to ensure that the sample size is appropriate within the external constraints imposed (e.g. ethical, financial, time). A clear theoretical and methodological rationale for the sample size should be given. In the case of quantitative studies, confirmation is needed that the assistance of a statistician has been sought, and that a power

analysis has been undertaken if the study is evaluating an intervention. Pointing out both the attrition rate and non-response rate and examining the effects on the findings are also imperative to recognizing any limitations posed by the size of the sample. In qualitative designs, evidence that there are sufficient informants to describe and explain the phenomena under investigation (but not too numerous to obscure the issues) needs to be considered.

You will need to consider if the researcher has made known any possible sources of bias, and what steps have been taken to minimize that bias. As we have seen, the strength of the probability sample resides in the reduction of sampling error and sampling bias to a known minimum. Inaccessible populations, unavailability of chosen sample, incomplete sampling frames and high attrition rates compound sampling biases. In qualitative studies researchers must maintain a delicate balance between using themselves as research instruments, and ensuring that their views do not bias, lead or inhibit the participants (Ingleton & Seymour 2001). For this reason it is imperative that the researcher makes explicit their background and credentials.

Finally, and perhaps most important, are the issues of consistency of findings and conclusions with the sampling strategy used. In other words, how transparent is the researcher about the inferences and conclusions drawn from the data and is there recognition of the limitations of the study (bearing in mind that there is no such thing as the 'perfect sample')? In the case of quantitative studies, how reliable (consistent), valid (true) and therefore generalizable are the findings from the sample to the population?

Box 9.7 Critiquing the sampling plan

- Are the population (target and accessible) and study setting clearly stated?
- Does the type of sample fit with the overall purpose of the study and type of design?
- Is the sample size underpinned by a sound methodological, ethical and theoretical rationale which is clearly explained and justified?
- Are all known and probable sources of bias made explicit and minimized? Can you identify others which are not?
- Are the findings, conclusions and generalizations (if made) appropriate and consistent with the sampling strategy used?

For qualitative studies, these criteria can be considered as analogous to transferability, credibility, confirmability and truth value (see Behi & Nolan 1995). These points are also discussed in Chapter 7. In the real world of health research it may not be feasible, or indeed appropriate, to fulfil all these criteria. Possibly more relevant is that you remain alert to claims that cannot be substantiated.

CONCLUSION

In this chapter we have seen that sampling considerations are central to the research process no matter what research strategy or investigatory technique is used. Each sampling strategy has different advantages and limitations and therefore each is best suited to a specific type of study aim and design. In many nursing studies, the sampling plan is the weakest facet of the study design. The sampling plan therefore warrants particular scrutiny because if it is flawed in some way, the findings and conclusions may be misleading. For this reason it is important that research consumers have an understanding of both the process of sampling and the rationale behind the sampling plan. They will then be able to make sound judgements on the rigour of the research and the applicability of the findings to health care practice.

Questions for your reflection

1. Which sampling method(s) would you adopt if you were planning a qualitative study looking at the meaning of incontinence to young and middle aged women?

2. How would you develop a sampling plan for a study of quality of life of people with chronic obstructive airways disease? First, identify the population parameters and then suggest how best to obtain a sample.

3. How would you design a sampling strategy to examine touch between nurses and elderly patients in a continuing care setting? Consider the population and set criteria for inclusion/exclusion. How would you minimize bias in your chosen design?

References

Bjorkstrom M and Hamrin E (2001) Swedish nurses' attitudes towards research and development within nursing. *Journal of Advanced Nursing* **34**(5): 706–714.

Bland M (1995) *An Introduction To Medical Statistics*, 2nd edn. Oxford: Oxford University Press.

Bryman A (2001) *Quantitative Data Analysis for Social Scientists*. London: Routledge.

Burns N and Grove SK (1997) *The Practice of Nursing Research: Conduct, Critique and Utilization*, 3rd edn. Philadelphia: WB Saunders.

Cohen J (1977) *Statistical Power Analysis for the Behavioral Sciences*. New York: Academic Press.

Coyne IT (1997) Sampling in qualitative research: purposeful and theoretical sampling; merging or clear boundaries? *Journal of Advanced Nursing* **26**: 623–630.

Creswell J (1998) *Qualitative Inquiry and Research Design: Choosing Among Traditions*. Thousand Oaks: Sage.

Depoy E and Gitlin L (1994) *Introduction to Research: Multiple Strategies for Health and Human Services*. St Louis: Mosby.

Faithfull S (2001) How many subjects are needed in a research sample in palliative care? In: Field D, Clark D, Corner J and Davis C (eds) *Researching Palliative Care* (Chapter 3 pp37–42). Buckingham: Open University Press.

Glaser B and Strauss A (1967) *The Discovery of Grounded Theory: Strategies for Qualitative Research*. Chicago: AVC.

Gomm R, Needham G and Bullman A (eds) (2000) *Evaluating Research in Health and Social Care*. London: Sage.

Grbich C (1999) *Qualitative Research in Health: an Introduction*. London: Sage.

Ingleton C and Seymour J (2001) Analysing qualitative data: examples from two studies of end-of-life care. *International Journal of Palliative Nursing* **7** (5): 227–233.

Ingleton C, Clark D and Field D (1998) Formative evaluation and its relevance to palliative care. *Palliative Medicine* **12**: 197–203.

Kenney J (2000) Women's inner balance: a comparison of stressors, personality traits and health problems by age groups. *Journal of Advanced Nursing* **31**(3): 639–650.

Kumar R (1999) *Research Methodology: a Step-by-Step Guide for Beginners*. London: Sage.

Lo-Biondo Wood G and Haber J (2000) *Nursing Research: Methods, Critical Appraisal, and Utilization*, 4th edn. St Louis: Mosby.

Marsland L and Murrell T (2000) Sampling for a longitudinal study of the careers of nurses qualifying from the English pre-registration diploma course. *Journal of Advanced Nursing* **31**(4): 935–943.

May T (1997) *Social Research: Issues, Methods and Process*. Buckingham: Open University Press.

Mays N and Pope C (1995) Rigour and qualitative research. *British Medical Journal* **331**: 109–112.

McCann T and Baker H (2001) Mutual relating: delivering interpersonal relationships in the community. *Journal of Advanced Nursing* **34**(4): 530–537.

Nolan M and Behi R (1995) Alternative approaches to establishing reliability and validity. *British Journal of Nursing* **4**(10): 587–590.

Payne S, Hardey M and Coleman P (2000) Interactions between nurses during handovers in elderly care. *Journal of Advanced Nursing* **32**(2): 277–285.

Payne S, Jarrett N, Sheldon F et al (2002) Differences in understanding of specialist palliative care amongst service providers and commissioners in South London. *Palliative Medicine* **16**: 395–402.

Polit DF and Hungler B (1999) *Nursing Research: Principles and Methods*, 4th edn. Philadelphia: Lippincott.

Robson C (1993) *Real World Research: a Resource for Social Scientists and Practitioner Researchers*. Oxford: Blackwell Science.

Schofield W (1997) Data collection and analysis. In: Sapsford R and Jupp V (eds) *Survey Sampling*, Chapter 2 pp25–54. London: Routledge.

Schwandt T (1997) *Qualitative Inquiry: a Dictionary of Terms*. Thousand Oaks: Sage.

Seymour JE (2001) *Critical Moments – Death and Dying in Intensive Care*. Buckingham: Open University Press.

Silverman D (2001) *Doing Qualitative Research: a Practical Handbook*. London: Sage.

Strauss A and Corbin J (1990) *Basics of Qualitative Research*. Newbury Park: Sage.

Teasdale K, Brocklehurst N and Thomas N (2001) Clinical supervision and support for nurses: an evaluation study. *Journal of Advanced Nursing* **33**(2): 216–224.

Further reading

Creswell J (1998) *Qualitative Inquiry and Research Design: Choosing among Traditions*. Thousand Oaks: Sage.

Chapter 7 (pp109–137) discusses locating a site or individual, gaining access and making rapport, and sampling in the five following traditions: Biography, Phenomenology, Grounded Theory, Ethnography and Case Study.

Faithfull S (2001) How many subjects are needed in a research sample in palliative care? In: Field D, Clark D, Corner J et al (eds) *Researching Palliative Care*. Buckingham: Open University Press.

Although this paper relates to palliative care it has relevance for other areas of research practice. Chapter 3 (pp37–42) gives an overview of the number of subjects needed to determine treatment effectiveness and suggests that sample size is important but is only one of four factors that increase the statistical power of a study.

Gomm R, Hammersley M and Foster P (2000) *Case Study Method*. London: Sage.

This text provides a detailed appraisal of sampling logic in case study design which is an increasingly popular approach to health services research.

Kumar R (1999) *Research Methodology: a Step-by-Step Guide for Beginners*. London: Sage.

Chapter 12 (pp148–166) describes the principles of sampling using a table of random numbers and calculation of sample size. The author describes the determinants and procedures for calculating sample size. Although difficult for the beginner, this chapter does allow insights into the determinants involved as questions relating to this area are commonly asked.

Schofield W (1997) Survey Sampling. In: Sapsford R and Jupp V (eds) *Data Collection and Analysis*. London: Routledge in association with Open University Press.

Chapter 2 (pp25–54) provides a useful overview about the problems and methods of designing uncertain sample surveys. The chapter also examines problems in applied survey sampling, for example, non response, unreliable or invalid measurement, sample loss, incomplete data and the ways of reducing the effect of these on the findings.

Schwandt T (1997) *Qualitative Inquiry: A Dictionary of Terms*. Thousand Oaks: Sage.

This book is a collection of selected works in a specific research language and their definitions. The short section on sampling (pp140–143) discusses selecting a field site or case and sampling *within* the case or field site.

Silverman D (2002) *Doing Qualitative Research: A Practical Handbook*. London: Sage.

Chapter 8 (pp102–111) describes how cases can be selected and discusses the poorly understood concept of generalizability in qualitative research. The chapter also examines how combining qualitative sampling with qualitative measures of population can be usefully employed.

Chapter 10

Critiquing ethical issues in published research

Liz Matthews, Gordon Grant

INTRODUCTION

Health care research raises many questions about what is right or wrong, good or bad, what is acceptable or not acceptable. With advances in health care technology, doctors and professionals in allied fields can aid conception, manipulate the human gene pool and breed animals with transgenic qualities (Carlin 1995), thus providing the possibility of a brave new world where disease is conquered, people live longer and suffer less. Although such pursuits may in themselves appear worthy, the route taken to solve such problems can at times be perceived by the general public to be unacceptable, thus raising the question 'should we do this?' rather than 'can we do this?'

The question 'should we do this?' has been debated at length in the media in relation to the use of animal organs such as pigs' kidneys in human transplantation. More recently, the 'can or should we do this?' debate has taken a further twist with the apparent arrival of human cloning, raising fundamental moral and ethical issues about the 'engineering' of the human species to suit what some might call the designer whims and fancies of prospective parents (Dickens 2002, Suvalescu 2002). In the case of transplant research, lives may be saved or improved by increasing the number of organs available for transplant though many people find this unacceptable from a religious or moral perspective. With human cloning there appear to be major questions to be asked not only about its acceptability from an ethical point of view but also about its viability as a scientific procedure and its long-term consequences for the human species. In both cases, fundamental issues are raised about how boundaries come to be established by communities and individuals who differ in their moral perspectives (Scully 2001).

The question 'can we do this?' is essentially concerned with identifying and solving the potential and actual consequential risks of such procedures and the scientific problems associated with the process. For instance, if we transplant the organs of an animal into a human, will this result in the possibility of transferring potentially dangerous bacteria or viruses from one species (pigs) to another (man)? If we do, what are the possible long-term implications for that individual and indeed society? However, health care research is generally perceived as being an overall good, providing benefits for society at large (see Further reading, p142).

The introduction of local research ethics committees (LRECs) in 1991 and multicentre research ethics committees (MRECs) in 1997 across the United Kingdom provided a screening system by which ethically questionable studies requiring access to patients and clients of health services can be sifted out before they start. This may lead the critical reader of research to surmise that published research is ethical because of the degree of scrutiny it has endured during the process from its original inception to its publication. However, a number of authors identify diversity of practice in the approval process for research which may result in the same study being approved by the LREC in one district health authority but not in another. While (1995), for example, describes the variation she experienced when gaining approval for a multicentre study focusing on the needs and provision of care to children who might be expected to die during childhood. Oakley (1992) highlights similar problems in the USA during the process of gaining approval for a multicentre study of social support and motherhood. The screening processes provided by LRECs and MRECs are therefore fallible and the assumption that all published research is ethically sound is questionable, given the degree of variation and subjective appraisal during the approval process.

It has been argued that, in its manifold forms, qualitative research is not well enough understood by LRECs and MRECs. Reasons for this appear to include lack of LREC/MREC members with experience of qualitative research, a prevailing view that qualitative research is less than scientific, and an inability to accept that research methods cannot necessarily be prescribed in advance for some qualitative research because of its serial or evolutionary character. This last reason helps to explain why

calculating the 'benefit to risk' ratio of qualitative research in advance of it taking place can be so problematic, leading one set of commentators to propose an 'ethics as process' model of decision making about the ethics involved (Ramcharan & Cutcliffe 2001).

THE CHALLENGE FOR HEALTH WORKERS

The critical reader of research requires sufficient knowledge of ethical principles to be able to decide for him or herself whether a research project has been carried out in an ethical manner. This requires some insight into ethical theories which can inform and solve the ethical dilemmas associated with research. This chapter describes one particular ethical framework which will aid the reader of published research to draw their own conclusions about the integrity of a study. This is the Four Principles and Scope of Application approach advanced by Beauchamp and Childress (1989) and Gillon (1994). Each of the four ethical principles is discussed in relation to different research designs, highlighting the inherent ethical implications. Issues are highlighted concerning each principle, which can then be applied to different types of research study. A fundamental point to recognize is that a research project which is completely sound in ethical terms is very hard to achieve and so is very hard to find. The aim must be to establish that the researcher has done all in their power to protect the rights of their research subjects, balanced against the need for rigour in the processes followed.

Key issues

- The ethical nature of research
- Research and promoting respect for autonomy
- Beneficence and non-maleficence and research
- Justice and research
- Critical appraisal of the ethical issues in research reports

ETHICAL PRINCIPLES TRANSCEND RESEARCH APPROACHES

There are many issues to consider in an evaluation of the ethical component of published research. Variations in research approaches mean that quantitative designs may raise ethical difficulties not apparent in qualitative designs and vice versa. However, similar questions should be asked about ethical issues in research, irrespective of the approaches used during the research process. Unfortunately, it may be difficult to consider the ethical issues within published work, as information on ethical considerations tends to focus on how the researcher overcame ethical problems which they themselves identified. The information needed to establish whether the researcher systematically considered *all* potential difficulties and took appropriate action to enable them to act ethically is often inadequate or even missing.

A straightforward approach to this task is provided by the Four Principles plus Scope of Application approach advocated by Beauchamp and Childress (1989) and Gillon (1994). This framework provides a 'simple, accessible and culturally neutral approach' (Gillon 1994) to inform the evaluation of the ethical dimensions of research reports. Also referred to later is an alternative 'three approaches' framework proposed by Foster (2001) which is equally applicable as a means of reviewing the ethical principles of research.

THE FOUR PRINCIPLES PLUS SCOPE OF APPLICATION APPROACH

The Four Principles plus Scope of Application approach is a complete moral theory in itself encompassing the application of various rules or principles that should be upheld. Beauchamp and Childress (1989) and Gillon (1994) claim that whatever our personal philosophy, politics, religion, moral theory or life stance, we will find no difficulty in committing ourselves to four *prima facie* (absolute) moral principles (Gillon 1994). *Prima facie* refers to those principles which ought to be upheld in any situation. Should any one of those principles be breached, clear justification for that action must be provided if an act is to be perceived as morally justifiable. The remaining principles must also be upheld.

The four *prima facie* moral principles are:

- Respect for autonomy (the obligation to respect the decision-making capacities of autonomous people)
- Beneficence (the obligation to provide benefits and balance these benefits against risks)
- Non-maleficence (the obligation to avoid causing harm)
- Justice (the obligation of fairness in the distribution of benefits and risks).

The approach does not provide a method for ranking these principles in order of importance but it can help health care workers make decisions about moral issues when critically appraising published research. As a result, this model provides a set of moral commitments, a common moral language and a common set of moral issues (Gillon 1994) . The following discussion examines the four principles along with their scope of application when reading published research. Autonomy and justice are considered separately. Beneficence and non-maleficence are discussed together for ease of explanation and brevity.

AUTONOMY

Respect for persons incorporates at least two fundamental ethical considerations in research, namely:

respect for autonomy – which requires that those who are capable of deliberation about their personal choices should be allowed to exercise their capacity for self determination; and

the protection of persons with impaired or diminished autonomy, which requires that those who are dependent or vulnerable be afforded security against abuse.

CIOMS/WHO 1993, p10

The need for research subjects to have a choice about whether or not they participate in a research study is a fundamental obligation in relation to respect for autonomy (Beauchamp and Childress 1989) and this is a question that should be asked in any research critique. However, it is debatable whether, in the context of research, choice or consent can be ever be fully informed in practice. Silverman (1989) argues that the obligation to uphold the primacy of informed consent to participate in research studies should be no different from the notion of the patient who consents for any health care intervention. However, there are differences in practical terms between gaining consent for treatment and gaining consent to participate in a research study.

Consent to treatment differs from consent to participate in research

Consent to treatment indicates that a patient is accessing that treatment for their own benefit. For example, they may undergo diagnostic tests because of symptoms they have experienced or treatment to alleviate symptoms or cure disease. Whatever the reason, the patient has something to gain from consenting (Association of Community Health Councils (ACHC) 1990). Consent to participate in research is different, in the sense that the researcher usually wants something from the patient. The purpose of the consent approach is also different in that researchers need the research subjects to participate and so need to provide the relevant information to enable them to reach an informed decision (ACHC 1990). This is important as it may mean that they agree to participate in clinical trials where outcomes are uncertain; for example, to test new drug regimens, to identify adverse effects or evaluate new treatments to determine their effectiveness. In qualitative research projects they may be asked to explore sensitive and emotive topic areas such as feelings about a partner's sudden death, or experiences of a life-threatening disease (Cowles 1988, Ramos 1989), which may make participants uncomfortable or lead to feelings of vulnerability.

Whatever the reason, a research subject is to some degree being used as a 'means to an end'. In practical terms the result is that tighter controls are applied to the process of gaining consent from individuals who are participating in research studies, when compared with the processes of gaining consent from people to participate in health care interventions. There are a number of issues to be considered when evaluating the autonomy of research subjects. These can be broadly categorized along the following dimensions identified by Faden and Beauchamp (1986):

- Disclosure and non-disclosure of information
- Understanding
- Voluntariness.

We consider it necessary to explore the notion of veracity (truth-telling) under the heading of disclosure and non-disclosure of information, as a cornerstone of the relationship between the professional and the patient/client is the existence of trust. Such trust is dependent upon the idea that professionals will tell the truth. Bok (1984) identifies that health care professionals are the only group afforded the privilege of withholding information from their patients, as the motive behind such an action could be justified as being in the patient's best interests. In research, if we cannot rely on the truthfulness of the researcher, we cannot rely upon the body of knowledge generated by that research, which in turn underpins clinical practice.

The concept of 'broad consent'

Legally, the gaining of broad consent is necessary in both treatment and research situations (NHSME 1990), in that the individual needs to be aware that they:

- Have the choice to refuse to participate
- Can withdraw from treatment or the study at any particular stage which they (rather than the clinician or researcher) identify
- Can refuse or withdraw without fear of any form of retribution or punishment.

Broad consent also implies an autonomous deliberate judgment on the basis of sufficient and comprehensible information (Neuberger 1992). In health research, fairly tight controls mean that the researcher must demonstrate to an independent body (in the UK the LREC or MREC) the process of gaining consent to participate in a research study before the study begins. This allows scrutiny of the process to determine whether respect for persons will be upheld.

In practical terms this means that a researcher must produce and use a consent form (Neuberger 1992). The consent form should ensure that potential subjects know that they are participating in a research study as opposed to a normal treatment (NHSME 1990), are over the age of 18 years (Dimond 1995) and have the capacity to understand the information given to them (Faden and Beauchamp 1986). The researcher must also provide a written protocol which specifies in advance both the individual characteristics required within the sample group to be studied and what, in precise terms, will happen to each participant during the study (ACHC 1990). Every published research report should include a clear description of the way in which subjects have consented to participate. There should also be an indication that the study was approved by an independent review body (usually the LREC or MREC), as this indicates that the process of gaining consent has been scrutinized.

Disclosure/non-disclosure of information

A research report should indicate that approval was gained from an independent review body (LREC or MREC) and that consent to participate was gained from each respondent. In itself this would indicate that the respondents were made aware of the fact that they were part of a research study. However, as a critical reader it is important to consider whether the researcher has disclosed the information necessary to enable subjects to make an informed choice. For example, to encourage participation a researcher might selectively control information given to potential subjects. To a certain degree this can be justified by the application of the doctrine of therapeutic privilege – to disclose all the known risks may induce too much anxiety or distress for the respondent. Thus, a researcher may be allowed to determine what is in the respondent's interests to know concerning reasonable risks (NHSME 1990). Another justification for the selective withholding of information is that the purpose of the study may be to identify unknown risks. In such cases the risk is assumed not to be expected and therefore need not be disclosed. This aspect will be discussed later in this chapter. (see *Beneficence and non-maleficence*, page 136).

When considering the selective disclosure of information, some research methods are more vulnerable than others in relation to the manipulation of information. These methods include experimental treatments such as previously untried surgical procedures (e.g. various forms of organ transplantation; Pence 1990), epidemiological studies which monitor the natural progress of diseases such as the Tuskagee Study (Burns & Grove 2001) and the cervical dysplasia study described by Paul (1988), as well as comparative studies of treatment within randomized controlled trials, such as the management of screening-detected ductal carcinoma in situ as discussed by Thornton (1993).

In such research the type of information given by the researcher to the respondent may be biased towards the positive aspects of the study, with the negative aspects underemphasized (Pence 1990). Ideally, written *and* verbal information should be provided to ensure that a balanced explanation is given. Since all written information for participants in a study should be evaluated in advance by an external body such as the LREC or MREC, there is some degree of control of selective disclosure of information. Within the UK, REC application forms and advice about information sheets and consent forms are downloadable from the Department of Health's website about research ethics committees (www.corec.org.uk). These are an integral part of the new research governance arrangements in the UK (Department of Health 2001a).

A further safeguard would be for an independent observer to be present during the consent interview. This person may be a relative, a health care worker or a legal guardian (Dimond 1995, Department of Health 2001b, Neuberger 1992). The critical reader should be alert to evidence of the presence or absence of such mechanisms in research reports. Involving others as proxy respondents can present some additional challenges, as we discuss later.

Another indicator of good practice is that consent is obtained from the respondent before their enrolment within the study. This allows the respondent time to reflect on the information given. A minimum reflection time of 24 hours should be allowed by the researcher to give the person time to think about and formulate questions they may wish to raise about the study and their participation in it (Pence 1990). Depending on the length or periodicity of a respondent's involvement in a research project, it may also be good practice to review or renegotiate consent from time to time. This can be especially important when research falls into natural stages when different kinds of demands are to be made upon respondents. In the case of some qualitative studies where the design of subsequent stages of research depends very much on the completion of earlier stages, it will be especially important to renegotiate consent at these points.

Selective non-disclosure

Veracity and disclosure/non-disclosure of information are also associated with the imparting of filtered information by the researcher to the respondent. In such instances, consideration must be given to whether planned, intentional non-disclosure of information to research participants is ever acceptable. Some examples of the types of research design which may consider this acceptable are randomized controlled trials, trials involving the use of placebos, and 'blind' experiments where deception is considered acceptable (even necessary) in an attempt to compensate for, or reduce, possible bias. Similarly, in social and behavioural research complete disclosure of information may jeopardize the study in that the participants may alter their behaviour to that which they think the researcher requires. This is often referred to as a socially desirable response (Burns & Grove 2001, Polit & Hungler 2001).

In randomized controlled trials there is no justification for failing to disclose that the research design includes the use of placebos or a non-treatment group. Similarly, there is no justification for failing to disclose the method of assignment to an arm of such a trial (Beauchamp & Childress 1989, Neuberger 1992). This is because it is only with such information that research respondents can give consent to participate which is informed. However, this only supplies them with the information needed to decide whether or not to participate. It is not necessary to inform them of the arm of the trial to which they have been assigned (Neuberger 1992), for example control or therapy.

Beauchamp and Childress (1989, p99) identify that deception may be acceptable in research if the following criteria are adhered to:

- Deception is essential in order to obtain important information
- No substantial risk is attached
- Other moral principles are not violated such as autonomy or beneficence/non-maleficence
- Subjects are informed that deception is part of the study before they consent to participate.

When deception is used, the risks to the respondent should be minimal and outweighed by the expected benefits. One of the classic psychological experiments which has been heavily criticized for the degree of deception used by the researcher is Stanley Milgramme's study of obedience (Faden & Beauchamp 1986). To reduce the social response bias, Milgramme deliberately lied to the respondents about the aim of the research study. Respondents were informed that the study was to explore their ability to recall information during times of stress when in fact the study was designed to explore the respondents' willingness to comply with authority. The consequences of Milgramme's action to deceive have meant that the findings from this study are open to constant criticism from his peers, at least from an ethical perspective.

Understanding

In the context of negotiating consent to participate in research, it is necessary to consider not only the extent of disclosure of information, but also whether that information was understood by the potential research subject. In a classic article, Beecher (1966) concludes that ordinary patients will not knowingly risk their health or their life merely for the sake of science. In studies associated with high and/or substantial risks, one indication that respondents may not have understood the significance of those risks is a high rate of agreement to participate. When this occurs it may suggest that understanding was insufficient to support the notion of informed consent or that these risks were not disclosed – otherwise it is likely that fewer people would have agreed to

participate. At this point, it is important to acknowledge that the assessment of the respondent's degree of understanding is as difficult in research as it is in clinical practice. Improved information sheets and good communication skills may not necessarily mean that all patients understand what is said to them (Neuberger 1992). Certain individuals and within-sample populations are particularly vulnerable in this respect. Vulnerable populations include:

- Ethnic minority groups (especially where English is a second language)
- Children (especially neonates)
- Individuals with mental health problems
- Individuals with cognitive disabilities
- Educationally disadvantaged persons.

Helpful guidelines about the seeking of consent were recently produced by the Department of Health (2001b) in relation to people with learning disabilities. This guidance makes very clear that, in the case of people *with* capacity, for consent to be valid the person must be:

- Capable of taking that decision ('competent')
- Acting voluntarily (not under pressure or duress from anyone)
- Provided with enough information to enable them to make a decision.

Hence, the experience must be seen as part of a respectful relationship, and a process rather than a one-off event. Importantly, adults are always presumed to be capable of taking health care decisions unless the opposite has been demonstrated. Therefore, irrespective of any labels that might be applied to individuals, capacity must be presumed unless there are demonstrative counter-indicators. Preconditions for capacity are suggested as including a person's ability to:

- Comprehend and retain information relevant to the decision, especially as to the consequences of participating or not participating in the intervention
- Use and weigh this information in the decision-making process.

This looks straightforward, but in practice:

- Decision-making capacity is context-dependent and is likely to reflect the nature and complexity of the issue requiring a decision, and how important it is to the person

- Capacity, or lack of it, may be temporary
- Capacity is not the same as the perceived reasonableness of a person's decision.

When adults *lack* capacity, the guidance suggests that the person's 'best interests' must be the overriding consideration, referring to their health, general well-being, close relationships and spiritual/religious welfare. In this connection it is made clear that it is not lawful to balance these interests (the person's own) against those of other parties; decisions should be made that those close to the person and the health/social care team agree are in the person's best interest. Courts can be asked what is in the person's best interests and second additional opinions should be offered. With research:

> it is not appropriate to carry out research on adults who cannot give consent for themselves, if the research can instead be carried out on adults who are able to give or withhold consent. The only exception to this rule would be where clinicians believe that it is in the person's own best interests to be involved in research

(Department of Health 2001b, p15)

There is a possible danger here that researchers might use such guidance to exclude persons who cannot give consent for themselves simply because it is easier to do so. Persons 'without voice' have as much right as anyone else to be involved in research.

Eighteen years of age is used as a chronological indicator of maturity for competence to broad consent to participate in research studies (Dimond 1995). However, guidelines from the British Paediatric Association (1992) indicate that a child from the age of seven years may make a competent decision about whether to participate in a research study. From an ethical perspective, researchers should involve the parent or legal guardian of a child in the consent process. However, it is considered unethical for the parents' views to override those of the child if the child does not want to participate (British Paediatric Association 1992). Since most children want to please their parents, the difficulties with this issue remain complex. Such issues have resulted in discussions as to whether children should participate in non-therapeutic research studies at all (Dimond 1995, Neuberger 1992).

Voluntariness

When respondents participate in a research study, there is an assumption that they are doing so of their own free will and are not coerced into the process

by force or threat or by monetary or material gain (Pence 1990). In some instances, healthy volunteers may be paid a nominal sum of money (for instance, when testing a new vaccine) in early clinical trials. However, any monetary gain must be seen as that which would *not* greatly influence their decision to participate. It should be noted that coercion to participate may be implied by psychological perception rather than physical threat or material gain. The respondent may believe that by participating in the research they may have their chances of a positive health outcome enhanced (Neuberger 1992, Pence 1990) or at least avoid the negative implications of being viewed as uncooperative.

The relationship between the researcher and the respondent can be of particular importance in certain areas of enquiry. In educational research, for instance, projects may involve accessing a 'convenient' sample of respondents who are enrolled on an educational programme managed by the researcher. As a result there may be a fear of reprisal if prospective respondents do not participate and this may influence their decision to take part in the study. In turn, this may influence the nature of the respondents and hence the data obtained within the study. For example, respondents wishing to find favour with the lecturer may be the ones who volunteer and who may give socially desirable answers to any questions asked (Hughes 1990).

Some issues associated with voluntariness can be difficult to overcome within the context of a particular study, given the nature of the study and the characteristics of the respondents. For example, studies which test new drugs or treatments which may reduce mortality and morbidity can influence the voluntariness of participants. Patients may feel that the only way to access a particular drug or treatment is to volunteer to participate in a research study (Walley & Barton 1995). This may mean that a researcher is overwhelmed by volunteers wishing to participate. In such studies clear criteria need to be identified with regard to who will or will not be selected and why. This allows the researcher to demonstrate that groups or individuals have been selected fairly and that they are not favouring one individual or group over another. This issue will be discussed later in the chapter.

The characteristics of some individuals may mean that they have unrealistic expectations about the benefits of participating in a study. For example, they may wish to participate with the false hope of a cure or may be so desperate to improve the quality of their lives that they underestimate the risks involved with participation. To reduce this possibility, researchers must be able to demonstrate that they have not misled participants. This can be achieved by providing clear information sheets, identifying the risks and benefits and involving a third party in the consenting process.

Summary

When evaluating published research in relation to the principle of autonomy, consideration should be given to the idea of broad consent, the degree of information disclosed to the research participants and whether the individuals or groups involved were likely to have understood the information given. It is important to be aware of the meaning of capacity and its preconditions and how, in the case of persons unable to give consent for themselves, their 'best interests' can be considered. If there was selective non-disclosure of information, it is important to consider whether this was justifiable. The relationship between the researcher and the respondent should also be considered to determine whether this could have affected the voluntariness of the respondent.

BENEFICENCE AND NON-MALEFICENCE

In the context of research, beneficence and non-maleficence refer to the ethical obligation to maximize benefits and to minimize harm.

This principle gives rise to norms requiring that the risks of research be reasonable in the light of expected benefits, that the research design be sound, and that the investigators be competent both to conduct the research and to safeguard the welfare of the research subjects. Beneficence further proscribes the deliberate infliction of harm on persons; this aspect of beneficence is expressed as a separate principle – non-maleficence (to do no harm).

CIOMS/WHO 1993, p10

In this section we consider the issues of risk/benefit ratios and inclusion/exclusion criteria as they are generally perceived – in terms of societal benefit.

The risk–benefit ratio

The terms beneficence and non-maleficence are used to describe the idea of maximizing benefits

and minimizing harm (Beauchamp & Childress 1989). In research, these terms are often applied in what is known as the risk–benefit ratio. Research ethics committees seek to evaluate risks and benefits by considering the balance of overall benefit that may be accrued to society by the outcome of the research. This involves an evaluation of the associated risks for individual respondents and, to a lesser degree, the risks to society in general. Within health care, the intention of research is generally perceived in terms of societal benefit (the outcome of any study should increase medical, nursing or social knowledge in some way) but it may not benefit individual respondents participating in the research. This is especially so in non-therapeutic (descriptive) research.

In practical terms, the main problem when considering the risk–benefit ratio of a study is the subjectivity in distinguishing a minimal risk from a substantial risk. Baum et al (1989) define minimal risk as the level of risk that would normally occur within the individual's own social environment. In other words, risks would be comparable to the treatment regimen that the individual would be prescribed in 'normal' circumstances. Substantial risk, on the other hand, would be defined as that which could cause death or hospital admission or dramatically alter the individual's quality of life (ACHC 1990) when this would not normally be expected.

Risk can also be associated with the degree of pain experienced by a subject, or, as in psychological studies, the degree of distress. Qualitative studies which seek to explore and describe respondents' feelings or experiences of illness or bereavement may also cause distress. In such cases psychological harm may be caused, as the researcher may ask probing questions which force respondents to confront areas of personal trauma they would rather not revisit.

Cowles (1988) reflects on this issue in discussing her research which involved interviews with adult relatives of homicide victims during the first four months following the murder. She suggests that ethical issues commonly considered by individual researchers and ethics committees may not be enough to evaluate the moral appropriateness of the research, which tends to be compared against the risks and benefits associated with scientific values. More practical concerns need to be considered, such as the degree of emotional response and the impact this may have on both the researcher and subject. It should also be acknowledged that such research can be viewed as helpful or even therapeutic by some research subjects. For example, Crookes (1996) found that a number of the bereaved nurses he interviewed in a study of personal bereavement in nurses were grateful for the opportunity to tell their story. For some it was the first time they had been given the chance to do so.

Strategies for maintaining objectivity and making decisions about what information may be too personal to use as data, need to be identified before the study begins, as well as during the study. Certainly, in studies requiring observational data collection, the researcher needs to establish when they would intervene if it appeared that the situation was in danger of harming the subject in some way. Ramos (1989) suggests that in this instance the researcher becomes the subject's advocate, in that they are acting in their interests by protecting them from harm.

The researcher's obligation is to respect the privacy of participants and uphold confidentiality. This aspect is exemplified by the notion of 'promise-keeping' between the researcher and the participant. However, it is important for the researcher to consider in advance any aspects of the study which may mean that they (the researcher) would need to breach confidentiality in order to protect members of the public. For example, although the researcher must be able to assure the participant that information is confidential, what if the participant discloses information that, if not acted upon, may endanger other individuals? In such instances, clear boundaries must be established between the researcher and the participant and the action that would be taken if sensitive situations arise should be made explicit.

In epidemiological research, the risks associated with observing patterns or the nature of a disease process mean that criteria for withdrawing respondents from a study should be identified before the study begins. The research question may consider the natural course of a disease such as syphilis (Pence 1990), or cervical dysplagia (Paul 1988). In such circumstances, it is important to determine in advance the percentage or number of respondents needed to progress to a given point in the disease process in order to answer the question posed by the research.

Inclusion and exclusion criteria

When reading published papers it is important to consider whether the author has taken into account the up-to-date knowledge base associated with a particular research question. This should be addressed within the literature review and in turn should establish the criteria for exclusion and withdrawal of the respondents involved in the study, as well as justifying the continuing inclusion of subjects within the study. Criteria for inclusion and exclusion of research respondents are also relevant when considering the risks and benefits associated with clinical trials and randomization as already discussed.

Neuberger (1992) discusses the problems of patients understanding the concept of randomization. This method of selection may be perceived as unfair if the trial is considered to have great benefits to the individuals involved in the 'experimental' group. Individuals may wish only to participate in those areas of the study that they perceive to be in their interests. Consent to participate in randomized controlled trials can therefore be problematic from both the researcher's and respondent's perspectives. Neuberger (1992) identifies a variety of models that have been proposed to make the process of randomization easier to explain and administer (see Table 10.1).

There is no ideal model for gaining consent to participation in a randomized controlled trial. However, this design is generally considered ethically sound because randomization is the only fair way to distribute the risks and benefits of the study fairly across the sample group.

Summary

Beneficence and non-maleficence refer to the imperative to do good and to do no harm. When evaluating published research with regard to these principles, a number of questions should be considered, including:

- What was the risk–benefit ratio (i.e. was the risk to participants acceptable in that it was minimal or congruent with normal treatments)?
- Was any risk equally distributed across the sample?
- Were there mechanisms to protect the privacy and confidentiality of individual participants?
- Were inclusion and exclusion criteria discussed fully with potential research subjects?

Table 10.1 Models for randomizing subjects in experimental studies (reproduced with permission from Neuberger 1992)

Model	Disadvantage
Patients could be prerandomized and then asked to consent to one arm of the trial only	Misleads patients as they may not fully understand that they are participating in a trial
Patients could be prerandomized and not told	Unethical unless there are exceptional circumstances. It is difficult to imagine what those circumstances might be
Patients could be given an information sheet which explains that taking part in the trial is likely to be of benefit to patients	May be dishonest because the whole point of a trial is that no-one knows which treatment group the patient is in

JUSTICE

In the context of research, justice refers to:

... the ethical obligation to treat each person in accordance with what is morally right and proper – to give each person what is due to him or her.
CIOMS/WHO 1993, p10

Gillon (1994, p185) claims that:

justice is synonymous with fairness and can be summarized as the moral obligation to act on the basis of fair adjudication between competing claims.

This section covers:

● Distributive justice (via randomization)
● Vulnerability of research subjects
● Scientific fraud
● Publication bias.

Distributive justice

In research ethics, the principle of justice refers primarily to ensuring that the benefits and burdens of participation are equally distributed across the sample group. The idea of justice also requires that there should be some indication of 'fairness' in the selection of the sample group identified. This will indicate the degree of vulnerability associated with the sample group. Some groups in society are more vulnerable to possible manipulation by the researcher than others. This may be because of impaired or diminished ability to understand what is expected of them (as in persons with mental health or learning difficulties), or because they do not understand

what is being said to them (for example, people who do not speak English as a first language). Other groups of individuals are more vulnerable to manipulation due to the nature of their occupation (such as armed service personnel and students). They may participate in research because of the fear of reprisal such as losing their job, reduced chances of promotion or perhaps exam failure. One should look out for evidence of all these issues when reading and evaluating research papers.

Randomization

The process of randomization is perceived as the fairest way of achieving distributive justice. In certain cases randomization is advocated not only to adhere to theories of probability (see Chapters 6 and 8) but also for ethical reasons. However, the distribution of risk can be seen as a narrow interpretation of the concept of justice because, for some researchers, participants' *needs* may be of equal importance (Warnock 1994). Imagine that some form of drug has shown astonishing results in clinical trials, in that anyone who takes it within 48 hours of having a heart attack appears to have a substantial chance of total recovery. Is it then appropriate that individuals who have had a heart attack have the possibility of being randomized into a control arm, receive a placebo and thus reduce the possibility that they will recover totally? Similarly, if respondents are chronically sick with no hope of a cure but there is a treatment that will alleviate their suffering in some way, is it fair that the treatment is withheld in the pursuit of the objectivity which randomized controlled trials afford? Certainly in these examples, distributive justice (as in randomization) should be seen as secondary to the needs of respondents. In these instances the vulnerable nature of the sample group must be considered in the context of the type of research design posed to address the question. It may be more appropriate from the perspective of need that the design of such trials affords a degree of treatment for *all*, rather than merely *some* respondents.

Vulnerability of subjects

Some groups are particularly vulnerable with respect to the principle of justice or fair treatment within research studies. It has been suggested, for example, that women are vulnerable because of their general acceptance of the medicalization of their health (Turner 1987), especially in studies relating to reproduction. In reviewing a study of cervical dysplasia, Paul (1988) suggested that women may ask fewer questions about their progress whilst involved in a study. Children may be more vulnerable because of their restricted autonomy in choosing to participate in research studies, the decision being made by the parent or legal guardian for children under the age of 7 years (Neuberger 1992) and often for much older children (see earlier discussion, pages 134–135). Whatever the reason, the nature of the sample group will provide some indication of their degree of vulnerability to manipulation by the researcher and the reader should be keenly aware of this. When reading published research, the critical reader should look for criteria for inclusion and exclusion of individuals from the study, along with a clear rationale for such choices.

An example of a study where a vulnerable group was apparently not protected is the Tuskagee Study. This study began in 1932 and concluded in 1972 (Pence 1990). A sample group of black respondents in a southern state of the USA were recruited with the intention of examining the progress of syphilis in male respondents, in order to determine the degree of mortality and morbidity associated with the disease (Burns & Grove 2001, Pence 1990). Since syphilis can affect any individual across the whole breadth of socio-economic backgrounds, the obvious question raised is why were only black respondents chosen to participate in the study? The answer appears to be bound up in the fact that the black population of the state were mainly uneducated and poor and therefore particularly vulnerable to manipulation.

One group that might be at risk of exploitation in research is people who are unable to give consent to participation themselves. In research this is likely to lead to the involvement of allies, advocates or proxies whose ostensible role is to ensure that the person's voice is heard. On the one hand, this can be seen as a way of simultaneously protecting individuals whilst also empowering them through facilitating their inclusion by speaking with or for them. On the other hand, there can be some risks. At the time of writing, the nature and extent of the possible risks of using allies, advocates or proxies as spokespersons for individuals who cannot speak for themselves are still largely unknown, but might be seen as including the following:

- Since allies may be well known to the person because of a preexisting relationship (family member, friend, support worker, for example), it is possible that there may be role conflicts if the ally begins to feel that the research threatens some element of that role relationship.
- People close to the person such as their allies or advocates may, in some contexts, also be their abusers.
- For some groups, like persons with severe learning disabilities, there is a tendency to understate their true capacity. This may lead to the involvement of allies or advocates in research where it is not really necessary. This might be termed the conservatism corollary.
- Little is known about the reliability of evidence from allies or advocates as proxy respondents, especially when there is a premium on eliciting subjective data.
- The costs and benefits of allies and advocates as a possible intrusive factor in people's lives need to be better understood.
- There are ethical issues about whether allies and advocates of individual participants in research should be paid.
- There appears to be no code of conduct about the involvement of allies and advocates as proxy respondents in research.

Fraud or deliberate deception

In research, deliberate deception is fundamentally wrong in that the researcher intentionally manipulates or even invents data to suit their own ends. Burns and Grove (2001) describe such activities as scientific fraud and see this as encompassing fabrication, falsification, plagiarism or other practices that depart significantly from norms accepted by the research community. Unfortunately, as Neuberger (1992) identifies, research ethics committees have no legal jurisdiction in the matter of continuous monitoring of studies once approval has been granted. Much of the responsibility therefore lies with the individual researcher or research team.

The critical reader may be able to discern some aspects of scientific fraud, by virtue of having advanced knowledge in areas such as research design and data analysis or perhaps the specific area of research. However, there is no foolproof way of establishing whether a scientific fraud has been committed from reading a research report. To protect against the publication of questionable research, articles submitted for publication in refereed journals are vetted by experts before acceptance for publication. However, no amount of 'critical analysis' can entirely circumvent such deception.

If fraud is suspected, the author may be asked to produce raw data for scrutiny – for example, research journals, interview recordings and completed questionnaires. If they are unable to do so the research would not be published and an investigation might be carried out by the relevant professional body. In the USA independent regulatory bodies monitor the possibility of research fraud and have the authority to prosecute in such cases. However, no such body exists in the UK; professional groups involved in health care are responsible for regulating their own research practice. In some cases, medical practitioners found guilty of research fraud have been removed from the medical register (Miller 1997).

Publication bias

Publication bias refers to the general trend of positive bias in published research material. Readers of research must always consider that for every research study which is published, another unpublished study may exist. This is due in part to a reluctance to publish studies that are inconclusive or do not demonstrate significant results. A true overall picture of the current state of knowledge may therefore be difficult to determine.

There are compensatory mechanisms in some areas of research to ameliorate positive publication bias. For example, within the UK, before studies are approved pharmaceutical companies must provide LRECs or MRECs with an assurance that *all* results will be published, whatever the findings. However, there are various ways in which studies can be published without these necessarily being disseminated through scientific journals, for example in company publications. For papers reporting studies involving metaanalysis (see Chapter 11) authors need to demonstrate a balance of studies from which the data are drawn for analysis and this should include published and unpublished sources.

A framework similar to the one elaborated here has more recently been proposed by Foster (2001). Her 'three approaches' framework is based on a series of goal-based, duty-based and rights-based questions, all of which address the ethics of research. The attraction of her framework is that it emphasizes the complementarity of the dimensions exposed, as well as possible points of conflict between them. Together they offer a formulation of motives for acting rather than a definitive prescription or checklist for achieving success. Examples of the kinds of questions highlighted by this framework are given below, from which it will be seen that they share important common features with the Four Principles plus Scope of Application approach.

Goal-based questions

- What question is the research addressing?
- Is the research addressing a good and desirable goal?
- How will the research achieve reliable results?
- How will the results be disseminated?

Duty-based questions

- Are the research procedures unacceptably risky?
- If therapeutic research, is there equipoise, i.e. a mindset in which clinicians do not know which treatment option is best for their patients, so they are content that 'best interest' is served by random allocation?
- If non-therapeutic research, are the risks greater than minimal?

Rights-based questions

- What procedures to obtain consent will be followed, and at what stages?
- How will confidentiality be respected?
- How will research participants be involved in confirming the authenticity of accounts?

(adapted from Foster 2001)

Summary

When evaluating published research and the principle of justice, consideration should be given to the following:

- Whether the sample population is vulnerable to manipulation by the researcher
- Whether the limitations of the study are clearly identified and discussed
- Whether the population sample was selected fairly
- Whether the sample was appropriate to answer the research question.

The justness of the published research should also be considered in relation to the degree to which the findings can be seen to be supported by the data and whether the research report or publication has been subject to external scrutiny (i.e. refereed).

CONCLUSION

Evaluating ethical issues in published research can be a difficult task for the reader. The purpose of this chapter is to provide an ethical framework that can be used to identify the ethical problems associated with different research approaches. An ethical framework provides 'clues' on what to look for when reading published research and this may make the evaluation less daunting. The framework also provides the reader with a structure upon which to base moral judgments. The principles inherent within the framework are common to all ethical theories and underpin professional codes of conduct. When using the framework, it is important that consideration is given to each of the four principles. This allows all areas of research practice (such as sampling techniques, reducing risks and maximizing benefits) to be examined.

The application of the principles identified within the ethical framework may give the reader a more critical insight into the 'world' of the research participant, enabling them in some way to put themselves into the research participants' shoes to consider what is or is not acceptable. Unfortunately, history has provided us with examples of how research participants may be manipulated and abused by researchers. In response to such examples, tighter controls are now applied to the process of research, through the establishment of local research ethics committees. This may lead us to assume that published research need not be critically examined for ethical weaknesses. However, published research is not necessarily good research and should not be accepted at face value. It is for this reason that an understanding of how to evaluate the ethical nature of published research is required. There is no definitive way of achieving this though we believe that the Four Principles plus Scope of Application approach or the Three Approaches Framework both offer productive ways of addressing the ethical nature of published research.

Acknowledgement

The authors would like to thank Angela Venables for her contribution to the version of this chapter that appeared in the first edition of this book.

References

ACHC (Association of Community Health Councils Working Party on Local Ethics Committees) (1990) *Information Resource Pack for Lay Members of Local Research Ethics Committees*. London: Community Health Council.

Baum M, Zikha J and Houghton J (1989) Ethics of clinical research: lessons for the future. *British Medical Journal* **229**(7): 251–253.

Beauchamp TL and Childress JF (1989) *Principles of Biomedical Ethics*, 3rd edn. Oxford: Oxford University Press.

Beecher H (1966) Ethics and clinical research. *New England Journal of Medicine* **274**(24): 1354–1360.

Bok S (1984) *Secrets: on the Ethics of Concealment and Revelation*. London: Oxford University Press.

British Paediatric Association (1992) Ethics Advisory Committee: *Guidelines for the Ethical Conduct of Medical Research Using Children*. London: British Paediatric Association.

Burns N and Grove S (2001) *The Practice of Nursing Research: Conduct, Critique and Utilisation,* 4th edn. Philadelphia, PA: WB Saunders.

Carlin (1995) US/*Genetic engineering: religious leaders take on scientists who play God*. Independent on Sunday 4 June:16.

CIOMS (Council for International Organisations of Medical Sciences)/WHO (1993) *International Ethical Guidelines for Biomedical Research Involving Human Subjects*. Geneva: CIOMS.

Cowles K (1988) Issues in qualitative research on sensitive topics. *Western Journal of Nursing Research* **10**(2): 163–179.

Crookes PA (1996) *Personal Bereavement in Registered General Nurses*. Unpublished PhD thesis. Hull: University of Hull.

Department of Health (DoH) (2001a) *Research Governance Framework for Health and Social Care*. London: Department of Health. Available online at: www.doh.gov.uk/research

Department of Health (DoH) (2001b) *Seeking Consent: Working with People with Learning Disabilities*. London: Department of Health. Available online at: www.doh.gov.uk/consent

Dickens, BM (2002) Guest editorial. Can sex selection be ethically tolerated? *Journal of Medical Ethics* **28**(6): 335–336.

Dimond BC (1995) *Legal Aspects of Nursing*, 2nd edn. London: Prentice Hall.

Faden R and Beauchamp TL (1986) *A History and Theory of Informed Consent*. Oxford: Oxford University Press.

Foster C (2001) *The Ethics of Medical Research on Humans*. Cambridge: Cambridge University Press.

Gillon R (1994) Medical ethics: four principles plus attention to scope. *British Medical Journal* **309**: 184–188.

Hughes P (1990) Evaluating the impact of continual professional education (ENB 941). *Nurse Education Today* **10**: 428–436.

Miller B (1997) Honesty on trial. *Nursing Times* **93**(35): 10–11.

Neuberger J (1992) *Ethics and Health Care: The Role of Research Ethics Committees in the United Kingdom*. London: King's Fund Institute.

NHSME (National Health Service Management Executive) (1990) *Consent to Treatment Guidelines*. London: HMSO.

Oakley A (1992) *Social Support and Motherhood*. Oxford: Blackwell.

Pappworth MH (1968) *Human Guinea Pigs*. Beacon: Boston.

Paul C (1988) The New Zealand cervical cancer study: could it happen again? *British Medical Journal* **297**: 533–538.

Pence GE (1990) *Classic Cases in Medical Ethics*. London: McGraw-Hill.

Polit DF and Hungler BP (2001) *Essentials of Nursing Research: Methods, Appraisal and Utilization*, 5th edn. Philadelphia: Lippincott.

Ramcharan P and Cutcliffe JR (2001) Judging the ethics of qualitative research: considering the 'ethics as process' model. *Health and Social Care in the Community* **9**(6): 358–366.

Ramos MC (1989) Some ethical implications of qualitative research. *Research in Nursing and Health* **12**: 57–63.

Royal College of Psychiatrists (1990) Guidelines for Research. Ethics Committees on Psychiatric Research involving Human Subjects. *Psychiatric Bulletin* **14**: 48–61.

Scully JL (2001) Drawing a line: situating boundaries in genetic medicine. *Bioethics* **15**(3): 189–204.

Silverman WA (1989) The myth of informed consent: in daily practice and clinical trials. *Journal of Medical Ethics* **15**: 6–11.

Suvalescu J (2002) Deaf lesbians, 'designer disability' and the future of medicine. *British Medical Journal* **325**(7367): 771–773.

Thornton H (1993) Whose interests: patients' or researchers'? *Bulletin of Medical Ethics* XX: 13–19.

Turner BS (1987) *Medical Power and Social Knowledge*. London: Sage.

Walley T and Barton S (1995) A purchaser perspective of managing new drugs: interferon beta as a case study. *British Medical Journal* **311**: 796–799.

Warnock M (1994) Comments: principles of health care ethics. *British Medical Journal* **38**: 988–989.

While AE (1995) Ethics committees: impediments to research or guardians of ethical standards? *British Medical Journal* **311**: 661.

Further reading

Council for International Organizations of Medical Sciences (CIOMS)(2002) *International Ethical Guidelines for Biomedical Research Involving Human Subjects*. Geneva, Switzerland: World Health Organization.

Department of Health (1997) *Report of the Review of Patient Identifiable Information*. The Caldicott Committee. London: HMSO.

Department of Health (2001) *Governance Arrangements for NHS Research Ethics Committees*. London: DoH. Available online at: www.doh.gov.uk/research

Department of Health (2001) *Research Governance Framework for Health and Social Care*. London: DoH. Available online at: www.doh.gov.uk/research

Department of Health (2001) *Seeking Consent: Working with People with Learning Disabilities*. London: DoH. Available online at: www.doh.gov.uk/consent

General Medical Council (1998) *Seeking Patients' Consent: the Ethical Considerations*. Available online at: www.gmc-uk.org

Medical Research Council. *Guidance on Ethical, Legal and Management Issues Concerning Human Tissue and Biological Samples for use in Research*. Available online at: www.mrc. ac.uk

World Health Organisation (2000) *Operational Guidelines for Ethics Committees that Review Biomedical Research*. Available online at: http://who.int/tdr/publications/publications

Chapter 11

Reviewing and interpreting research: identifying implications for practice

Sue Davies

INTRODUCTION

Where is the knowledge we have lost in information?
(from *Choruses From the Rock*, a poem by T S Eliot)

One of the most difficult tasks for any health care practitioner wanting to ensure that their practice is research based is synthesizing the evidence from a mass of literature into clear indicators for practice. Most of us have, at some time or another, sat beside a pile of research papers and articles with pen poised thinking 'where do I begin?' The purpose of this chapter is to provide some practical suggestions for extracting the relevant information from the literature, organizing that information and presenting it in a way that clearly identifies the implications for practice, education and further research. The chapter is designed to complement the contribution from Peter Bradley (Chapter 12) who provides an excellent description of systematic reviews – a highly structured approach to reviewing literature. This chapter focuses on more wide-ranging literature reviews that incorporate both qualitative and quantitative research studies as well as non-empirical sources.

At points within the chapter, reference is made to a published literature review which I carried out as part of a research project funded by the English National Board for Nursing, Midwifery and Health Visiting (Nolan et al 2001, 2002). This project aimed to evaluate the extent to which educational programmes in nursing prepare nurses to work effectively with older people and their families. The review outlined here focused on the needs of frail older people who need some form of continuing care. Some of the tools and techniques used by the project team to review this large body of literature are included within this chapter in the hope that readers will be able to modify and adapt our approach to suit their own purposes.

Key issues

- The importance of critical reviews of literature
- Types of literature review, systematic review and metaanalysis
- Purposes of a literature review
- Stages in the literature review process
- Structuring and writing a review.

SYNTHESIS: A COMPLEX SKILL

If the current emphasis on self-directed professional education is to be successful in enhancing the quality of health care, practitioners need to develop the habit of critically evaluating and integrating literature early in their careers. Research modules on nursing programmes across the country, and indeed this book, have been developed with this aim in mind. Unfortunately, it remains the case that many published reviews of nursing and health care literature present a largely narrative description rather than a critical evaluation of existing material and there are few good examples to act as a guide. In Chapter 6, Jan Draper makes reference to an excellent article by Nicky Cullum (1994) who summarizes the pitfalls commonly found in published literature reviews (p71). You may find it helpful to refer to this section again before you read on.

In recent years, there are signs that the review of published and unpublished research literature is developing a methodology in its own right (Cooper et al 2000, Hek et al 2000, Roe 1994), raising the hope that the limitations identified by Cullum may become a thing of the past. With the establishment of centres for the systematic review and dissemination of research evidence, such as the NHS Centre for Reviews and Dissemination in York and the Cochrane Collaboration, research synthesis is being recognized as a rigorous and scientific process. In order to appreciate how literature reviews might contribute to health care practice, it is important to recognize the range of possible approaches to reviewing material and these will now be discussed.

TYPES OF REVIEW

Reviews of research-based evidence and other literature can be broadly divided under three headings:

- Literature review
- Systematic review
- Metaanalysis.

The more general term *literature review* is used to describe the process of synthesizing the results and conclusions of a number of items of literature on a given topic. This type of review will incorporate all types of literature relating to the topic, not just those based upon empirical research, and will include both qualitative and quantitative studies. *Systematic review* refers to the process of comprehensively identifying all the research on a given topic and synthesizing the findings. Systematic reviews are normally based on research that meets strict inclusion criteria such as random allocation to experimental and control groups (see Chapter 12). Examples of published systematic reviews include Hignett's review of the evidence underpinning guidelines for safe moving and handling of patients (Hignett et al 2003) and McDonnell et al's review of the effectiveness of pain teams in the management of postoperative pain (McDonnell et al 2003).

In recent years, there has been a growing interest in the process of combining empirical evidence from studies conducted in a similar way. This process, known as *metaanalysis*, involves transforming the findings of reviewed studies to a common metric and then using statistical tests to determine whether there are overall effects, subsample effects and associations among attributes of studies and particular findings (Ganong 1987). In other words, the review incorporates a specific statistical technique to assemble the results of several studies into a single estimate. As the number of studies relevant to nursing and health care using an experimental design increases, the number of metaanalyses of substantive bodies of literature is also likely to increase. One example is Brodaty et al's (2003) metaanalysis of psychosocial interventions for caregivers of people with dementia (see Box 11.1).

The remainder of this chapter will focus on the development of the more comprehensive type of literature review, which is likely to incorporate a range of types of material and evidence. For a more in-depth discussion of systematic reviews and metaanalyses, the interested reader is referred to

Box 11.1 An example of metaanalysis

Brodaty H, Green AB, Koschera A (2003) Metaanalysis of psychosocial interventions for caregivers of people with dementia. *Journal of the American Geriatrics Society* 51(5): 657–664.

Aim: To review published reports of interventions for caregivers (CGs) of persons with dementia, excluding respite care and provide recommendations to clinicians.

Design: Metaanalytical review. Electronic databases and key articles were searched for controlled trials, preferably randomized, published in English from 1985 to 2001 inclusive. Thirty studies were located and scored according to set criteria and the interventions' research quality and clinical significance were judged.

Setting: Home or non-institutional environment.
Participants: Informal caregivers (CG) – persons providing unpaid care at home or in a non-institutional setting.

Measurements: The primary measures were psychological morbidity and burden. Other varied outcome measures such as CG coping skills and social support were combined with measures of psychological distress and burden to form a main outcome measure.

Results: The quality of research increased over the 17 years. Results from 30 studies (34 interventions) indicated, at most current follow-up, significant benefits in CG psychological distress (random effect size (ES) = 0.31; 95% confidence interval (CI) = 0.13–0.50), CG knowledge (ES = 0.51; CI = 0.05–0.98), any main CG outcome measure (ES = 0.32; CI = 0.15–0.48), and patient mood (ES = 0.68; CI = 0.30–1.06), but not CG burden (ES = 0.09; CI = −0.09–0.26). There was considerable variability in outcome, partly because of differences in methodology and intervention technique. Elements of successful interventions could be identified. Success was more likely if, in addition to CGs, patients were involved. Four of seven studies indicated delayed nursing home admission.

Conclusion: Some CG interventions can reduce CG psychological morbidity and help people with dementia stay at home longer. Programmes that involve the patients and their families and are more intensive and modified to CGs' needs may be more successful. Future research should try to improve clinicians' abilities to prescribe interventions.

Chalmers and Altman (1995), Droogan and Song (1996), Cooper et al (2000) and Hek et al (2000).

PURPOSES OF A LITERATURE REVIEW

The broad aim of any literature review is to synthesize the critical evaluation of existing work on a topic. More specifically, a literature review should perform some or all of the following functions:

- Identify the context in which the problem or topic is being explored
- Outline what is known about a topic
- Identify and define concepts and variables of relevance to the topic
- Review the methods used to study the topic
- Identify theoretical and conceptual frameworks within which the topic can be explored
- Suggest appropriate indicators for practice, education and further research.

These functions may be covered to different degrees depending on the overall purpose and focus of the

review. For example, a literature review prepared for a course assignment is likely to focus more on the findings of the review and implications for practice. In comparison, a literature review conducted as a stage in a research process, and which therefore needs to provide the foundation for empirical work, is likely to place more emphasis on the definition of concepts and variables. However, a good review will perform all the functions listed to a greater or lesser extent and each will now be considered in more detail.

IDENTIFY THE CONTEXT IN WHICH THE PROBLEM OR TOPIC IS BEING EXPLORED

Whatever the focus of the review, it is essential that the reviewer identifies the rationale underpinning their efforts. They should identify reasons for undertaking the review at this time and how it will contribute to an understanding of the topic. It is likely that this will necessitate a consideration of the professional and political factors, including government policies, influencing developments relating to the subject area (see Chapter 2). It may also be appropriate for the author to indicate their personal motivation for undertaking the review. Limitations and boundaries of the review should be acknowledged: for example, the scope and coverage of a focused essay will be different to that of a major work or thesis.

OUTLINE WHAT IS KNOWN ABOUT THE TOPIC

Research needs to build upon existing work if knowledge about health care, and as a consequence health care practice, is to move forward. In contrast to the physical sciences, single studies in the social and behavioural sciences rarely provide definitive answers to research questions. Rather, progress is accomplished through the identification of trends from the synthesis of findings from a number of studies. A review of the literature needs to indicate the current 'state of the art' in relation to the topic being investigated. It is important to be clear about the aim(s) or intention(s) of the paper.

IDENTIFY AND DEFINE RELEVANT CONCEPTS AND VARIABLES

In identifying what is already known about a topic, it is important to define key concepts and variables. For example, a review of research to evaluate the impact of social activities on the quality of life of nursing home residents would need to indicate how the concept *quality of life* had been defined and described by the authors of relevant research reports. It may be that key concepts have been measured in different ways by different researchers, leading to apparently contradictory findings.

Identifying themes in the literature contributes to this process. Also, sometimes outlining what is *not* known or covered well in the literature, is important/useful to note.

REVIEW THE METHODS USED TO STUDY THE TOPIC

The main consideration is whether the research methods were sufficiently rigorous to produce valid information (see Chapters 6–9). The methods of study will also provide an indication of the type of information and the level of knowledge created by the body of literature to date.

IDENTIFY THEORETICAL AND CONCEPTUAL FRAMEWORKS WITHIN WHICH THE TOPIC CAN BE EXPLORED

A literature review should identify the current state of knowledge with reference to the development of theory in relation to the topic under consideration. This will involve the identification and critique of conceptual and theoretical frameworks that have provided the basis for empirical study (see Chapter 5). It is important that any literature review on a particular topic identifies assumptions upon which the body of literature has been developed as these may influence the applicability of the findings of the review.

IDENTIFY APPROPRIATE INDICATORS FOR PRACTICE, EDUCATION AND FURTHER RESEARCH

In a seminal paper on nurses' use of research findings, Hunt (1981) suggests that research in nursing provides three types of practice indicator: what nurses should do, what nurses should try and indicators of practices and procedures for which there is no sound basis. By identifying the level of knowledge in relation to the topic under consideration (see Chapter 6), critical readers can determine which type of indicator is produced by the body of literature under review. Implications for education and gaps in knowledge suggesting the need for further research should also be identified.

Summary

The ability to synthesize information from the critical evaluation of research reports on a given topic is an important skill for all engaged in health care practice. There are a number of approaches to reviewing literature including systematic review and metaanalysis as well as the more all-encompassing review that will also include non-empirical literature. The choice of approach depends on the purpose of the review. Functions of the literature review include summarizing the current state of knowledge in relation to a given topic, defining key concepts and variables, examining the conceptual and theoretical frameworks which have been used to study the topic, reviewing methods to indicate the existing level of knowledge in relation to the topic and identifying implications for practice, education and research.

Literature reviews have the potential to inform health care practice in a whole host of ways. However, in order to make an impact, reviews need to demonstrate a systematic and logical method. The rest of this chapter will be devoted to describing the stages in this process in more detail. First, the arguments for adopting an organized approach will be revisited.

A METHODOLOGY FOR REVIEWING LITERATURE: THE IMPORTANCE OF A SYSTEMATIC APPROACH

The process of identifying and retrieving literature relevant to a particular topic has been comprehensively discussed in Chapters 3 and 4. However, it is worth reiterating here that whatever the purpose of the review, it is essential that the approach to collecting, organizing and reviewing material is as systematic as possible. Ganong (1987) suggests that the approach to reviewing a research-based body of literature needs to be as systematic as an empirical research process. Unfortunately, relatively few published literature reviews meet the standards of primary research (Lederman 1992).

STAGES IN THE REVIEW PROCESS

Jackson (1980) proposes that the methodology of literature reviewing involves six stages:

1. Selecting the hypotheses or questions for the review
2. Sampling the research to be reviewed
3. Representing the characteristics of the studies and their findings
4. Analysing the findings
5. Interpreting the results
6. Reporting the review.

An important first step is to describe the aims and objectives for the review (or as Jackson suggests, the hypotheses or questions). These should be carefully stated and reviewed regularly in order to make sure that the review does not lose focus. The aims and objectives for the continuing care review mentioned

earlier for example were:

> ... to draw together literature describing experiences of older people living in care homes, their families and staff working in these environments, in order to identify a framework to guide practice that will help ensure a good quality of life for older people living in care homes

(Davies 2001, p75)

Important components of this broad aim were the focus on experiences and the desire to produce a framework for change. This helped me both in the identification of relevant literature and in structuring the review to produce clear indicators from practice.

The analysis of material can also be divided into three stages:

1. Classifying material
2. Identifying themes and concepts
3. Critiquing methods and theoretical frameworks.

Before considering each of these steps in more detail, it is important to think about the best way of recording information for the review. Some of these points are also covered in Chapter 3. It is also important to remember that literature review is often an iterative process: if gaps in knowledge are found it may be necessary to rerun searches using different key words.

RECORDING INFORMATION

Perhaps the most fundamental rule is to avoid recording references or useful quotes on bits of paper that can easily be lost or separated. Once again, the key is to be systematic in your approach. In a useful paper on how to survive writing a thesis, Johanson (1985) compares the virtual impossibility of writing a literature review from pages of notes and photocopies of articles with the ease of writing using an organized system which has extracted the relevant information.

With the ready availability of computer technology, an important decision facing the would be literature reviewer is whether to record information on a computer database or to use a manual system. A number of packages are now available to assist in the process of recording and retrieving information for a literature review. These bibliographic tools can take the chore out of adding references to a review: most link to word-processing packages in order to automatically build a complete list of references as each reference is inserted in the text. Some allow sophisticated manipulation of information: Endnote and Reference Manager are examples. However, data entry for all these packages can be time-consuming, particularly for anyone unfamiliar with their use. In making a decision about the most appropriate system, the following points are worth taking into account.

The size of the database

If the database is going to be very large it is probably worth investing the effort into computerizing the information, particularly if data can be copied across to the text file for word processing.

The level of manipulation required

If the records will require frequent and highly sophisticated manipulation that cannot easily be done manually, then use of a computer package may be preferable.

The main source of references

If the literature search is being carried out mainly via online databases and information can be downloaded and incorporated into the review data-base, this may be the most efficient way to store information.

Use of a computerized database for storing the information extracted during the review process does have a number of disadvantages. Access to a computer terminal may be limited, although the availability of lightweight laptop computers that can be taken into libraries is now widespread. Another limitation of computerized databases for storing records is that it may be necessary to rely on printouts to compare entries since only one record is displayed at a time. It is also worth bearing in mind that computer disks can be corrupted and hard disks do occasionally crash. However, it is also possible to lose manual records.

If using a computer package, it is essential to maintain a back-up which is stored separately from the main computer. Whichever system is used, it should be kept as simple as possible, otherwise recording references becomes time consuming and tedious. Finally, it is important to organize photocopies of items within the database, for example by numbering each item and cross-referencing, either to cards or to each computerized entry. It is extremely frustrating to be in the final stages of writing and having to search for an elusive item in order to check a quote or page number.

CLASSIFYING MATERIAL

One of the first steps in reviewing a collection of literature is to categorize the information contained within individual papers and articles. Polit and Hungler (1999) have provided a very useful classification based upon five types of information. These are:

- Facts, statistics and research findings
- Theoretical discussion
- Research methods and procedures
- Opinions and viewpoints
- Anecdotes and clinical descriptions.

Different types of information can contribute to a literature review in different ways. However, a research-based review should focus mainly upon information in the first three categories listed above. Opinions and anecdotes can be used to illustrate points and are also useful in suggesting concepts and ideas for new research. They can also be useful in helping to demonstrate the context, background and motivation for undertaking the review.

A second helpful step in classifying material is to rate each item according to its value and relevance to the focus of the review. For example, a report of a study that has investigated a similar topic might be awarded three points whereas a paper of only marginal relevance to the topic under investigation might be awarded only one point. This type of rating approach helps to identify quickly those items that will contribute most significantly to the review.

It is also useful to classify each item of literature in relation to the field of study, particularly for reviews where a consideration of a broad body of literature is indicated. For example, when reviewing the literature relating to the continuing care needs of frail older people and their families, I explored the social science and social work literature in addition to nursing and medical literature (Davies 2001).

Exercise 11.1

- Choose a topic relevant to your own practice.
- Identify at least 10 references related to the topic using any resources to which you have access (e.g. OVID, abstracting indexes).
- Using the abstract for each item, attempt to classify the items using Polit and Hungler's five-point classification system.

IDENTIFYING THEMES: DEVELOPING A THEME MATRIX

It is important to identify themes and concepts within the literature in order to determine the appropriate structure for the review. These should emerge from the literature rather than being imposed by the reviewer. In fact, some authors have suggested that synthesizing material for a literature review can benefit from an approach similar to content analysis used in qualitative research (Cooper et al 2000, Nolan et al 1997). The simplest way to approach this process is to read through each item and identify the major themes or issues covered within the paper. A list of themes can then be developed and these can be condensed into broader themes once all the material for review has been considered.

A simple method for identifying themes is to record information on a theme matrix (Table 11.1). This consists of two axes with numbered items on the vertical axis and categories/themes on the horizontal axis. Items can be classified according to categories relevant to the review and themes identified, simply extending the x-axis as new themes emerge. The cells of the matrix can be used to incorporate additional information or reminders about the way in which each theme features within the paper. Once all the literature has been categorized in this way, themes can be condensed into broader categories as appropriate. Computerized databases such as Excel can help in this process.

Exercise 11.2

- Develop a theme matrix on the basis of the 10 papers identified in the previous exercise.
- What are the major themes?
- How could these help you to synthesize the material you have collected?

You should find the approach suggested in this exercise just as useful (and necessary) for shorter 'essays' as it is for longer and more detailed literature reviews.

CRITICAL ANALYSIS

Having classified the material for review and identified the major themes within the body of literature as a whole, the reviewer is ready to begin a more detailed critical analysis of the material. Critical review of literature broadly involves two aspects: theoretical critique and methodological critique. Theoretical critique is perhaps the most difficult and most commonly neglected aspect of literature reviewing and will be dealt with first.

Theoretical critique

In Chapter 5 the various ways in which theoretical and conceptual frameworks and assumptions contribute to research design were outlined. However, as the authors point out, it is not uncommon for researchers to fail to make these assumptions explicit when writing research reports. This may be the first challenge for the reviewer: to identify the assumptions and theoretical ideas upon which a study has been developed. The second challenge is to question these assumptions and consider alternative theoretical explanations for the phenomena under investigation. Examples of theoretical frameworks identified within the review of continuing care literature are considered in Table 11.2.

Theories can be tentatively accepted if there is a substantial body of evidence demonstrating their legitimacy. However, it is the researcher's responsibility to present this evidence in support of their own theoretical perspective. Most importantly, perhaps, as a practitioner, you should 'beware the dominant ideology' which could 'blinker' you to alternative theoretical perspectives which might offer greater illumination of the topic under review (Abbott & Sapsford 1997).

Exercise 11.3

- Select two of the papers identified during Exercise 11.1 for more detailed study.
- Try to identify the conceptual or theoretical framework on which each study is based.
- Has the researcher presented sufficient evidence in support of the theoretical assumptions underpinning the study?
- Does the theoretical or conceptual basis of the study suggest ideological assumptions which may have influenced the findings?

Methodological critique

Most readers of this chapter will probably have had experience of critiquing individual research reports, particularly since the research critique appears to be a common assessment strategy for research modules on educational programmes in nursing and health care. It is important that nurses and other health practitioners are encouraged to develop skills in critiquing research reports as this 'critical' culture has long been absent in the 'softer' caring disciplines.

Table 11.1   Extract from a theme matrix for a literature review on the continuing care needs of older people and their families

Classification						Themes				
Author/date	No.	Ty	Or	Fi	Use	Managing the transition	Threats to identity	Vulnerability/ powerlessness	Maintaining links to family	Creating a sense of community
Rader et al 1996	223	2	US		**		X Lack of an individualized approach to care	X Residents sometimes show aggression when their wishes are ignored		
Rantz et al 1999	224	1	US	Nur	**			X Staff and residents identify different priorities	X Family involvement seen as crucial	
Reed et al 1999	225	1	UK	Nur Res	***			X Potential for residents to be involved in quality assurance processes		
Reed and Payton 1996	226	1	UK	Nur Res	***	X Requires extensive social activity by resident	X Residents need to create a degree of familiarity following admission			X Importance of relationships with other residents
Reinardy 1995	227	1	US	Nur	**	X Practitioners need to recognize coping styles of individuals		X Relationship between perception of control and satisfaction		
Richardson 1992	228	2	US	Nur	*			X Residents lack access to health screening		X Need to offer full range of services to care home residents
Ross et al 1997	229	1	Can	CCF	***				X Family members as a resource	X Wife's role changes over time

Key:

Ty = Type   Or = Origin   Fi = Field   Use = Usefulness   X = Major theme

1. Facts, statistics and research findings
2. Literature review/theoretical discussion
3. Research methods and procedures
4. Opinions and viewpoints
5. Anecdotes and clinical descriptions

Nur = Nursing homes
Res = Residential homes
CCF = Chronic care facility
Com = Community

*** = Highly relevant to review focus
** = Fairly relevant to review focus
* = Marginal to review focus

Table 11.2 Application and critique of theoretical frameworks pertaining to experiences of nursing home entry

Theoretical framework	Examples	Definition/description	Typical application within the literature	Critique
Caregiving as a career	Cosbey 1994 Aneshensel 1995 Murphy et al 1997 Ross et al 1997	Career is defined as 'a series of statuses and clearly defined offices held throughout the life course in which there are typical sequences of position, achievement and responsibility'	The notion of the caregiving career can be used to explain the motivations of community-dwelling spouses at different stages in the care-giving career and their feelings associated with visiting	Relatives often describe the move to a nursing home and subsequent changes in role and identity in the context of their caregiving relationship as a whole. Whether they perceive this as a 'career' is less clear
Locus of control	Morgan and Zimmerman 1990 Brown and Furstenberg 1992 Chen and Snyder 1996	Locus of control construct has three foci: internal control, external control and the influence of powerful others. Intervention of practitioners can result in changes in LOC orientation in client	Shifting the locus of control in decision-making towards older people and family members will enhance satisfaction with care and ease adjustment	Numerous studies have demonstrated that feeling in control of events is associated with positive experiences at all stages of the move to a care home
Life crisis and transition	Oleson and Shaddick 1993 Meleis and Trangenstein 1994 Schumacher and Meleis 1994	Transition is defined as *the passage or movement from one state, condition or place to another.* Effective coping with transition/crisis requires understanding and effective management of the event	Older people and their families relocating to a nursing home experience a life transition that they often perceive as a crisis. People experiencing transition are usually able to discern discrete phases in the process	The potential for family members themselves to take action to influence outcomes is under-explored in the literature
Continuity theory	Elliot 1995 Gladstone 1995 Reed and Payton 1995 Ghusn et al 1996 Onega and Tripp Reimer 1997	Continuity theory is concerned with '*maintaining a continuous sense of self in the face of the many internal and external disruptions accompanying old age.*' (Becker 1993)	Continuity is maintained not only by performing familiar activities, but also by engaging in a subjective process that brings about a feeling of order, consistency and a restoration of personal meaning in situations marked by physical, psychological or environmental change	Attempts to maintain continuity for the older person appear to be a key function for relatives and staff within the new care environment
Social exchange theory	Clarke 1993 Nelson 2000	Relationships are rooted in reciprocity	Delayed reciprocity is an important concept for understanding why relatives continue to engage in seemingly unbalanced relationships with nursing home residents	Relatives within a number of studies acknowledge the foundations of the caregiving relationship and their commitment to reciprocating for a lifetime of love and care
Family systems theory	Kaplan and Ade-Ridder 1991 Bogo 1987 Drysdale 1993	The family is perceived as a unitary group with the consequence that change affecting one member will bring about change in the rest of the family unit. The implication is that the family as a whole will need additional support and information to re-establish equilibrium	Family systems theory has been used to explain the impact of relocation on family caregivers and to suggest interventions which may assist families to preserve and enhance relationships following the move	A number of studies provide evidence that the relocation of an older family member has a significant impact on other close family members resulting in an ongoing need for guidance and support

However, the value of a detailed review of one research paper for informing practice is questionable since it is unlikely to be appropriate to change nursing practice on the evidence of one study. Detailed checklists for critiquing individual research reports also become somewhat redundant in the context of reviewing a large body of literature.

Numerous checklists for reviewing individual research reports are available (see, for example, Burns & Grove 2001). However, in order to review a *body* of literature, a more pragmatic approach is required. In a very useful book on writing for social scientists, Cuba (1993) suggests that the following information should be extracted for each item in the review:

- A complete bibliographic reference
- The major questions posed in the study
- The method of investigation
- The major variables/concepts of interest and their operational definition
- The study population and sampling strategy
- The findings
- The author's conclusions.

The methodological critique for each item can then be framed around the following questions adapted from Depoy and Gitlin (1994) in conjunction with material presented in earlier chapters of this book:

1. What is the existing level of knowledge in relation to the topic and the population of interest? (see Chapters 1, 3, 4, 5, 6)
2. Does the research design used within the study reflect the existing level of knowledge and are the resultant findings at the level of exploration, description or prediction? (Chapters 4, 5, 6)
3. Consider the research strategy or design used in each study (Chapter 6):
   - Is it appropriate for the existing level of knowledge?
   - Is it appropriate to answer the question? (Chapters 6, 7, 8, 9)
   - Is there compatibility between procedures, findings and conclusions? (Chapters 6, 7, 8, 9)
4. Consider the boundaries of each study – what level of knowledge exists for the population and setting you are interested in? (Chapter 9)

These can be seen as the 'basic notes' recommended for an entry into a personal references database.

Once this information has been extracted for each item and entered into the database (see Figure 11.1

for an example), a useful next step is to develop a methodological matrix for each theme (Table 11.3). This approach enables easy comparison of studies relating to similar themes and issues. A similar approach can be used to extract the relevant information from non-empirical sources and suggested criteria are included in Box 11.2 on page 154.

Summary

The key to a successful literature review is a systematic approach. Items should be classified and relevant information extracted and stored in a database. The development of theme and method matrices is one approach to the classification and categorization of information. Evaluating each item of literature from a theoretical and methodological perspective is a crucial element in the review process.

Reference Type: Journal Article
Record Number: 93
Author: Gentili A; Weiner D; Kuchibhatla M; Edinger JD
Year: 1997
Title: Factors that disturb sleep in nursing home residents
Journal: Aging-Clinical and Experimental Research
Volume: 9
Issue: 3
Pages: 207–213
Themes: Poor sleep quality in nursing homes
Sleep-wake cycle of elderly residents frequently does not coincide with the institution's schedule.
Questions/objectives: To determine the prevalence of sleep complaints in cognitively intact NH residents and identify particular features associated with poor sleep.
Boundaries: 48 cognitively intact residents in two nursing homes,US.
Methods: Pittsburgh Sleep Quality Index
Depression Scale
Subjective Health Indicator
Duke University Severity of Illness Scale
Rapid Disability Rating Scale
Findings: 73% of subjects were identified as poor sleepers
Most common causes of disturbance were nocturia, noise or light, pain
Predictors of poor sleep were co-morbidity and depression
Recommendations: More individualized night-time care practices
Minimize levels of light and noise at night
Level of knowledge: Description
Keywords: Elderly patients, quality index, care, depression, patterns, health, complaints, insomnia, facility, illness
Points of critique: Use of validated tool – the PQSI
Sample only generalizable to cognitively intact residents

Figure 11.1   Example of a database entry.

Table 11.3 Extract from a methodological matrix for the theme Vulnerability/Powerlessness from a literature review on the continuing care needs of older people and their families

Author/year/ paper number	Level of knowledge	Focus/ boundaries	Methods/ critique	Findings/ compatiblity
Rantz et al 1999	Exploratory	To develop a conceptual model of nursing home care quality from the perspective of consumers 11 groups involving 16 residents and 80 family members drawn from five Missouri communities – two urban, three rural	Focus group interviews video-taped and transcribed	Two core variables: staff and care. Staff attitudes are crucial to experiences of care. Family involvement can help to ensure that staff 'follow through' Importance of continuity of staff
Reed et al 1999	Descriptive	To describe an initiative for involving older people in service quality specification. Single health authority, residents of five care homes, UK	Literature review and descriptive account of practice-based initiative	Older residents of care homes can make valuable and meaningful contributions to determining service quality specifications. Practical challenges to involvement need careful consideration
Reinardy 1995	Descriptive	To study the effect of deciding to move and wanting to move to a nursing home on the initial reactions of nursing home residents 502 residents of 10 nursing homes	Secondary analysis of data from Geriatric Nurse. Practitioner project. Face-to-face structured interviews using 3 scales. Limited to 3–4 weeks following admission	Deciding to move and wanting to move associated with satisfaction and participation in activities. Only 41% said that they had made the decision to relocate themselves
Stirling and Reid (1992) 296	Predictive	Can the caregiving practices of nurses influence the well being of patients when they try to facilitate the control felt by patients? 28 patients, 28 primary care nurses	3 experimental groups: skills training (7 pairs); attention control (6 pairs); no treatment control (7 pairs) Sample limited to residents without cognitive impairment	Significant differences for treatment group but not for control groups on three main outcome measures (residents' perception of environment and self-concept, nurses' self-perception of control)

PUTTING IT ALL TOGETHER

There is no 'recipe' for writing a literature review and the most appropriate format will often be determined by the literature under consideration and the aims of the review. However, there are some general points that will help to ensure that the review remains focused and succeeds in identifying clear research-based indicators for practice. The following outline is intended as a guide to ensure that all relevant information is included. As with any research-based paper, it is essential that the review has a clear introduction, a middle section where the main arguments are developed, and a concise summary. Within these broad parameters, the final structure of the review will be determined by the nature of the topic, in particular the themes which have emerged from the consideration of the literature.

Have a plan

A good review requires structure and organization. It is worth mapping out a plan of the review before you start writing, including key points to cover within each section. The appropriate structure will

> **Box 11.4 Extract from main body of literature review on continuing care needs of older people and their families**
>
> **Effects of different staffing levels and skill mix on quality of care**
>
> A common suggestion for improving the quality of care in nursing homes is to increase the ratio of qualified nurses and reduce the reliance on unqualified health care assistants. However, the literature review revealed a dearth of studies which consider the issue of skill mix within the context of nursing homes. Certainly, few studies have addressed the central issue of whether resident outcomes are affected by the skill mix of the nursing team or whether similar outcomes can be achieved by varying skill mix combinations. In a carefully designed study, Pearson et al (1992) surveyed 200 non-government homes in four Australian states and found no relationship between the proportion of qualified nursing staff and quality of care or quality of life for residents. However, there was a significant positive relationship between access to therapy staff and the variety of experience of residents. Exposure to in-service training for staff and the leadership style of the most senior nurse within each facility were also found to influence quality of care.
>
> There is some evidence to suggest that the attitude of carers may be a more significant factor than staffing levels in determining resident experiences (Booth 1985, Reed & Payton 1998). Certainly, increasing the proportion of qualified nursing staff alone appears to have little impact on quality of care. Sixsmith et al (1993) studied staff activity in six nursing homes for the elderly mentally ill, three of which had received additional resources as part of an initiative aimed at promoting 'positive care'. The researchers found that the extra resources available within the experimental homes were used largely for routine care, such as resident hygiene, rather than 'positive', life-enhancing care such as social interaction and group activities. They conclude that, in order to increase 'positive care', it is necessary to employ staff with that specific function.
>
> Zinn (1993) found no consistent relationship between staffing levels and selected quality indicators including prevalence of catheterization, restraint usage and incidence of pressure sores. Data were drawn from 10 metropolitan areas in the US and also revealed wide variation in staff to resident ratios. A large retrospective survey of more than 12 000 nursing home residents in one state in the US (Bliesmer et al 1998) did find a relationship between licensed nursing hours (i.e. the amount of nursing time provided by qualified nurses) and resident outcomes, including functional ability, probability of being discharged home and death. However, the sample included acutely ill residents and when limited to chronic residents, this relationship virtually disappeared.
>
> In one of the few qualitative studies to consider issues related to staffing within nursing homes, Grau et al (1995) explored residents perceptions of their quality of care by asking 46 residents to describe both their best and worst experiences since nursing home placement. Of particular relevance to the current discussion is the finding that the most frequently reported worst experiences concerned care provided by unqualified nursing aides. However, an important limitation of this study is the researchers' failure to acknowledge that residents will have had more experience of care provided by nursing aides and are therefore more likely to recall critical incidents related to them.

SOME POINTS ABOUT STYLE

As with any piece of writing, it is important to ensure that a literature review is written in a clear and readable style and is structured to maintain the reader's interest. It is also important to maintain a balanced approach. Structured checklists for critiquing research reports can make reviewers very cynical about the literature by encouraging a focus on weaknesses and

limitations of a study rather than strengths. However, rigorous research is very difficult to achieve and there is a danger that structured checklists may be over-critical. A balanced view is required which acknowledges the validity of current knowledge in addition to any limitations.

Downs (1994) highlights the issue of balance in relation to citation of references within a review of the literature (Box 11.6). She suggests that some

Box 11.5 Concluding sections of literature review on the continuing care needs of older people and their families (from Bowsher (1994) A theoretical model of independence for nursing home elders. © Springer Publishing Company, Inc., New York 10012, used by permission)

Theoretical and methodological critique

Most of the research reviewed is cross-sectional with few longitudinal studies tracing the experiences of older people over time. There is also evidence of sampling bias in a number of studies, the majority using purposive or accidental sampling. Overall, the body of research evidence examined revealed a limited focus on the perceptions of older people themselves, particularly those with any degree of cognitive impairment. The views of minority groups such as gay and lesbian older people and older people from ethnic minorities are notable by their absence. Research carried out in the UK, particularly in nursing homes is limited, with most work originating from the US and Canada, the Scandinavian countries and Australia.

In terms of the development of theory in relation to the needs of older people living in care homes and their families, a number of conceptual and theoretical frameworks are identified in the literature. However, these are mostly derived from research carried out in settings other than care homes and there is a need for more explicit empirical testing of a range of theoretical ideas within this setting.

In spite of these limitations, the literature reveals a remarkable consensus about the factors which contribute to enabling older people to maintain their quality of life after moving into a care home. These factors will now be summarized.

Conclusions

The literature demonstrates the complexity of ensuring that older people residing in nursing homes enjoy a good quality of life. However, a consistent theme is the need to ensure that nursing care is tailored to individual needs. This requires comprehensive and regular assessment of needs in collaboration with the older person and their family. The significance of interpersonal relationships, both within and outside the home, also seems clear. Enabling continuity of resident/staff relationships through the retention of a stable workforce is likely to enhance quality of care and quality of life. Nonetheless, it is likely that the benefits of a stable workforce will not be fully realized in the absence of regular training and clinical supervision. In particular, unqualified staff need access to education which encourages them to value the older person's individuality and unique contribution to the life of the home. Stability among the staff of a home is likely to be enhanced by the introduction of a career structure for care assistants and the development of senior care assistant roles is already taking place within some homes, although systematic evaluation of such roles is limited. Such initiatives are likely to proliferate as the recommendations of the most recent strategy for nursing (DoH 1999) come into effect. In particular, the proposal for more flexible programmes of nurse education and training are likely to encourage more care assistants to study for vocational qualifications.

Collectively, the evidence reviewed here suggests that we need to develop new cultures of care within care homes, which involve and value older people and their families, as well as valuing the providers of care. Willis and Linwood (1994), for example, contrast the medical and holistic models of care prevalent within services for older people, with what they term the emancipatory model of care. This model assumes a horizontal relationship between the care provider and the older person and their family, with the role of the care provider being a supportive one. The emphasis is on interpersonal relationships and achieving a balance between preventive, curative and restorative care in full consultation with the older person.

At the beginning of the 21st century, no older person living in a care home should be subject to the 'personalized warehousing' approach to care first described so vividly by Miller and Gwynne in 1972, yet still so prevalent in many care homes today. It is no longer acceptable for any resident to merely have their physical needs met, particularly when the potential for enhancing quality of life through simple interventions is so enormous.

In summary, the aims of long-term care should include for older people to be able to:

- continue to develop competencies in new and different ways
- contribute to the development and maintenance of positive social support networks and social climates within their own social groups and nursing facility

- attain from their environment some of the things that are important or valued by them
- maintain some degree of congruence between desired and achieved goals
- experience satisfactions and positive affects even in their frailty
- generate some stories to tell about this time of their lives that are as interesting as those of their younger years.

Achieving these objectives, even with the most frail older person, should not be beyond our resources.

Box 11.6 How not to include references! (Downs 1994)

Researchers (Findings and Lookin 1990; Seeker, Findings, Lookin & Arena, 1991; Wiseman, Searcher & Findings, 1992) often know a lot about their subject by the time they complete a study (Finis, Enders, Dunn, Over & Caput 1990; Terminus, Complete, Enders, Dunn & Last, 1989). For instance, Findings and Lookin (1990) and Seeker et al (1991) believe it is difficult, if not impossible, to sum up that much information. Oodles, Much and Complex (1922) documented this in their seminal work, which was replicated by More, Less and Somme (1942). Social influence (Complete, Overmuch & Somme, 1952; Push, Pull & Shake, 1967), anxiety (Worried, Shook & Rattled, 1987), and weariness (Tired, Worn & Shot, 1978) all play a role in the problem of condensing findings. Lost, Worried, Shook and Rattled (1988) confirmed these results. Given the plethora of information (Complete, Overmuch & More, 1952; Push, Pull and Heave, 1967; Worried, Shook and Catalysis, 1987), we definitely have sufficient evidence to indicate immediate action is necessary.

Klausner and Green (1991) suggest a series of criteria for evaluating literature reviews which can be helpful in attempting to construct your own review. An adapted version is included as Box 11.7.

Summary

As with any academic paper, a literature review should be clearly structured. The introduction should identify the focus and rationale for the review as well as the methods and boundaries. The main body of the review should be structured according to the key themes to emerge from the literature examined. Within each section, individual studies can then be compared and contrasted to identify consistent and contradictory findings. The final section should summarize the key points to emerge from the theoretical and methodological critique of individual items and identify implications of the review for practice, education and further research.

Exercise 11.4

Using one of the literature reviews listed at the end of this chapter, apply the criteria in Box 11.7 to critique the review. Alternatively, apply the criteria to a literature review which you have written yourself. How could the review be improved?

PUTTING REVIEWS INTO PRACTICE

Issues relating to the use of research to inform practice are covered in detail in Chapters 13 and 14. However, an interesting suggestion for ensuring that systematic reviews inform nursing practice described by Swanson et al (1990) is worth mentioning here. The authors describe a research teaching strategy

statements are so obvious that they do not need to be supported with references. General comments can be used to introduce a paragraph without an accompanying string of citations. Authors can then be referred to one by one in the subsequent paragraph and the context of the opening statement is made clear. Downs suggests that it is generally unnecessary to cite more than four references to support previously established relationships. You should use the most recent and credible work as evidence. A literature review dominated by a laundry list of citations is boring reading and signals the author's inability to synthesize the content (Downs 1994). It is also important to be concise and to summarize. In other words: review the literature – do not reproduce it.

> ### Box 11.7 Criteria for evaluating literature reviews (Klausner & Green 1991)
>
> #### Introduction
>
> - Is the rationale stated clearly so that the relevance of the review is determined quickly?
> - Is the rationale important (significant)?
> - Is the purpose of the review stated clearly?
> - Is the policy context for the review clearly identified?
>
> #### Methodology
>
> - Were the criteria for the selection of references clearly identified?
> - Did the author(s) critically assess the studies included in the review?
> - Are the limits of the review clearly identified (in terms of time period covered, databases searched)?
>
> #### Discussion or conclusions
>
> - Did the author(s) integrate the selected references or merely restate the individual findings and conclusions?
> - Were the conclusions supported by the references reviewed?
> - Application
> - What information have you learned from this article that can be applied to practice?

whereby nursing students are attached to nurses in a practice setting and collaborate to review the literature relating to a clinically defined problem. The resulting information is then shared with the practice team. Such initiatives can ensure that the work invested in reviewing the literature on a particular topic or problem has a direct impact on practice.

CONCLUSION

With the current emphasis on evidence-based practice, the ability to review and synthesize the available literature on a particular topic is an essential skill for all those involved in health care. This chapter has outlined a systematic, step-by-step approach to reviewing literature that should enable 'beginning' reviewers to overcome the first hurdle of knowing where to start. By following the steps outlined here, the critical reviewer should be able to produce a concise summary of the literature that evaluates both the theoretical basis of knowledge in a particular topic area and the methods used to generate that knowledge. Appropriate indicators for practice, education and research can then be identified in the light of the strengths and limitations of the body of literature reviewed. The next step is to ensure that these indicators are translated into action, where appropriate, and this particular challenge forms the focus of the final two chapters of this book.

References

Aneshensel CS, Pearly LI, Mullan JT et al (1995) *Profiles in Caregiving: the Unexpected Career.* San Diego: Academic Press.

Becker H (1986) *Writing for Social Scientists: How to Start and Finish your Thesis, Book, or Article.* Chicago: University of Chicago Press.

Bliesmer MM, Smayling M, Kane RL et al (1998) The relationship between nursing staffing levels and nursing home outcomes. *Journal of Aging and Health* **10**(3): 351–371.

Bogo M (1987) Social work practice and family systems in adaptation to homes for the aged. *Journal of Gerontological Social Work* **10**(1/2): 5–20.

Booth T (1985) *Home Truths. Old Peoples' Homes and the Outcome of Care.* Aldershot: Gower.

Bowsher JE (1994) A theoretical model of independence for nursing home elders. *Scholarly Inquiry for Nursing Practice* **8**(2): 207–224.

Brown J and Furstenberg A (1992) Restoring control: empowering older patients and their families during health crisis. *Social Work in Health Care* **17**(4): 81–101.

Burns and Grove (2001) The practice of nursing research: conduct critique and utilisation, 4th edn. Philadelphia, PA: WB Saunders.

Caris Verhallen W, Kerkstra A and Bensing J (1997) The role of communication in nursing care for older people: a review of the literature. *Journal of Advanced Nursing* **25**(5): 915–933.

Chalmers I and Altman D (1995) *Systematic Reviews.* London: BMJ Books.

Chen K and Snyder M (1996) Perception of personal control and satisfaction with care among nursing home elders. *Perspectives* **20**(2): 16–19.

Clarke E (1993) *Family ties between nursing home residents and their relatives: a comparative perspective.* University of York: Unpublished PhD thesis.

Cosbey J (1994) *Letting go: how caregivers make the decision for nursing home placement.* The University of Akron: Unpublished PhD thesis.

Cuba L (1993) *A Short Guide to Writing about Social Science,* 2nd edn. New York: Harper Collins.

Cullum N (1994) Critical reviews of the literature. In: Hardey M and Mulhall A (eds) *Nursing Research: Theory and Practice*. London: Chapman & Hall.

Davies S (2001) Caring for older people with continuing care needs and their families. In: Nolan M, Davies S and Grant G (eds) *Working with Older People and their Families*. Buckingham: Open University Press.

Department of Health (1999) *Making a Difference: strengthening the nursing, midwifery and health visiting contribution to health and healthcare*. London: The Stationery Office.

DePoy E and Gitlin L (1994) *Introduction to Research: Multiple Strategies for Health and Human Services*. St Louis, MO: Mosby.

Downs FS (1994) Information processing. *Nursing Research* **43**(6): 323.

Droogan J and Song F (1996) The process and importance of systematic reviews. *Nurse Researcher* **4**(1): 15–26.

Drysdale AE, Nelson CF and Wineman NM (1993) Families need help too: group treatment for families of nursing home residents. *Clinical Nurse Specialist* **7**(3): 130–134.

Elliott K (1995) Maintaining cultural and personal continuity in a Danish nursing home. *Journal of Women and Ageing* **71**(1/2): 169–185.

Ganong LH (1987) Integrative reviews of nursing research. *Research in Nursing and Health* **10**: 1–11.

Ghusn HF, Hyde D, Stevens ES et al (1996) Enhancing satisfaction in later life: what makes a difference for nursing home residents? *Journal of Gerontological Social Work* **26**(1/2): 27–47.

Gladstone JW (1995) The marital perceptions of elderly persons living or having a spouse living in a long-term care institution in Canada. *The Gerontologist* **35**(1): 52–60.

Grau LB, Chandler B and Saunders C (1995) Nursing home residents' perceptions of the quality of their care. *Journal of Psychosocial Nursing and Mental Health Services* **33**(5): 34–43.

Hek G, Langton H and Blunden G (2000) Systematically searching and reviewing literature. *Nurse Researcher* **7**(3): 40–57.

Hignett S (2003) Systematic review of patient handling activities starting in lying, sitting and standing positions. *Journal of Advanced Nursing* **41**(6): 545–552.

Hunt J (1981) Indicators for nursing practice: the use of research findings. *Journal of Advanced Nursing* **12**(1): 101–110.

Jackson GB (1980) Methods for integrative reviews. *Review of Educational Research* **50**: 438–460.

Johanson L (1985) Ten hints for thesis survival. *Nursing Outlook* **33**(4): 206, 208.

Kaplan L and Ade-Ridder L (1991) The impact on the marriage when one spouse moves to a nursing home. *Journal of Women and Ageing* **3**(3): 81–101.

Klausner LH and Green TG (1991) An instructional method for teaching literature evaluation. *Journal of Continuing Education in the Health Professions* **11**(4): 331–339.

Lederman R (1992) Reviews of research literature: meta-analysis for synthesising. *American Journal of Maternal and Child Nursing* **17**(3): 157.

McDonnell A, Nicholl J and Read S (2003) Acute pain teams and the management of post-operative pain: a systematic review and meta-analysis. *Journal of Advanced Nursing* **41**(3): 261–273.

Meleis AI and Trangenstein PA (1994) Facilitating transitions: redefining the nursing mission. *Nursing Outlook* **42**(6): 255–259.

Miller EJ and Gwynne GV (1972) *A Life apart: a pilot study of residential institutions for the physically handicapped and the young chronic sick*. London: Tavistock.

Morgan M and Zimmerman M (1990) Easing the transition to nursing homes: identifying the needs of spousal caregivers at the time of institutionalisation. *Clinical Gerontologist* **9**: 1–7.

Murphy KP, Hanrahan P and Luchins D (1997) A survey of grief and bereavement in nursing homes: the importance of hospice grief and bereavement for the end-stage Alzheimer's disease patient and family. *Journal of the American Geriatrics Society* **45**(9): 1104–1107.

Nelson HW (2000) Injustice and conflict in nursing homes: towards advocacy and exchange. *Journal of Aging Studies* **14**(1): 39–61.

Nolan M, Nolan J and Booth A (1997) *Preparation for Multi-Professional/Multi-Agency Health Care Practice:The Nursing Contribution to Rehabilitation within the Multi-Disciplinary Team. Literature Review and Curriculum Analysis*. Final Report to the English National Board for Nursing, Midwifery and Health Visiting, London.

Oleson M and Shadick KM (1993) Application of Moos and Schaefer's (1986) model to nursing care of elderly persons relocating to a nursing home. *Journal of Advanced Nursing* **18**(3): 479–485.

Onega LL and Tripp Reimer T (1997) Expanding the scope of continuity theory: application to gerontological nursing. *Journal of Gerontological Nursing* **23**(6): 29–35.

Pearson A, Hocking S, Mott S et al (1992) Skill mix in Australian nursing homes. *Journal of Advanced Nursing* **17**: 767–776.

Polit DF and Hungler BP (1999) *Nursing Research: Principles and Methods*. Philadelphia, PA: Lippincott.

Rader J, Lavelle M, Hoeffer B et al (1996) Maintaining cleanliness: an individualized approach. *Journal of Gerontological Nursing* **22**(3): 32–38.

Rantz MJ, Zwygart-Stauffacher Popejoy L, Grando VT et al (1999) Nursing home care quality: a multidimensional theoretical model integrating the views of consumers and providers. *Journal of Nursing Care Quality* **14**(1): 16–37.

Reed J and Payton VR (1995) *Working to create continuity: older people managing the move to the care home setting*. Newcastle-upon-Tyne: Centre for Health Services Research, University of Northumbria.

Reed J and Payton VR (1996) Constructing familiarity and managing the self: ways of adapting to life in nursing and residential homes for older people. *Ageing and Society* **16**(5): 543–560.

Reed J and Payton VR (1998) Understanding the dynamics of life in care homes for older people: implications for de-institutionalising practice. *Health and Social Care in the Community* **5**(4): 261–268.

Reed J, Cook G and Stanley D (1999) Promoting partnership with older people through quality assurance systems: issues arising in care homes. *NT Research* **4**(5): 257–267.

Reinardy JR (1995) Relocation to a new environment: decisional control and the move to a nursing home. *Health and Social Work* **20**(1): 31–38.

Richardson JP (1992) Health promotion for the nursing home patient. *Journal of the American Board of Family Practitioners* **5**(2): 127–136.

Roe B (1994) Undertaking a critical review of the literature. *Nurse Researcher* **1**(1): 35–46.

Ross HM, Rosenthal CJ and Dawson P (1997) Spousal caregiving in the residential setting – visiting. *Journal of Clinical Nursing* **6**(6): 473–483.

Sapsford R (1994) Making sense of the literature. *Nurse Researcher* **1**(1): 23–30.

Schumacher KL and Meleis AI (1994) Transitions: a central concept in nursing. *Image: Journal of Nursing Scholarship* **26**(2): 119–127.

Sixsmith A, Hawley C, Stilwell J et al (1993) Delivering positive care in nursing-homes. *International Journal of Geriatric Psychiatry* **8**(5): 407–412.

Stirling G and Reid DW (1992) The application of participatory control to facilitate patient well-being: an experimental study of nursing impact on geriatric patients. *Canadian Journal of Behavioural Science* **24**(2): 204–219.

Swanson J, Easterling P, Costa L et al (1990) Student-staff collaboration in identifying nursing problems and reviewing the literature. *Western Journal of Nursing Research* **12**(2): 262–266.

Willis LD and Linwood ME (1994) *Measuring the Quality of Care*. New York: Churchill Livingstone.

Zinn J (1993) Inter-SMSA a variation in nursing home staffing and resident care management practices. *The Journal of Applied Gerontology* **12**(2): 206–224.

Further reading

Articles and chapters about writing literature reviews

Cuba L (1993) *A Short Guide to Writing about Social Science.* New York: Harper Collins.

Cullum N (1994) Critical reviews of the literature. In: Hardey M and Mulhall A (eds) *Nursing Research: Theory and Practice*. London: Chapman & Hall.

Hek G, Langton H and Blunden G (2000) Systematically searching and reviewing literature. *Nurse Researcher* **7**(3): 40–57.

Examples of literature reviews

When writing a review for the first time it can be helpful to look at published examples and some useful reviews are listed here. Bear in mind, though, the limitations of many published reviews identified by Cullum (1994).

Aspinal F, Addington-Hall J, Hughes R et al (2003) Using satisfaction to measure the quality of palliative care: a review of the literature. *Journal of Advanced Nursing* **42**(4): 324–339.

Caris Verhallen W, Kerkstra A and Bensing J (1997) The role of communication in nursing care for older people: a review of the literature. *Journal of Advanced Nursing* **25**: 915–933.

Davies S, Laker S and Ellis L (1997) Promoting autonomy and independence for older people within nursing practice: a literature review. *Journal of Advanced Nursing* **26**(2): 408–417.

Holden J, Harrison L and Johnson M (2002) Families, nurses and intensive care patients: a review of the literature. *Journal of Clinical Nursing* **11**(2): 140–148.

Kelly M and May D (1982) Good and bad patients: a review of the literature and a theoretical critique. *Journal of Advanced Nursing* **7**: 147–156.

McMullan M, Endacott R, Gray M et al (2003) Portfolios and assessment of competence: a review of the literature. *Journal of Advanced Nursing* **41**(3): 283–294.

Chapter 12

Evidence–based practice and critical appraisal of quantitative review articles (systematic reviews)

Peter Bradley

INTRODUCTION

WHAT IS EVIDENCE-BASED PRACTICE?

Evidence-based practice emphasizes a philosophy where health professionals' decisions are based on research results, their clinical expertise and patient preferences. In the context of medical care, evidence-based practice has been defined as follows:

> *Evidence based medicine (EBM) is the integration of best research evidence with clinical expertise and patient values.*
>
> (Sackett et al 2000)

Evidence-based practice is therefore seen as a means to improve clinical practice, where scientific literature (evidence) forms the basis for clinical decisions. It is not the intention that research results will be able to replace professional skills and negate patient choice. Quite the reverse, in fact, only by using clinical knowledge and listening to patients can practitioners use research results appropriately.

The five basic steps in evidence-based practice are described as follows:

1. **Ask a clear question** – a specific clinical problem forms the basis for a clear question
2. **Search for evidence** – the question identified is used as a basis to search for evidence (scientific articles)
3. **Critically appraise evidence** – the research articles found are judged in terms of quality (critically appraised)

4. **Use evidence in practice** – the results from the 'good quality' articles are used to supplement clinical expertise and patient opinion in the management of the original clinical problem
5. **Evaluate practice** – the effect of clinical management is noted, and refined.

Steps 1 and 2 are covered in Chapters 3 and 4 of this text. In this chapter, we will concentrate on steps 3 and 4 – how to critically appraise evidence and use the results in practice. Before we do this, it is important to note that there are many reasons why health care professionals do not use research results in clinical practice. This topic is expanded upon in Ann McDonnells's chapter (13). Research on the implementation of evidence-based practice identifies the following as important barriers: clinicians' lack of time, lack of financial incentive and lack of confidence and skills in evidence-based practice and lack of support from employers. One further barrier is limited access to information (NHS CRD 1999). It is estimated that thousands of new articles are produced every week, which for many professionals leads to 'information overload'. Review articles are seen as one way of increasing accessibility to research. These summarize the results from several articles and thereby increase the accessibility of research evidence. However, the production of review articles alone is not enough to promote evidence-based practice. Before health care workers' behaviour can be influenced, review results need to be disseminated and implemented (NHS CRD 1999).

Key issues

- What is evidence-based practice?
- The purpose of review articles
- Critically appraising a systematic review using an evaluation tool

REVIEW ARTICLES

The main purpose of review articles is to present the results of several *primary studies* in one article to present more valid evidence than is available from individual studies. Reviews can consist of studies using any type of study design, but this chapter will concentrate on reviews consisting of controlled trials and reporting on the *effect* of interventions (see question 2 below). In other words, reviews which answer the following type of question: does

this treatment, rehabilitation or preventive measure work? What are the effects and side-effects? The majority of systematic reviews currently published (including those available in the Cochrane Library) consider questions about effect.

Some reviews use a methodology which aims to give a balanced assessment of all available evidence. These are known as *systematic reviews* because they use an explicit and systematic methodology to find available studies and evaluate the quality of studies before including their results in the final review. (It is, however, possible for a poor quality review to give an unbalanced, biased view of available evidence).

The evidence-based approach emphasizes that research of poor quality should not be used to inform clinical decisions and it is important to differentiate between good- and bad-quality research. The process which sorts the 'wheat from the chaff', i.e. identifies trustworthy (*valid*) and untrustworthy (*invalid*) studies is referred to as *critical appraisal*. Concerning quantitative studies, or studies containing numbers, there are three main reasons for rejecting studies as invalid. The first reason is that the article does not have a clear objective or question which it is trying to answer. The second reason is that the scientific method used to carry out the study contains systematic errors (*bias*) which are likely to lead to false conclusions. The methodological quality of the study is referred to as its *internal validity*. The third reason for rejection is that the results of the study are not easily implemented in practice. The ease with which results can be used in practice is

Summary

Systematic reviews are able to provide condensed, summarized information on specific topics, which help answer specific clinical questions (Egger & Davey-Smith 1998). The majority of systematic reviews consider whether health interventions are effective and are based on controlled trials. Systematic reviews are of variable quality and critical appraisal is an important skill in differentiating between poor- and high-quality reviews. Poor quality systematic reviews should not be used to inform future policy as they may advise the use of ineffective or even harmful interventions. High-quality systematic reviews will always help decision making, even if only to highlight the paucity of existing research.

You have been contacted by a self-help group for depression. The group has read and become interested in an article which reports the benefits of St John's wort in improving the symptoms of depression. The article has the following reference:

Linde K, Ramirez G, Mulrow CD, Pauls A, Wiedenhammer W and Melchart D (1996) St John's wort for depression – an overview and meta-analysis of randomised controlled trials. *British Medical Journal* **313**: 253–258

The group wants to know what you think about the use of St John's wort and about the article's conclusions.

1. Does St John's wort help people with depression?
2. If you were depressed would you take St John's wort?

known as the *external validity* or *generalizability* of the study. The rest of this chapter will discuss critical appraisal, using a sample systematic review.

CRITICAL APPRAISAL OF A SYSTEMATIC REVIEW: AN EXAMPLE

In this section we will critically appraise a systematic review (Linde et al 1996), by using a checklist which systematically assesses the review's quality. The checklist is based on one produced by the Critical Appraisal Skills Programme (CASP 2003). This is one example of a checklist; further examples are given at the end of the chapter in the Further reading section. Before we continue, consider the scenario in Box 12.1. Take some time to read the systematic review by Linde et al (1996) provided as an appendix to this chapter (this should take about 45 minutes) and answer the questions asked in the scenario presented in Box 12.1. Having done that, read to the end of this chapter and then return to these questions and compare your answers with those presented in the text.

The checklist consists of 10 questions, which are designed to help us think about these issues systematically. The checklist is split into four main parts and helps us decide:

- Whether the article is worth critically appraising (screening questions: 1 and 2) – the first two

questions are screening questions and should be answered quickly. If you can answer 'yes' to both questions it is worth continuing with a detailed critical appraisal of the article.
- Whether the study's methodology can be trusted to give a reasonably valid answer (questions on internal validity: 3 to 5)
- What the results are (questions on effect size: 6 and 7)
- Whether the results can be used in your local situation (questions on external validity: 8 to 10).

SCREENING QUESTIONS

1. Did the systematic review address a clearly focused question?

Consider whether the question is 'focused' in terms of:

- *The population studied*
- *The intervention given (or exposure)*
- *The outcomes considered.*

We need to be sure what central question is being addressed when we read any type of study. There is no point in appraising an article with a poorly focused question, which does not define the population (study participants), intervention (e.g. treatment) or outcomes considered. A fourth helpful but non-essential element is that the treatment under consideration is compared with an alternative treatment. These three (four) elements should be identifiable in the article and are referred to as a '*three (or four)-part question*'.

In Linde et al (1996), the study population, intervention and outcomes are described in the section 'objectives' in the abstract. The questions addressed in the study can thus be formulated as follows.

Is St John's wort (*intervention*) effective in treating depression (*population – people with depression, outcome – treating depression*) when compared to (1) placebo or (2) other antidepressants (*alternative treatments*)?

This four-part question is a satisfactory beginning to the critical appraisal of the systematic review.

2. Did the systematic review include the right type of study?

Consider whether the included studies:

- *Address the review's question*
- *Have an appropriate study design.*

As mentioned earlier, systematic review articles can in theory include any type of study design.

Table 12.1   Which study design is appropriate to answer which question

Question	Preferred design(s)
Why do some people become ill, whilst other remain well? (questions about cause)	Cohort studies Case-control studies
How can we decide whether a person is ill? (questions about diagnosis)	Diagnositic studies (comparison with a gold standard)
How can an illness be prevented, treated or rehabilitated? (questions about effect)	Controlled trials
What do we expect to happen with someone who is ill? (questions about prognosis)	Cohort studies
What is it like being ill? (questions about experiences)	Qualitative studies
How many people are ill? (questions about prevalence/incidence)	Cross-sectional studies

However, the studies included in the systematic review must be appropriate to answer the question(s) identified.

Table 12.1 categorizes the questions most frequently asked in health care and considers which study design is usually considered most appropriate to answer them. The choice of study design is, of course, somewhat more complex in practice, being dependent on many issues – ethical, medical, scientific, economic and political. There is usually more than one study design capable of answering a specific question and Table 12.1 should only be used as a guide.

In order to assess whether the authors in Linde et al (1996) have included the right type of study, we need to find a statement where the reviewers explicitly state inclusion and exclusion criteria for the systematic review, with respect to population, intervention, outcome and study design. The exclusion criteria, listed under 'criteria for trial inclusion' under 'methods', provide this information. Studies will be included if they compare treatment using St John's wort (as a single preparation or in combination) with (1) inactive treatment (placebo) or (2) other established antidepressants. The authors considered the following reported outcomes as relevant to the systematic review – the number of participants with depression, the number of participants who drop out of the studies and the reported side-effects. In addition, the authors have chosen to look for randomized controlled trials and quasi-controlled trials. Since the research question was about the effect of St John's wort, this appears to be an appropriate choice (see Table 12.1).

Randomized controlled trials (RCTs) are considered an appropriate study design, because they (1) do not rely on before and after measurements but are able to compare outcomes after treatment with a control group (receiving no treatment or a different treatment) and (2) measure the actual effects of the treatments under study by minimizing the effects of external factors which may influence the results.

In the *controlled trials* included in the Linde et al (1996) systematic review, researchers have compared treatment outcomes in two study groups (e.g. St John's wort and placebo) *after* treatment. If the review had included *uncontrolled* trials which measured depression before and after treatment with St John's wort *with no control group comparison*, it would have been much more difficult to judge the effectiveness of St John's wort. Before-and-after measurements alone would not have allowed us to judge whether St John's wort produces changes in depression symptoms or whether the changes were due to other factors (for example, spontaneous improvement of depression as part of the natural progression of the disease).

The trials included in the Linde et al systematic review (1996) were *randomized* controlled trials. Randomization means, in practice, that every individual study participant has an equal chance of receiving active treatment or being in the control group regardless of whether they are male or female, old or young, how ill they are, etc. In other words, the randomization process is an attempt to ensure that *patient characteristics* (sex, age, etc.) and other factors which may influence the results of the trial are randomly distributed between study groups, whether or not those factors are known to the researcher.

In contrast, *non-randomized* controlled trials can produce a systematic imbalance in patient characteristics or other factors, which can affect the result of the study. For example, a non-randomized trial might compare St John's wort and placebo as treatments for improving depression for 200 patients, of whom 100 have mild depression and 100 have moderate depression. Clinicians may, unwittingly, have allocated patients to treatments according to the severity of their illness or for other reasons.

If 90% (i.e. 90 patients) of those with moderate depression were allocated to receive more active treatment, namely St John's wort, and 90% (90 patients) of those with mild depression were allocated to receive placebo, the two study groups would no longer be similar in terms of disease severity. The participants in the St John's wort group, who were more severely depressed, would then have more potential for improvement. If St John's wort was an ineffective treatment but depression improved spontaneously, the active treatment group would show a greater improvement than the control group, falsely showing St John's wort to be effective. If there was no spontaneous improvement of depression, St John's wort would be falsely shown to be harmful because the treated group would end up with more severe depression, purely because they were more severely depressed to begin with. Non-randomized trials can theoretically give us false results in either direction but tend to exaggerate the *treatment effect* (see questions 6 and 7) (Kunz & Oxman 1998).

In order to randomize and allocate participants to the study groups, researchers usually use computer generated random numbers or paper-based random number tables. Other, less robust methods can also be used, for example, using day of the week or the participant's date of birth to decide group allocation or simply allocating every other participant to the intervention group. These trials are known as *quasi* or *pseudo-randomized* trials. Such trials were included in the systematic review by Linde et al (1996). In theory, such randomization methods can lead to unbalanced study groups if patient characteristics or other factors affect both the study outcomes *and* the likelihood of being allocated to one of the study groups, e.g. if every second person on the recruitment list is a woman. However, this is not normally regarded as a major methodological problem (threat to *internal validity*).

If the inclusion of quasi-randomized trials in a systematic review is considered of potential importance, the results from randomized and quasi-randomization designs can be compared using statistical techniques (*sensitivity analysis*). The choice to include all types of controlled trials in the Linde et al systematic review should not prevent us looking at the rest of the article. More information about sensitivity analysis can be found in a handbook by the Australian National Health and Medical Research Council (NHMRC 1999).

QUESTIONS ON INTERNAL VALIDITY

3. Did the authors identify all relevant studies?

Consider:

- *Which bibliographic databases and search terms were used*
- *Whether personal contact was made with experts*
- *Whether the reviewers searched for unpublished studies*
- *Whether the reviewers searched for non-English language studies*
- *Whether the reviewers obtained relevant articles referred to in other included studies.*

An important attribute of systematic reviews is that they are able to produce a comprehensive and balanced view of the available research. It is therefore necessary for systematic reviews to be based on extensive literature searches, which represent a balanced range of studies. This can present a considerable challenge. MEDLINE, one of the largest bibliographic databases in medicine, indexes in the region of 8000 journals but represents a fraction of the total number of journals produced worldwide (Egger & Davey-Smith 1998). Many journals are not indexed in any databases and many studies are never published. It might seem more practical in systematic reviews to concentrate on literature available from the main bibliographic databases. However, empirical research has shown that articles which show 'positive' results in trials are more likely to get published per se, more likely to get published in journals which are indexed in databases and more likely to get published if they are in English (Egger & Davey-Smith 1998). Studies which show negative or inconclusive results are therefore underrepresented in indexed literature. This concept is known as *publication bias*. An additional problem is that articles are indexed in databases in a somewhat untidy way, which means that several *search terms* need to be included in a search strategy to ensure that the majority of relevant articles have been found. The aim of a search is to find a balanced set of studies for assessment.

In practice, this means that systematic reviewers wishing to present a balanced view of available literature need to:

- perform comprehensive searches in several databases using several search terms
- obtain relevant articles referred to in other studies and include non-English language and unpublished studies
- contact experts, who may know of unpublished trials.

In Linde et al (1996), further details are given of their 'search strategy' under 'methods'. Published and unpublished studies were sought in databases and by contact with experts. The following databases were searched: MEDLINE (Silver Platter), Psychlit, Psychindex, EMBASE, Phytodok. The bibliographies of obtained articles were checked. Pharamaceutical companies and study authors were also contacted. There were no language restrictions on the search and it is interesting to note that many of the included trials were published only in German language journals (look in the reference list). The search terms used for database searching are also described. In conclusion, the search strategy is fairly thorough and more comprehensive than we would usually see for an article published in 1996. However, the search is not perfect. Journals could have been searched by hand, as studies about herbal preparations are poorly indexed in the bibliographic databases. If the article had been written today, the Cochrane Controlled Trials Registry (CCTR) would need to be searched, as this is now the world's most comprehensive register of controlled trials.

So what is good enough? It is sometimes difficult to judge whether a systematic review's search strategy is sufficient to answer the question posed, but the following omissions should make us suspicious: restriction to one bibliographic database, to one language or to published articles only, no contact with experts and no details of the search terms used. A 'biased' selection of studies can sometimes be the result of even a thorough search strategy. If this is suspected, statistical methods, such as *funnel plots*, can also be used to assess whether a balanced selection of studies has been found by the reviewers. Further information on funnel plots can be found in a handbook by the Australian National Health and Medical Research Council (NHMRC 1999). The Council looked at the systematic review by Linde

et al (1996) and considered that there was a suggestion of publication bias in the review. In practice, this may mean that the quoted treatment effect (see questions 6 and 7) is exaggerated, because studies showing equivocal results may have been missed (NHMRC 1999).

4. Did the reviewers assess the quality of the included studies?

Consider whether a clear, predetermined strategy was used to determine which studies were included. Look for:

- *use of a prevalidated checklist*
- *more than one assessor.*

First, the authors of any systematic review should exclude all primary studies found in the search which do not meet the predetermined inclusion criteria, e.g. those that do not address the question or use a different study design. The authors of the systematic review then need to critically appraise the remaining articles with respect to their internal and external validity and results. Data from studies of poor quality can then be excluded or analysed separately. Since critical appraisal can become a somewhat subjective process, especially when deciding which studies are of good enough quality to include in the systematic review, it is desirable that two independent assessors appraise the articles using a *prevalidated* checklist, i.e. one that has been pilot tested and has been shown statistically to measure what it is supposed to. There are several checklists which can be used to assess study quality which share many common elements (NHMRC 1999). Prevalidated generic checklists can be supplemented with 'locally-adapted' checklists, which look at methodological issues of particular importance to the topic under review.

In Linde et al (1996), the section 'assessment of methodological quality' under 'methods', describes how each study included in the systematic review was assessed by at least two independent reviewers. The reviewers used a prevalidated scale developed by Jadad (see [8] in Appendix) and a locally developed scale to carry out critical appraisal. The Jadad scale considered some of the most important elements in critically appraising randomized controlled trials – random allocation, blinding and description of dropouts and withdrawls) – and the locally developed scale looked at other issues of importance, e.g. *allocation concealment*, which refers to how the randomization was carried out in practice, for example whether opaque envelopes were used and the characteristics of study groups at *baseline* (start of the study). This in principle seems to have been a satisfactory process. A further description of how to critically appraise RCTs is not possible in this chapter, but a detailed checklist is available from the Critical Appraisal Skills Programme (CASP).

5. If the results have been combined, was it reasonable to do so?

Consider whether:

- *The results of each study are clearly displayed*
- *The results were similar from study to study (look for tests of heterogeneity)*
- *The reasons for any variation in results are discussed.*

Reviewers can decide to describe the results of included primary studies individually without trying to combine them numerically. However, reviewers often choose to do this so that a single quantitative measure of effect can be quoted for each outcome. This method is called metaanalysis, which is essentially a statistical method for combining numeric data from several primary studies. This method presupposes that the studies combined are sufficiently similar (for example, in terms of their study populations, interventions and outcomes) to allow metaanalysis to produce meaningful results.

Two issues allow us to decide whether it was reasonable to combine the results from primary studies in a metaanalysis. The first issue is whether it appears acceptable, using clinical common sense, to combine the results of the primary studies in a metaanalysis (considering the populations, interventions and outcomes used). The second issue is whether statistical tests indicate *heterogeneity* (i.e. considerable variation in the results of the various studies). If the results indicate heterogeneity, further investigation of the reasons for this is required. What is it about the primary studies that might make their results so different from each other? Is there an obvious reason for discrepancies?

In the systematic review by Linde et al (1996), the results of several studies are combined in metaanalyses. The results from the metaanalyses are shown in their Figure 2 and the characteristics of the individual studies in their Table 1. Table 1 describes studies which have considered different populations in terms of diagnosis, method of diagnosis (clinical impression, depression scales), disease severity, treatment setting, dose of St John's wort, treatment duration, follow-up time and, where applicable, comparison treatment. From a clinical point of view, we might then have some concerns that all these very different studies are included in a metaanalysis.

To consider whether there is statistical heterogeneity, we need to look at Linde et al's Figure 2, in which we see four separate metaanalyses which compare St John's wort to *placebo* (inactive treatment) or other preparations. Figure 2 first compares St John's wort alone with placebo (look under 'placebo controlled trials of single preparations'). We see here that the results from the different primary studies, at first sight, do seem to differ, but how can we assess whether this is important?

If differences in treatment effect are seen in individual studies, statistical tests for heterogeneity can be used to investigate whether differences are due to chance variation or other factors, which require further investigation. A statistical test for heterogeneity was not carried out by Linde et al (1996), but such a test ('Cochrane Q') has been calculated by the Australian National Health and Medical Research Council for the first comparison (St John's wort as a single preparation versus placebo) (NHMRC 1999). The results of this test show significant heterogeneity, indicating that the treatment effect of St John's wort compared to placebo varies in the different studies to such an extent that further investigation is warranted. It seems that the investigation of heterogeneity between studies is inadequate in the Linde et al (1996) review and it is probable that it was not appropriate to combine *all* the study results of St John's wort versus placebo in one metaanalysis. This methodological weakness may mean that the size of the treatment effect cannot be completely trusted, as dissimilar studies have been combined. A more detailed approach to the consideration of heterogeneity between study results has been described by the Australian National Health and Medical Research Council (NHMRC 1999).

QUESTIONS ON EFFECT SIZE

6. How are the results presented and what is the main result?

Consider:

- *How the results are expressed (e.g. odds ratio, relative risk, etc.)*
- *How large the size of result is and how meaningful it is*
- *How you would sum up the bottom-line result of the systematic review in one sentence.*

Many people with depression are treated in primary care settings.[2,3] Given the complexity of differential diagnosis and treatment of depression, it is often difficult for primary practitioners if antidepressant drugs are indicated. Some practitioners and patients are reluctant to use antidepressants because of associated side effects. Additional treatment modalities with little risk, credible benefit, and moderate costs could be a useful addition to depression management in primary care settings.

Extracts of the plant Hypericum perforatum (popularly called St John's wort), a member of the Hypericaceae family, have been used in folk medicine for a long time for a range of indications including depressive disorders (fig. 1). Extracts of St John's wort are licensed in Germany for the treatment of anxiety and depressive and sleep disorders. In 1993 more than 2.7 million prescriptions were counted for the seven most popular preparations in Germany.[4] Hypericum extracts contain at least 10 constituents or groups of components that may contribute to its pharmacological effects. These include naphthodi-anthrons (for example, hypericins, on whose content most of the available preparations are standardised), flavonoids (for example, quercetin), xan-thones, and bioflavonoids.[5] The mechanism of action of the postulated antidepressant effects is unclear.[6]

In the past 10 years several randomised clinical trials have compared the effects of pharmaceutical preparations of St John's wort with placebo and common antidepressants. Recently, a systematic review on these trials has been published in a phytomedical journal[7]; this review, however, focused on the assessment of methodological quality and did not include an analysis of effect sizes. Our objective was to provide a comprehensive overview including a quantitive meta-analysis of the existing evidence of the antidepressant activity of extracts of St John's wort. Specifically we investigated whether extracts of hypericum are more effective than placebo in the treatment of depression, are as effective as standard antidepressive treatment, and have fewer side effects compared with standard antidepressant drugs.

Methods

Search strategy

Published and unpublished eligible trials were searched for by full text searches in Medline Silver-Platter CD-ROM 1983–94 (screening titles and available abstracts of all hits from searches for the terms "St John's wort", Johanniskraut, "hyperic*"); full text

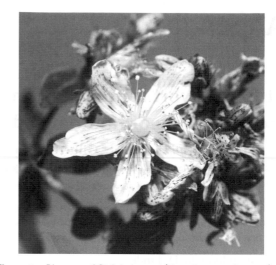

Figure 1   Blossom of St John's wort (Hypericum perforatum)

searches in Psychlit and Psychindex 1987–94 CD-ROM; additional online searches in Medline (1966 onwards) and Embase (1974 onwards); searches in the private database Phytodok, Munich; checking bibliographies of obtained articles; and contacting pharmaceutical companies and authors. There were no language restrictions.

Criteria for trial inclusion

The following parameters had to be met for study inclusion: firstly, design-randomised or quasi-randomised (for example, alternation) controlled trials; secondly, types of participants–people with depressive disorders; thirdly, types of interventions–comparison of preparations of St John's wort (alone or in combination with other plant extracts) with placebo or other antidepressants; and, finally, outcome measures – all clinical outcome measures such as depression scales or symptoms. Trials which measured physiological parameters only were excluded. At least two reviewers assessed the eligibility of each trial, and there were no disagreements. A complete list of all of the included trials is available from us.

Assessment of methodological quality

The methodological quality of each trial was assessed by at least two reviewers using a scale developed by Jadad et al[8] (with items on random allocation, blinding, and description of dropouts and withdrawals) and a scale developed by ourselves (additional items on concealment of randomisation and comparability at baseline).

Data extraction and summarising study results

Primary study characteristics and results were extracted by at least two independent reviewers. Questionnaires were then sent to authors or sponsors, or both, of all studies for checks of the correctness of extracted data and to obtain missing information (response rate 13/23 from both authors and drug manufacturers).

The trials used various methods to measure treatment effects. The most consistently used instruments were the Hamilton depression scale[9] (used in 17 trials) and the clinical global impressions index[9] (used in 12 trials).

The Hamilton depression scale is an observer rated scale focusing mainly on somatic symptoms. The original version includes 17 items, but a more recent one with 21 items is also in use. Most studies using this scale also report the number of "treatment responders" (patients with a score less than 10 or less than 50% of the baseline score, or both). If available, we extracted means (SD) before, during, and after treatment as well as the number of "responders".

The clinical global impressions index is an observer rated instrument with three items (severity of illness, global improvement, and an efficacy index). We extracted the number of patients rated as "much improved" or "very much improved" for global improvement.

Additionally, we extracted all reported means (SD) for other rating scales and numbers for "treatment responders" from other global assessments.

Analyses

For analyses comparing hypericum with placebo and standard antidepressants, numbers of treatment responders and treatment failures according to the Hamilton depression scale (first preference), the clinical global impressions index subscale for global improvement (second preference), or another global responder criteria were entered in a 2 × 2 table. Odds ratios and rate ratios (relative risks) were calculated on an intention to treat basis (with ratios greater than 1 representing a superiority of hypericum v control). A Mantel-Haenzsel method was used for odd ratio measures and a variance weighted procedure for rate ratios. Estimations of summary estimates were preceded by homogeneity testing by using an (alpha) level of 0.10. Summary measures of both fixed effects and random effects were estimated. For the present report the rate ratio represents the effect estimate.

Cohen's d (standardised mean difference) was calculated for all studies contributing to a continuous data hypothesis with a pooled SD. The summary effect sizes from these analyses were converted to rate ratios by using techniques for converting effect sizes to a binominal effect size display.[10] Additionally, variance weighted mean differences were calculated for scores on the Hamilton depression scale.

Results

We originally identified 37 randomised or possibly randomised trials that evaluated preparations containing extracts of hypericum (V Wienert et al, third phytotherapy congress, Lubeck-Travemunde, 1991; M Bernhardt et al, fifth phytotherapy congress, Bonn, 1993).[11-45] Most of the trials were identified through reviews (especially through that of Harrer and Schulz[46]), bibliographies of papers, and the complementary database Phytodok, while our original online and CD-ROM searches in Med-line, Embase, Psychlit, and Psychindex revealed less than one third of the trials. Fourteen trials were excluded from our analysis as they included only healthy volunteers and investigated physiological parameters[34-38] (V Wienert et al, third phytotherapy congress, Lubeck-Travemunde, 1991); studied disorders other than depression[39-42]; investigated only pharmacodynamics[43]; or did not include a placebo or antidepressant control group[44,45] (M Bernhardt et al, fifth phytotherapy congress, Bonn, 1993).

Table 1 gives an overview of the 23 randomised clinical trials that compared extracts of hypericum with placebo or another treatment in depressive patients. Fifteen trials with 1008 patients were placebo controlled (14 on single preparations,[11-24] one on a combination with four other plant extracts[25]) and eight trials (six on single preparations[26-31] and two on a combination of hypericum and valeriana[32,33]) with 749 patients compared hypericum with other antidepressant or sedative drugs. With the exception of two trials,[30,31] all had treatment and observation periods of four to eight weeks.

A heterogeneous group of patients were included in the trials, and classification of depressive disorders was inconsistent. Most reports stated that patients suffered from mild to moderately severe depression, but this statement did not always correlate with the severity of symptoms according to the Hamilton depression scale or other scales (see, for example, Schmidt et al[22] in table 1). The trials were performed in private practices of psychiatrists (explicitly stated

Table 1   Description of randomised double blind controlled trials of hypericum for depression: patients and interventions (grouped for preparations)

Trial	Characteristics of patients			Mean (SD) severity of symptoms at baseline	Characteristics of interventions				
	No of patients	Centres*	Classification according to diagnosis		Compared treatment	Test preparation	Total hypercin/ day (mg)	Extract/ day in (mg)	Duration of treatment (weeks)
Placebo controlled trials of monopreparations									
Halama 1991[12]	50	1 Psy	ICD-9	Neurotic depression, adjustment disorder	HDS 18.0 (2.7)	Placebo	Jarsin	1.08	900	4
Hansgen 1994[11]	72	11 Psy/GP	DSM-III-R	Major depression	HDS 20.4 (3.4)	Placebo	Jarsin 300	2.7	900	4
Hubner 1994[15]	40	1 Int	ICD-9	Neurotic depression, adjustment disorder	HDS 12.4 (1.3)	Placebo	Jarsin 300	2.7	900	4
Lehrl 1993[17]	50	4 Practices	ICD-9	Neurotic depression, adjustment disorder+	HDS 21.6 (4.8)	Placebo	Jarsin	1.08	900	4
Schmidt 1993[23]	65	1 GP, 1 Int, 1 Psy	ICD-9	Neurotic depression, adjustment disorder	HDS 16.4 (2.6)	Placebo	Jarsin	1.08	900	6
Sommer 1994[24]	105	1 GP, 1 Int, 1 Psy	ICD-9	Neurotic depression, adjustment disorder	HDS 15.8 (4.3)	Placebo	Jarsin 300	2.7	900	4
Harrer 1991[13]	120	6 Int	ICD-9	Neurotic depression, adjustment disorder	HDS 20.9 (7.7)	Placebo	Psychotonin M	0.75	500	6
Osterheider 1992[18]	47	NA	NA	Moderately severe to severe endogenous, neurotic, or reactive depression	HDS 23.0 (NA)	Placebo	Psychotonin M	0.75	500	8
Quandt 1993[19]	88	4 Practices	ICD-9	Neurotic depression	HDS 17.3 (NA)	Placebo	Psychotonin M	0.75	500	4
Schlich 1987[21]	49	1 Practice	NA	Mild to moderately severe depression	HDS 24.0 (10.3)	Placebo	Psychotonin M	0.5	350	4
Schmidt 1989[22]	40	1 GP, 1 Int	ICD-9	Neurotic depression and various others	HDS 29.5 (12.9)	Placebo	Psychotonin M	0.75	500	4
Hoffmann 1979[14]	60	NA	NA	13 Psychogenic, 13 climacteric, 14 involution, 10 somatogenetic, 10 juvenile depressive patients	Only single symptoms presented	Placebo	Hyperforat	0.6	NA	6
Konig 1993[16]	112	50 GP	NA	Psychoaffective disorders with depressed mood	BfS 34.3 (7.6)	Placebo	Extract Z 90017	1.00–2.00	500–1000	6
Reh 1992[20]	50	1 Psy	ICD-9	Neurotic depression, adjustment disorder	HDS 20.0 (2.5)	Placebo	Neuroplant	1	500	8

	N	Specialty	Criteria	Diagnosis	Baseline	Comparator		Preparation	Dose	
Placebo controlled trial of combination										
Ditzler 1994[25]	60	1 Psy	DSM-III-R	Major depression	DSI 56.8 (3.75)	Placebo	0.48	Neurapas	600	8
Trials comparing single preparations and another drug										
Harrer 1994[27]	102	6 Psy	ICD-10	Single moderately severe depressive episode+	HDS 21.5 (3.9)	Maprotiline 75 mg	2.7	Jarsin 300	900	4
Trials comparing single preparations and another drug										
Harrer 1994[27]	102	6 Psy	ICD-10	Single moderately severe depressive episode+	HDS 21.5 (3.9)	Maprotiline 75 mg	2.7	Jarsin 300	900	4
Vorbach 1994[29]	135	20 Practices	DSM-III-R ICD-9	Major depression Neurotic adjustment disorders	HDS 19.4 (4.8)	Imipramine 75 mg	2.7	Jarsin 300	900	6
Kugler 1990[28]++	80	1 (Physician at research institute)	NA	Mild to moderately severe depressions (endogenous depression excluded)	DSI 44.2 (3.4)	Bromazepam 6 mg	0.75	Psychotonin M	500	4
Werth 1989[31]&	30	1 Surgery department	NA	Reactive depression after informing patients of necessity of amputation	HDS 26.7 (13.1)	Imipramine 50 mg	0.75	Psychotonin M	500	2
Bergmann 1993[26]	80	1 Psy	ICD-10	Single and recurrent mild and moderate severe depression episodes	HDS 15.4 (3.6)	Amitriptyline 30 mg	0.75	Esbericum	NA	6
Warnecke 1986[30]++	60	1 Gyn	NA	Climacteric (endogenous, involutive, reactive) depressive patients	NA	Diazepam 6 mg	0.4	Hyperforat	NA	12
Trials comparing combination of hypericum and valeriana with another drug										
Kniebel 1988[32]	162	19 GP, 8 Psy, 5 Int	DSM-III	Dysthymic disorders (ICD-9 adjustment disorders, neurotic depression, etc)	HDS 24.3 (5.0)	Amitriptyline 75–150 mg	0.45–0.90	Sedariston	300–600	6
Steger 1985[33]	100	1 Int	ICD-10*	Single, mild, and moderately severe depression episode	D-S 18.3 (5.6)	Desipramine 100–150 mg	0.60–0.90	Sedariston	400–600	6

*Official German specialties: GP = general practice, Int = internal medicine, Psy = neurology and psychiatry, Gyn = gynaecology and obstetrics.
+ According to information from sponsor, patients met diagnostic criteria for major depression (DSM-IIIR). ++ Open trials and single blind trials. ^No information given in the publication: according to coauthors originally classified according to ICD-9 and reclassified post-hoc.
HDS = Hamilton depression scale; BfS = Befindlichkeits-Skala (von Zerssen, adjective mood scale); DSI = depression status inventory; DS = depression scale (von Zerssen).
NA = no information available.

Table 2   Overview of effect size estimates for outcomes measured in randomised clinical trials of hypericum

| Outcome | Placebo controlled trials | | | | | | Trials comparing hypericum and another drug | | | | | |
| | Single preparations | | | Combination | | | Single preparations | | | Combination with valeriana | | |
	No of trials	Cohen's d	Rate ratio (95% confidence interval)	No of trials	Cohen's d	Rate ratio (95% confidence interval)	No of trials	Cohen's d	Rate ratio (95% confidence interval)	No of trials	Cohen's d	Rate ratio (95% confidence interval)
HDS score:												
After 2/3 weeks	9	0.51	1.66 (1.26 to 2.14)	0			3	−0.07	0.93 (0.74 to 1.17)	1	0.07	1.07 (0.78 to 1.46)
After 4 weeks	9	0.76	2.10 (1.58 to 2.76)	0			2	0.05	1.05 (0.81 to 1.36)	0		
After 6 weeks	3	0.59	1.79 (1.22 to 2.57)	0			2	0.14	1.15 (0.88 to 1.50)	1	0.17	1.19 (0.87 to 1.61)
After 8 weeks	1	1.00	2.62 (1.49 to 4.33)	0			0			0		
After treatment	9	0.77	2.12 (1.56 to 2.84)	0			3	0.08	1.08 (0.86 to 1.35)	1	0.17	1.19 (0.87 to 1.61)
DS score after treatment	4	0.84	2.26 (1.43 to 3.48)	1	0.81	2.20 (1.31 to 3.51)	2	0.07	1.07 (0.69 to 1.64)	1	0.00	1.00 (0.67 to 1.49)
BfS score after treatment	1	0.03	1.03 (0.70 to 1.49)	0			1	−0.01	0.99 (0.63 to 1.55)	1	0.28	1.32 (0.97 to 1.79)
BL score after treatment	2	0.89	2.37 (1.56 to 3.48)	1	0.24	1.27 (0.75 to 2.08)	0			1	0.18	1.20 (0.81 to 1.77)

HDS = Hamilton depression scale; DS = depression scale (von Zerssen), BfS = Befindlichkeits-Skala (von Zerssen, adjective mood scale), BL = Beschwerdeliste (von Zerssen, complaints list).

disorders than others, and neither do we know if different preparations of hypericum are equally effective or the optimum dosages. Hypericum preparations may work as well as other antidepressants, but the evidence is still insufficient because of the limited number of patients included in trials. Hypericum seems to have fewer short term side effects than some other antidepressants. Phototoxicity in animals has been reported after ingestion of extremely high doses of hypericum (about 30 to 50 times higher than therapeutical doses).[48] Drug monitoring studies suggest that side effects are rare and mild,[49–52] although observation periods did not exceed eight weeks. Information on long term side effects is lacking.

Future clinical trials on hypericum should compare its effects with those of other antidepressants and not with placebo. Different preparations of hypericum have to be compared and dose response investigations should be carried out. Longer trials with formal standard mechanisms for the assessment of side effects are needed to evaluate relative efficacy and safety compared with other antidepressants. Types of depression among study participants should be delineated better to determine whether hypericum works for milder forms of depression or for major and severe forms as well. Because available clinical trials suggest that hypericum might become an important tool for the management of depressive disorders, especially in primary care settings, such further research is highly desirable.

Funding: No specific funding.
Conflict of interest: None.

References

1. Kessler RC, McGonagle KA, Zhao S, Nelson CB, Hughes M, Eshleman S, et al. Lifetime and 12-month prevalence of DSM-III-R psychiatric disorders in the United States. Results form the national comorbidity study. *Arch Gen Psychiatry* 1994; 51: 8–19. [Abstract]
2. Regier DA, Narrow WE, Rae DS, Manderscheid RW, Locke BZ, Goodwin FK. The de facto US mental and addictive disorders systems: epidemiologic catchment area prospective 1-year prevalence rates of disorders and services. *Arch Gen Psychiatry* 1993; 50: 85–94. [Abstract]
3. Upmeyer HJ. Praxisproblem depressive Verstimmung. *Zeitschrift fur Allgemeinmedizin* 1990; 66(suppl 1): 33–35.
4. Lohse MJ, Muller-Oerlinghausen B. Psychopharmaka. In: Schwabe U, Paffrath D eds Arzneiverordnungsreport '94. Stuttgart: *Gustav Fischer* 1994: 354–370.
5. Wagner H, Bladt S. Pharmaceutical quality of Hypericum extracts. *J Geriatr Psychiatry Neurol* 1994; 7(suppl 1): 65–68.
6. Holzl J. Inhaltsstoffe und Wirkmechanismen des Johanniskrauts. *Zeitschrift fur Phytotherapie* 1993; 14: 255–264.
7. Ernst E. St. John's wort, an anti-depressant? A systematic, criteria-based review. *Phytomedicine* 1995; 2: 67–71.
8. Jadad AR, Moore RA, Carrol D, Jenkinson C, Reynolds DJM, Gavaghan DJ, et al. *Assessing the quality of reports of randomized clinical trials: is blinding necessary? Contr Clin Trials* 1996; 17: 1–12.
9. Association for Methodology and Documentation in Psychiatry (AMDP), Collegium Internationale Psychiatriae Scalarum (CIPS). Rating scales for psychiatry. Weinheim: Beltz, 1990.
10. Hedges LV, Olkin I. Statistical methods for meta-analysis. San Diego: Academic Press, 1985.
11. Hansgen KD, Vesper J, Ploch M. Multi-center double-blind study examining the antidepressant effectiveness of the Hypericum extract LI 160. *J Geriatr Psychiatry Neurol* 1994; 7(suppl 1): 15–18.
12. Halama P. Wirksamkeit des Johanniskrautextraktes LI 160 bei depressiver Verstimmung. *Nervenheilkunde* 1991; 10: 250–253.
13. Harrer G, Schmidt U, Kuhn U. 'Alternative' Depressionsbehandlung mit einem Hypericum-Extrakt. *Therapiewoche Neurologie/Psychiatrie* 1991; 5: 710–716.
14. Hoffmann J, Kuhl ED. Therapie von depressiven Zustanden mit Hypericin. *Zeitschrift fur Allgemeinmedizin* 1979; 55: 776–782.
15. Hubner WD, Lande S, Podzuweit H. Hypericum treatment of mild depression with somatic symptoms. *J Geriatr Psychiatry Neurol* 1994; 7(suppl 1): 12–15.
16. Konig CD. Hypericum perforatum L. (gemeines Johanniskraut) als Therapeutikum bei depressiven Verstimmungszustanden – eine Alternative zu synthetischen Arzneimitteln. Basel: University of Basel, 1993. (Thesis.)
17. Lehrl S, Woelk H. Ergebnisse von Messungen der kognitiven Leistungsfahigkeit bei Patienten unter der Therapie mit Johanniskraut. *Nervenheilkunde* 1993; 12: 281–284.
18. Osterheider M, Schmidtke A, Beckmann H. Behandlung depressiver Syndrome mit Hypericum (Johanniskraut) – eine placebokontrollierte Doppelblindstudie. *Fortschritte der Neurologie/Psychiatrie* 1992; 60(suppl 2): 210–211.
19. Quandt J, Schmidt U, Schenk N. Ambulante Behandlung leichter und mittelschwerer depressiver Verstimmungen. *Der Allgemeinarzt* 1993; 2: 97–102.
20. Reh C, Laux P, Schenk N. Hypericum-Extrakt bei Depressionen – eine wirksame Alternative. *Therapiewoche* 1992; 42: 1576–1581.
21. Schlich D, Braukmann F, Schenk N. Behandlung depressiver Zustande mit Hypericin. *Psycho* 1987; 13: 440–447.

present the pack in a jargon-free format which was appealing to practitioners. Given the response of some nurses to material produced by pharmaceutical companies, a grant was obtained from a commercial company who oversaw production of the packs. The impact of the pack on reported practice was assessed through an experimental study design. The information pack produced a significant increase in the knowledge scores of the experimental group.

Gerrish et al (1999) used an action research model to promote evidence-based practice in the assessment of pressure damage risk. Using a collaborative approach, a team of researchers, nurse managers and practitioners (including the Trust's clinical nurse specialist in skin care), adopted a three-stage approach. In the first stage, current research evidence was reviewed. This was followed by a survey and audit to describe existing knowledge and practice. Finally, top-down and bottom-up strategies were implemented to achieve change. The findings of the audit and survey were disseminated through a variety of mechanisms, then evidence-based practice groups were established, evidence-based protocols were developed, the role of the specialist nurse was developed further and a number of training initiatives were instituted.

Both of these examples illustrate the complexity of getting research into practice and highlight the importance of using strategies which take into account the unique characteristics of the practice setting and which are tailored to local needs.

Collaboration between clinicians and researchers to carry out research

Collaborative research of this nature is seen by many as a surefire way to ensure that subsequent research findings are seen as relevant by practitioners and therefore applied in practice. Many successful attempts at collaborative research are reported in the literature. For example, Koch et al (2001) describe a participatory action research study where a team of continence advisors and researchers carried out research to explore women's understandings of living with multiple sclerosis and urinary incontinence and Heslop et al (2000) describe a collaborative study to improve the care of patients with mental health problems attending emergency departments.

Much of the documented collaboration between clinicians and researchers involves innovations in clinical practice and the evaluation of change and is

described under the heading of *action research*. Although one of the principal features of action research is collaboration, the term also has other implications. Action research implies a different philosophical approach, in which research questions are generated by practitioners in response to problems 'on the ground' and local solutions are sought through the collaboration and participation of clinicians and researchers. Participation in the research process is thus seen as empowering for clinicians.

Action research is seen by many as a particularly appropriate approach to nursing research, not least because research results are immediately available and relevant to practitioners. Action research as a method has its critics, largely on the basis that research findings may not be generalizable across a wider population, the findings only being useful locally. Nonetheless, this approach represents a powerful way of ensuring that research is useful to clinicians not only in terms of the results produced but also in terms of the questions it seeks to answer. Action research is also discussed in Chapters 5 and 6.

Secondment of clinicians to research teams to acquire skills

Given the need to increase research capacity in nursing and allied health professions (HEFCE 2001), secondments for practitioners to academic departments to participate in funded research projects may provide valuable learning opportunities. Not only is it likely that these individuals will become more active in using research themselves, it is possible that they will become advocates for research in their own practice area, thus providing a further impetus for research-based practice. In my own area, two local research institutions, the Trent Institute and Trent Focus have set up a Research Secondment Opportunity Scheme, which aims to match health care professionals with some experience of research with appropriate research projects.

INITIATIVES TO OVERCOME BARRIERS RELATED TO THE SETTING

Policy initiatives

The policy context of health care research has changed markedly over recent years and is fully discussed by John Daly and colleagues in Chapter 2 of this book. The greater emphasis on the implementation as well as on the conduct of research is reflected not only in research strategy at governmental level, but also at trust level. Within the UK, national initiatives include the drive for clinical effectiveness (DoH 1996), the creation of NICE and the clinical governance initiative (DoH 1997). Documentary analysis of local trust policy documents indicates that the profile of research and development at an organizational level has also increased and is reflected in trust policies and business plans (FoNS 2001a).

Clinical leaders to promote research-based practice

Inspirational clinical leadership which encourages and empowers others has been identified as an important element in creating a positive research culture (FoNS 2001a). Recent work by Thompson et al (2001) indicated that for nurses working in acute settings, the most useful source of research-based knowledge to inform real-time clinical decision making, was not written texts or electronic information but a clinically credible and experienced human source.

Clinical leaders to promote research-based practice come in a variety of forms. Many NHS trusts employ practice development nurses with the promotion of research-based practice forming part of their remit. The lecturer–practitioner may also have the potential to facilitate research-based practice, given the nature of their remit to narrow the theory–practice gap. Some see the creation of new roles, including clinical nurse specialists (CNS) or nurse practitioners, as ideally suited to implementing research findings within their sphere of expertise. However, there is evidence to suggest that many nurses or members of the allied health professions experience difficulties with the research component of these new roles, possibly due to lack of research experience and training (Read et al 2001). New nurse consultant posts may also provide a valuable contribution in this area although as yet, little formal evaluation of these roles has taken place. A detailed examination of all these roles is beyond the scope of this text. However, it is important to highlight the value of positive role models and practical support for all clinicians wishing to make their practice as research-based as possible.

Establishment of research interest groups

In attempts to tackle research implementation 'on the ground', some practitioners are involved in journal clubs or research interest groups. Hunt and Topham (2002) describe establishing a multidisciplinary journal club in the field of learning disabilities to facilitate professional developments but note that support from management is vital to enable staff to attend and participate.

Journal clubs, where clinicians meet on a regular basis and take turns in presenting either a paper from a journal or an overview of a particular edition of a journal, represent a simple yet effective way of keeping up to date. They can provide peer support and a means of accessing literature and expertise within the group. When facilitated by members with the skills to critically evaluate research findings, they can provide a powerful springboard for ideas and increase the drive towards research-based care. Although the value of face-to-face contact should not be underestimated, local, national or even international electronic discussion groups can also work in a similar way.

There are many other simple steps which can improve accessibility to research findings such as providing journals in clinical areas, keeping a file of relevant research reports, and presentation of research at staff meetings or as part of a ward-based teaching programme. All of these can contribute to a more positive climate for evidence-based health care.

Initiatives to create a research culture at the organizational level

In the USA, the government has funded a number of nursing research utilization programmes – notably the Western Interstate Commission for Higher Education (the WICHE programme) and the Conduct and Utilization of Research in Nursing project (the CURN project).

The WICHE programme, carried out in the 1970s and reported by Loomis (1985) and Closs and Cheater (1994), involved collaborative workshops between researchers and clinicians at a number of sites. The intention was to identify patient care problems and work towards research-based solutions through planned change. Interestingly, the WICHE researchers note that the major barrier was lack of access to good nursing research and concluded that no further large-scale research utilization projects should be attempted until current research was made more accessible.

The CURN project viewed research utilization as an organizational rather than an individual

Mallett J (ed) (2000) The Royal Marsden Hospital Manual of Clinical Nursing Procedures, 5th edn. Oxford: Blackwell.

Mander R (1988) Encouraging students to be research minded. *Nurse Education Today* 8: 30–35.

Markham G (1988) Special cases. *Nursing Times* 84(26): 29–30.

Marsh G (2000) Strengthening evidence based-nursing and midwifery practice. Sheffield: Central Sheffield University Hospitals Trust.

Marshall M and Lockwood A (2002) Assertive community treatment for people with severe mental disorders. *Cochrane Database of Systematic Reviews*. Available online at: www. update-software.com/cochrane.

NHS Centre for Reviews and Dissemination (2001) Accessing the evidence on clinical effectivenss. *Effectiveness Matters* 5(1): 1–7.

Parahoo K (1999) A comparison of pre-Project 2000 and Project 2000 nurses' perceptions of their research training, research needs and their use of research in clinical areas. *Journal of Advanced Nursing* 29(1): 237–245.

Parahoo K (2000) Barriers to, and facilitators of, research utilization among nurses in Northern Ireland. *Journal of Advanced Nursing* 31(1): 89–98.

Parahoo K (2001) Research utilization among medical and surgical nurses; a comparison of their self-reports and perceptions of barriers and facilitators. *Journal of Nursing Management* 9(1): 21–30.

Pearcey P (1995) Achieving research-based practice. *Journal of Advanced Nursing* 22: 33–39.

Peters DA (1992) Implementation of research findings. *Health Bulletin* 50(1): 68–77.

Read SM, Lloyd-Jones M, Doyal L et al (2001) Exploring New Roles in Practice (ENRiP). Sheffield: University of Sheffield. Available online at: www.snm.shef.ac.uk/ research/enrip/enrip.htm.

Rizutto C, Bostrom J, Suter WN et al (1994) Predictors of nurses' involvement in research activity. *Western Journal of Nursing Research* 16(2): 193–204.

Rodgers S (1994) An exploratory study of research utilization by nurses in general medical and surgical wards. *Journal of Advanced Nursing* 20: 904–911.

Scott JT, Entwistle VA, Sowden AJ et al (2002) Communicating with children and adolescents about their cancer. *Cochrane Database of Systematic Reviews*. Available online at: www.update-software.com/cochrane

Sheldon T, Freemantle N, Grimshaw J et al (1994) The good guide to guides. *Health Services Journal* 8: 34–35.

Smith CA, Collins CT and Crowther CA (2002) Complementary and alternative therapies for pain management in labour. *Cochrane Database of Systematic Reviews*. Available online at: www.update-software.com/cochrane

Stetler CB and DiMaggio G (1991) Research utilization among clinical nurse specialists. *Clinical Nurse Specialist* 5(3): 151–155.

Thompson C, McCaughan D, Cullum N et al (2001) Research information in nurses' clinical decision-making: what is useful? *Journal of Advanced Nursing* 36(3): 376–388.

Titler MG, Kleiber C, Steelman V et al (1994) Infusing research into practice to promote quality care. *Nursing Research* 43(5): 307–313.

Walsh M (1997a) Perceptions of barriers to implementing research. *Nursing Standard* 11(19): 34–37.

Walsh M (1997b) How nurses perceive barriers to research implementation. *Nursing Standard* 11(29): 34–39.

Webb C and Mackenzie J (1993) Where are we now? Research-mindedness in the 1990s. *Journal of Clinical Nursing* 2(3): 129–133.

Williamson P (1992) From dissemination to use: management and organizational barriers to the application of health services research findings. *Health Bulletin* 50(1): 78–86.

Wilson-Barnett J, Corner J and De-Carle B (1990) Integrating nursing research and practice – the role of the researcher as teacher. *Journal of Advanced Nursing* 15(5): 621–625.

Further reading

The Foundation of Nursing Studies website provides access to four reports in a new dissemination series. The reports describe initiatives to improve the care of patients by using research findings and evidence to develop and change practice. The four subjects are: reducing patient falls in an acute general hospital, breaking bad news, self-administration of medicines and the re-use of patients' own drugs and implementing and validating guidelines to facilitate the involvement of carers in the care of people with dementia and other people requiring long-term care. http://www.fons.org/projects/dissemination/index.htm

Mallett J (ed) (2000) *The Royal Marsden Hospital Manual of Clinical Nursing Procedures*, 5th edn. Oxford: Blackwell.
   This manual, whilst describing clinical nursing procedures, provides a rationale for each step and includes relevant research findings which support or inform the process.

Dougherty L and Lister S (eds) (2004) *The Royal Marsden Hospital Manual of Clinical Nursing Procedures*, 6th edn. Oxford: Blackwell Science.

Vaughan B and Edwards M (1995) *Interface Between Research and Practice: Some Working Models*. London: King's Fund Centre.
   This book arose through the practical experience of promoting evidence-based practice in a number of Nursing Development Units. The strengths and difficulties of six models of research utilization are discussed.

Wye L and McClenahan J (2000) *Getting Better with Evidence. Experiences of Putting Evidence into Practice*. London: King's Fund.
   This report describes a study undertaken by the King's Fund to establish the effectiveness of different approaches to getting evidence into practice. Common lessons are drawn from 17 diverse projects in a range of clinical settings.

Chapter **14**

Techniques and strategies for translating research findings into health care practices

Patrick A. Crookes, Terry Froggatt

INTRODUCTION

Once the decision has been made about whether a body of research is rigorous and worthy of application to practice, plans need to be made regarding how best to go about introducing, managing and evaluating its implementation – even the best ideas are not self-executing. In Chapter 13, Ann McDonnell discussed barriers to research utilization, along with some solutions. In this chapter, we argue the need for a planned approach when implementing change of any kind. This is a view obtained from personal experience and the reviews of innovation research undertaken by authors such as Rogers (1962), Rogers and Shoemaker (1971) and Havelock (1972).

From reading, it would appear that in health care, systematic planning regarding services or care based on a clear theoretical framework is rather rare. Health journals are full of examples of keen and committed staff attempting to change and improve systems for patients and professionals alike, yet rarely do they overtly utilize any particular model of change to inform and structure their efforts. One of the principles of this chapter, therefore, is that much of the theory of 'managing change' can and should be applied to the implementation of research findings within health care settings. The five essential factors for change, identified within the document *Managing Change in Nursing Education* (ENB 1987), will be used as the framework for much of the rest of this chapter. Content will be categorized under the headings of:

- the attributes of the environment where change is to take place
- the users of proposed innovation

those which are not. Such thought processes not only maximize the chances of success of any proposed innovation, but also allow even the most junior of personnel to perceive *realistically* that they can make a difference – even if the impact is relatively small in the greater scheme of things. As Harvey (1990, p25) points out, 'you only learn to walk by taking baby steps'.

In practice, the clarification of what 'the problem' actually is can only take place if a thorough analysis of the *need* for a change has also been carried out. This involves, not merely an examination of the attributes of the innovation (Rogers & Shoemaker 1971) to be discussed later, but also a clear understanding of the problem that requires the change to be made and a consideration of *why* it needs to take place. If this diagnostic work has been done then the innovator should be in possession of a clearly defined and focused statement of what they wish to change and why, which can then be shared coherently with others. Havelock and Zlotolow (1995) also provide a useful model of such activity, as does Lewin's force field analysis, discussed later. This preparatory work should also ensure that the change(s) made address(es) the true problem. Finally it means that the innovator will find themselves at a point where the 'five essential factors' of change (ENB 1987) are of real relevance and use to them.

Summary

In order to occupy the role of change agent successfully, an individual needs both to perceive the need for change and to possess the belief that they can effect it – that they can make a difference.

One-dimensional 'problems' rarely exist. Instead we are usually confronted by amalgamations of interrelated issues. As a result, problem resolution should be seen as an alternative to problem solving as a basis for identifying the true nature of problems – including what should be the focus of innovation.

Exercise 14.1

Think about the following questions in relation to your own practice.

- Do you perceive the need for change within your area of work? Why? Name at least three factors.
- Do you perceive that it is possible for you to effect any of these changes?

- Think about the concept of 'problem resolution' and apply it to an issue that you view as 'a problem'. Try to identify the component parts of 'the problem' and some possible solutions to them.
- What rules or systems might/will impede your progress?

FIVE FACTORS CRUCIAL TO THE SUCCESS OF CHANGE MANAGEMENT

If you take the time to read the ENB *Managing Change* document, you will see that its authors discuss the five factors in a different order to the one we are using. Most notable is that they cover the attributes of the innovation first. We have chosen to discuss the situation where it is intended that change will take place (the change environment) and the people within it (the users) first. This is because it seems more logical to us to consider the importance of diagnosing a situation (e.g. a workplace) and the people within it (perhaps to the point of involving them in the processes of problem resolution and identification), before discussing the attributes of any solutions put forward (the innovation). In writing this it occurs to us that perhaps a consideration of the environment and those who will be affected by change is perhaps where the innovator should start. Otherwise there will always be a tendency to try to start the process at the point of implementation, rather than at the point of assessment and diagnosis. Models of change typically attempt to steer innovators away from this trap – a major indication for their use.

ATTRIBUTES OF THE ENVIRONMENT

No-one has yet come up with the definitive work on 'innovative environments' or what essentially characterizes a workplace where a 'research culture' can be said to exist. The team who developed the ENB document (1987) suggest that an environment is ripe for change when five conditions coexist:

- Openness
- Interpersonal and information linkages
- Freedom from organizational constraints
- Supportive leadership
- Trust.

Openness

This relates to the need for people within an organization to be willing to question the status quo and be prepared to accept that there is benefit in recognizing and constantly exploring the idea that there is always scope for improvement. Furthermore, they need to recognize that there is rarely only one answer to any particular question – what Pirsig (1974) refers to as 'value rigidity'. It is crucial that these 'truths' are recognized by staff at all levels of the hierarchy. Those at the top have a responsibility to encourage reflection, personal initiative and innovation, not least by avoiding the tendency to dismiss ideas and suggestions put forward by more junior colleagues. Meanwhile, those in subordinate positions need to accept that they have a responsibility to do more than 'just the job'. Such an ethos could be engendered in a number of ways, including the formation of quality circles to review and develop policies and procedures (Crocker et al 1984, Hatfield & Campbell 1987, King's Fund Centre 1992), the development of participatory action research groups (Street 1995) and practice development initiatives (McCormack et al 2002).

Interpersonal and information linkages

Effective channels of communication (both formal – meetings, team briefings, memos – and informal) need to exist. If they do not, then openness in the form of sharing of ideas and information, along with the opportunity to give and receive support and discuss issues openly, is lost. Numerous health authorities and trusts have formal mechanisms for cascading information throughout the organization. Perhaps more effort needs to be put into facilitating upward motion of feedback and ideas – again through quality circles, research groups and practice development mechanisms, for example. Clutterbuck (1999) poses the rhetorical question 'who can innovate in an unstimulating environment?'.

Freedom from organizational constraints

This again is a two-edged sword, in that organizations (in the form of managers) need to function so that individuals and groups are encouraged and *rewarded* for initiative, self-directedness and innovation. At the same time, 'subordinates' must accept the burdens of increased autonomy, responsibility and accountability.

Supportive leadership

The leadership within an organization must support innovation and be *seen* to be doing so by those in subordinate positions. Indeed, as stated above, they need to encourage and reward innovative thought and action. Fullan (1986, p77) sees leaders as being central to successful change, either in the role of supporter or as a director of the change effort. For individual innovation attempts, leaders can also help by exerting their influence and authority to sustain motivation and impetus, until such a time as the change has become 'custom and practice'. Perhaps the main point to be taken from this is that in an innovative environment, 'subordinates' must also take on the mantle of 'leader'. We will explore leadership further, later in the chapter.

Our discussions to date have been based upon the ENB document *Managing Change in Nursing Education* (1987). Argyris (1983) offers other interesting suggestions for managers on ways in which they can be more supportive of change. What appears to be fundamental from his point of view is the need for managers to acknowledge that they can and should learn from those around them, that they neither have, nor do they need to have, the answer to every problem. It is perhaps useful to point out here that leadership and authority may not always be a function of seniority. Rogers and Shoemaker (1971) and Havelock and Zlotolow (1995) identify that opinion leaders can be from any echelon of an organization. They also make the point that any would-be innovator should attempt to ensure that such people are 'on board' early in their planning, so as to benefit from their input and influence as well as avoiding the potential risk of being covertly undermined by them.

Trust

Change leads to an uncertain and unsettling time for most people, even those leading the way. If an air of trust and collegiality exists, then staff involved will be more likely to collaborate constructively and effectively towards achieving common goals. If it does not, then vested interests, rivalries and 'office politics' will conspire to ensure failure.

LEARNING ORGANIZATIONS

The establishment of 'learning organizations' and the essential requirements for this desired state have received much attention (Birleson 1998, Senge et al 1994, Slater & Narver 1995). A learning organization provides a stimulating climate for members to continually strive for new approaches in acquiring knowledge. Specifically, organizational learning can be

Exercise 14.4

Identify an innovation you have seen or been involved with and rate it against each of the criteria discussed above:

- relative advantage
- compatibility
- complexity
- trialability
- observability.

Come to some conclusion as to why it succeeded or failed based on its attributes as an innovation.

CHANGE AGENTS

Vaughan and Pillmoor (1992) characterize change agents as people (or groups of people) who can take an idea for change from the drawing board, carry it through all the stages of its implementation and finally evaluate its success (or failure). Given this view, without a change agent innovation will not take place. This can also be seen to be the case in action research (see Chapters 5, 6) where the team can be considered change agents.

In organizations such as modern health services, the responsibility for the role of change agent is typically invested with clinical or general managers and more recently 'practice developers'. This is not accidental. Change agents do not necessarily need to be senior but this can certainly help, not least because the ability to initiate and implement change is often a function of power. This is not to say that power is merely linked to position or rank and the ability to control resources. Charisma (personal power) and expertise (power of authority) also confer power on those who possess these traits or attributes (Handy 1986).

Whatever the source, it seems reasonable to suggest that a change agent needs power to implement change (Allen 1993), even if it is conferred vicariously through the support of someone with power. It is important, however, that such power is used constructively. Clutterbuck illustrates this when he says that many of today's successful leaders '… don't worry about what most professional managers worry about'; they (by contrast with professional managers) spend their time working on what is important to them, rather than spending a great deal of time 'preventing undesirable things from happening – usually by stopping other people from doing things' (Clutterbuck 1999, p71).

However, it should be recognized that power is not the 'be all and end all' to being able to lead successful innovation, not least because of the need for collaboration and ownership of the change by its 'users'. We have already discussed, for example, the importance of the innovator's 'mental set' (I *can* make a difference) and the need to have a clear vision of the problem and what they want to achieve. Again, having reviewed a range of studies, Rogers & Shoemaker (1971, p183–191) identify other attributes of effective change agents related to the success or otherwise of innovation. Interestingly, these relate less to the need for power (though credibility or 'authority' in the eyes of 'users' is seen as crucial) and more to their willingness to value and include input from prospective 'users' of the innovation. McCormack and Garbett (2003), in generating a taxonomy of attributes of effective practice developers, via focus groups and telephone interviews with clinicians with experience of such developers, come to much the same conclusion. They constantly came across the view that if anyone was going to be successful in changing clinical practice, then they would need to do so in concert with clinicians. They also found that effective practice developers need to be seen as being: independent of management (at least to the degree that changes advocated do not reflect a purely organizational agenda); clinically competent and/or credible to clinicians; and a skilled communicator and politician.

Real leadership, of course, has never been a matter of mere formal authority. What we do know from our personal experiences is that leaders are effective only when other people acknowledge them as such. The issue of leadership continues to take centre stage in any discussion about learning or innovative health care organizations. However, it seems to us, at least, that the attributes identified by Goleman (1998; see Box 14.4) are essential for leaders inclined towards creating an organizational culture conducive to innovation and entrepreneurialism.

Other specific attributes demonstrated by successful innovators include their empathy with 'users', along with the points encompassed within earlier discussions of the first three 'essentials for change' (ENB 1987). Another interesting point raised by Rogers and Shoemaker (1971, p183) is the issue of venturesomeness – the eagerness to take risks and try new ideas, while at the same time being willing to accept the occasional setback when one of the new ideas proves unsuccessful. This relates to the issue of 'reactance' and 'creativity' discussed earlier in this chapter.

Box 14.4 Goleman's attributes of effective leaders. Reprinted by permission of *Harvard Business Review*. From *What Makes a Leader?* by Goleman D (1998) 76(6). Copyright © 1998 by the Harvard Business School Publishing Corporation; all rights reserved.

Self-awareness – the ability to recognize and understand one's own moods, emotions and drives as well as their effect on others. This includes self-confidence, realistic self-assessment and a self-deprecating sense of humour.

Self-regulation – the ability to control or redirect disruptive impulses and moods and the propensity to suspend judgement – to think before acting. This includes trustworthiness and integrity, comfort with ambiguity and openness to change.

Motivation – a passion to work for reasons that go beyond money or status and a propensity to pursue goals with energy and persistence. This includes a strong drive to achieve, optimism, even in the face of failure, and organizational commitment.

Empathy – the ability to understand the emotional make-up of other people and the skill of treating people according to their emotional reactions. This includes expertise in building and retaining talent, cross-cultural sensitivity and service to clients and customers.

Social skill – proficiency in managing relationships and building networks and an ability to find common ground and build rapport. This includes effectiveness in leading change, persuasiveness and expertise in building and leading teams.

Lancaster and Lancaster (1982) take a slightly different track. In addition to the above, they highlight the need for a sound knowledge of human behaviour and group processes (p2 and 20), along with good interpersonal skills (both verbal expression and listening, p3). They reiterate the need for the change agent to possess an awareness of the general feel of the change environment and the 'users' within it (as in preceding discussions). In particular, they emphasize the need to be able to engender an atmosphere of trust and a willingness to work through the processes of change systematically and with clarity of mind – preferably with clear objectives and a strategic plan. Finally they and others (e.g. Open University 1991) make the crucial point that change agents must recognize that there are any number of factors outside their control which can influence the success or failure of any innovation. They therefore need to be politically astute, resilient, flexible, a risk taker and, perhaps most important of all, lucky.

Lancaster and Lancaster (1982, pp20–23 and Chapter 6 on Leadership), Hunt (1986), Havelock and Zlotolow (1995), Birleson (1998), Goleman (1998) and McCormack and Garbett (2003) all offer excellent further reading, in the form of research-based discussions of the attributes of leaders and change agents/practice developers.

The merits of being a change agent

Earlier in this chapter, in discussing health care culture and its possible ramifications for innovation, a fairly negative picture was painted of the change agent's lot. This was followed by a suggestion of indications that this may slowly be changing in the light of policy shifts at the highest levels, for example the increasing emphasis on innovation and evidence-based practice within purchasing agreements between health authorities and health providers and the advent of practice development initiatives.

It should also be acknowledged that being successful as an agent of change – being vindicated in the belief that you can indeed make a difference – is a heady potion. It does wonders for self-esteem and may even enhance how you are perceived by others – peers, managers and even prospective employers. It also makes any job more interesting and fulfilling, leading to a sense of self-efficacy and worth.

This brings us back to the issue of oppressed group behaviour (Freire 1971) which we discussed earlier in relation to 'culture'. It is interesting that those who offer solutions to the vicious cycle of horizontal violence and marginalization in nursing (Roberts 1983, 2000), rather than merely exposing and bemoaning it (Farmer 1993, Speedy 1987), suggest that such behaviours will disappear only when a critical mass of nurses possess such self-esteem and pride in their work and their profession.

Summary

Power to initiate and/or enforce change is a useful tool for any change agent. If this is combined with a clear sense of purpose, along with a willingness to invite and value input from the potential 'users' of the innovation, then the chances of success are increased.

Becker G (1993) Continuity after a stroke: implications of life-course disruption in old age. *Gerontologist* **33**: 148–158.

Benner P (1984) *From Novice to Expert: Excellence and Power in Clinical Nursing Practice.* Menlo Park: Addison Wesley.

Bennis WG, Benne KD, Chin R (1976) *The Planning of Change.* London: Holt Rinehart and Winston.

Birleson P (1998) Building a learning organization in a child and adolescent mental health service. *Australian Health Review* **21**(3): 223–240.

Burns N and Grove S (2001) *The Practice of Nursing Research: Conduct, Critique and Utilization,* 4th edn. Philadelphia: WB Saunders.

Clutterbuck D (1999) *Doing it Different. Lessons for the Imaginative Manager.* London: Orion Publishing Group.

Cooper H, Carlisle C, Watkins C et al (2000) Using qualitative methods for conducting a systematic review. *Nurse Researcher* **8**(1): 28–38.

Cornwell T (1996) Manual handling and the elderly. *The Lamp* **53**(2): 40–41, 44–45.

Coxon T (1990) Ritualised repression. *Nursing Times* **86**(31): 35–36.

Crocker OL, Chiu JSK and Charney C (1984) *Quality Circles: a Guide to Participation and Productivity.* New York: Methuen.

Crookes PA (1992) The politics of health care. In: Boddy J and Rice V (eds) *Health: Perspectives and Practices.* Palmerstone North, New Zealand: Dunmore Press.

Crookes PA (1996) Personal bereavement in registered general nurses (unpublished PhD thesis). Hull: University of Hull.

Davies S (2001) Caring for older people with continuing care needs and their families. In: Nolan M, Davies S, Grant G (eds) *Working with Older People and Their Families: Key Issues in Policy and Practice.* Buckingham: Open University Press.

English National Board for Nursing, Midwifery and Health Visiting Working Group 1987 *Managing Change in Nursing Education.* London: ENB.

Farmer B (1993) The use and abuse of power in nursing. *Nursing Standard* **7**(23): 33–36.

Freire P (1971) *Pedagogy of the Oppressed.* New York: Continuum.

Fullan MG (1986) The management of change. In: Hoyle E and McMahon A (eds) *The World Yearbook of Education.* London: Kogan Page, pp73–86.

Gilmartin MJ (1998) The nursing organization and the transformation of health care for the 21st century. *Nursing Administration Quarterly* **22**(2): 70–86.

Goleman D (1998) What makes a leader? *Harvard Business Review* **76**(6): 93–102.

Green GJ (1988) Relationships between role models and role perceptions of new graduate nurses. *Nursing Research* **37**(4): 245–248.

Grissum M and Spengler C (1976) *Women, Power and Health Care.* Boston: Little, Brown.

Gupta B, Lakshmi S and Aronson JE (2000) Knowledge management: practices and challenges. *Industrial Management Data Systems* **100**: 17–21.

Hagerman ZT and Tiffany CR (1994) Evaluation of two planned change theories. *Nursing Management* **25**(4): 57–62.

Handy J (1986) Considering organizations in organizational stress research: a rejoinder to Glowinkowski and Cooper to Duckworth. *Bulletin of the British Psychological Society* **39**: 205–210.

Harvey TR (1990) *Checklist for Change: a Pragmatic Approach to Creating and Controlling Change.* Boston: Allyn and Bacon.

Hatfield B and Campbell D (1987) Quality circles: tapping people power. *Nursing Management* **18**: 94.

Havelock R (1972) *Bibliography on Knowledge Utilisation and Dissemination.* Ann Arbor: Institute for Social Research.

Havelock RG and Huberman M (1978) *Solving Educational Problems: the Theory and Reality of Innovation in Developing Countries: a Study Prepared for the International Bureau of Education.* Paris: UNESCO.

Havelock RG and Zlotolow S (1995) *The Change Agent's Guide to Innovation in Education,* 2nd edn. Englewood Cliffs: Educational Technology Publications.

Hunt JW (1986) Changing organizations. In: *Managing People at Work,* 2nd edn. London: Institute of Personnel Management.

King's Fund Centre (1992) *Nursing Developments Network.* Guidance notes. London: King's Fund.

Laight SE (1995) A vision for eye care: a brief study of the change process. *Intensive and Critical Care Nursing* **11**: 217–222.

Lancaster J and Lancaster L (1982) *Concepts for Advanced Nursing Practice: the Nurse as a Change Agent.* St Louis: Mosby.

Larson DG (1987) Internal stressors in nursing: helper secrets. *Journal of Psychosocial Nursing* **25**(4): 20–27.

Lewin K (1951) *Field Theory in Social Science.* New York: Harper and Row.

Lippitt GL (1973) *Visualizing Change: Model Building and the Change Process.* Fairfax: NTL – Learning Resources Corporation.

Lutjens LRJ and Tiffany CR (1994) Evaluating planned change theories. *Nursing Management* **25**(3): 54–57.

Mabbett P (1987) From burned out to turned on: skills of personal energy management and 'caring'. *Canadian Nurse* **83**(3): 15–19.

Machiavelli N (1513) *The Prince* (trans Bull G 1961) Harmondsworth: Penguin.

Maslow AH (1971) *Attaining the Farther Reaches of Human Nature.* New York: Penguin.

McCormack B and Garbett R (2003) The characteristics, qualities and skills of practice developers. *Journal of Clinical Nursing* **12**(3): 317–325.

McCormack B, Kitson A, Harvey G et al (2002) Getting evidence into practice: the meaning of context. *Journal of Advanced Nursing* **38**(1): 94–104.

Miles MB (1995) Foreword. In: Havelock RG, Zlotolow S 1995 *The Change Agent's Guide to Innovation in Education* 2nd edn. Englewood Cliffe: Educational Technology Publications.

Milio N (1988) Strategic lessons for health-promoting policy. A meta-study of national case studies. Paper presented at the 2nd International Conference on Health Promotion, WHO and Commonwealth of Australia, 3–10 April, Adelaide.

Mink OG (1992) Creating new organizational paradigms for change. *International Journal of Quality and Reliability in Management* **19**(3): 21–35.

Moilanen R (2001) Diagnostic tools for learning organizations. *The Learning Organization* **8**(1): 6–20.

Morgan G (1986) *Images of Organization.* Newbury Park: Sage.

Nolan M, Davies S and Grant G (2001) *Working with Older People and their Families.* Buckingham: Open University Press.

Nolan M, Brown J, Davies S et al (2002) Advancing gerontological education in nursing: final report of the AGEIN project. Report to the English National Board for Nursing, Midwifery and Health Visiting, University of Sheffield.

Ollikainen L (1986) Towards a change in nursing practice. *International Nursing Review* **33**(2): 40–43.

Open University (1991) Managing health services, book 9 managing change. Buckingham: Open University Press.

Pirsig RM (1974) *Zen and the Art of Motorcycle Maintenance.* London: Vintage.

Polit DF and Hungler BP (1991) *Nursing Research: Principles and Methods.* Philadelphia: Lippincott.

Richman J (1987) *Medicine and health.* London: Longman.

Roberts SJ (1983) Oppressed group behaviour: implications for nursing. *Advances in Nursing Science* **5**(4): 21–30.

Roberts SJ (2000) Development of a positive professional identity: liberating onself from the oppressor within. *Advances in Nursing Science* **22**(4): 71–78.

Rogers EM (1962) *Diffusion of Innovations.* New York: Free Press.

Rogers EM and Shoemaker FF (1971) *Communication of Innovations: a Cross-cultural Approach.* New York: Free Press.

Rycroft-Malone J, Harvey G, Kitson A et al (2002) Getting evidence into practice: ingredients for change. *Nursing Standard* **16**(37): 38–43.

Salvage J (1985) *The Politics of Nursing.* London: Heinemann.

Schon D (1987) *Educating the Reflective Practitioner.* San Francisco: Jossey-Bass.

Seligman MEP (1975) *Helplessness: on Depression, Development and Death.* New York: WH Freeman.

Seligman MEP (1992) *Learned optimism.* Australia: Random House.

Senge PM (1990). *The Fifth Discipline: the Art and Practice of the Learning Organization.* New York: Currency/ Doubleday.

Senge PM (1992) Building learning organizations. *Journal for Quality and Participation* **15**(2): 30–38.

Senge PM, Roberts C, Ross RB et al (1994) *The Fifth Discipline Field Book: Strategies for Building a Learning Organization.* New York: Currency/Doubleday.

Shimko BW, Meli JT, Restrepo JC et al (2000) Debunking the 'lean and mean' myth and celebrating the rise of learning organizations. *The Learning Organization* **7**(2).

Skevington S (1984) *Understanding Nurses.* Chichester: John Wiley.

Slater S and Narver JC (1995) Market orientation and the learning organization. *Journal of Marketing* **59**(3): 63–75.

Smith PAC and Tosey P (1999) Assessing the learning organization; part 1 – theoretical foundations. *The Learning Organization* **6**(2): 70–75.

Speedy S (1987) Feminism and the profession of nursing. *Australian Journal of Nursing* **4**(2): 20–28.

Street A (1995) *Nursing Replay: Researching Nursing Culture Together.* Melbourne: Churchill Livingstone.

Vaughan B and Pillmoor M (1992) *Managing Nursing Work.* London: Scutari Press.

Waters M and Crook R 1990 *Sociology One: Principles of Sociological Analysis for Australians,* 2nd edn. Melbourne: Longman Cheshire.

Watkins S (1997) Introducing bedside handover reports. *Professional Nurse* **14**(4): 270–273.

Whitehouse DM (1991) Games of one-upmanship and sabotage. *Nursing Management* **2**(6): 46–50.

Wilkinson P 1994 Introducing a change of nursing model in a general intensive therapy unit. *Intensive and Critical Care Nursing* **10**: 267–231.

Wortman CB and Brehm JW (1975) Responses to uncontrollable outcomes: an integration of reactance theory and the learned helplessness model. In: Berkowitz L (ed) *Advances in Experimental Social Psychology,* Vol 8. New York: Academic Press.

Wright SG (1998) *Changing Nursing Practice.* London: Arnold.

Further reading

Open University (1991) Managing Health Services, Book 9 Managing Change. Milton Keynes: The Open University Press.

Roberts SJ (1983) Oppressed group behaviour: implications for nursing. *Advances in Nursing Science* **5**(4): 21–30.

Senge PM, Roberts C, Ross RB et al (1994) *The Fifth Discipline Field Book: Strategies for Building a Learning Organisation.* New York: Currency/Doubleday.

Wright SG (1998) *Changing Nursing Practice.* London: Arnold.

Glossary

With grateful thanks to W.B. Saunders Company for permission to reproduce adapted extracts from the glossary in Burns N and Grove S K (1997) *The Practice of Nursing Research: Conduct, Critique and Utilization*, 3rd edn.

A

abstract. Clear, concise summary of a study, usually limited to 100-250 words.

abstract thinking. Oriented towards the development of an idea without application to, or association with, a particular instance and is independent of time and space. Abstract thinkers tend to look for meaning, patterns, relationships, and philosophical implications.

accessible population. Portion of the target population to which the researcher has reasonable access.

accidental or convenience sampling. Subjects are included in the study because they happened to be in the right place at the right time; available subjects are simply entered into the study until the desired sample size is reached.

across-method triangulation. Combining research methods or strategies from two or more research traditions in the same study.

alpha (α). Level of significance or cut-off point used to determine whether the samples being tested are members of the same population or of different populations; alpha is commonly set at .05, .01, or .001.

alternate form reliability. Comparing the equivalence of two versions of the same instrument.

analysis of covariance (ANCOVA). Statistical procedure designed to reduce the error term (or variance within groups) by partialing out the variance due to a confounding variable by performing regression analysis before performing ANOVA.

analysis of variance (ANOVA). Statistical technique used to examine differences among two or more groups by comparing the variability between the groups with the variability within the groups.

analytic induction. Qualitative research technique that includes enumerative induction, in which a number and variety of instances are collected that verify the model, and eliminative induction, which requires that the hypothesis be tested against alternatives.

anonymity. Subject's identity cannot be linked, even by the researcher, with his or her individual responses.

applied research. Scientific investigations conducted to generate knowledge that will directly influence or improve practice.

associated key words. A set of words that could be allied with the topic area concerned.

associative relationship. Identifies variables or concepts that occur or exist together in the real world; thus, when one variable changes, the other variable changes.

assumptions. Statements taken for granted or considered true, even though they have not been scientifically tested.

attrition. The loss of participants during the course of a study: can introduce an unknown amount of bias by changing the composition of the sample initially drawn – particularly if more subjects are lost from one group than another; can thereby be a threat to the internal validity of a study.

auditability. Rigorous development of a decision trail that is reported in sufficient detail to allow a second researcher, using the original data and the decision trail, to arrive at conclusions similar to those of the original researcher.

B

backward stepwise regression analysis. Type of stepwise regression analysis where all the independent variables are initially included in the analysis. Then, one variable at a time is removed from the equation and the effect of that removal on variance is evaluated.

baseline measure. The measurement of the dependent variable before the introduction of an experimental intervention.

beneficence, principle of. Encourages the researcher to do good and above all, do no harm.

benefit–risk ratio. Researchers and reviewers of research weigh potential benefits and risks in a study to promote the conduct of ethical research.

bias. Any influence or action in a study that distorts the findings or slants them away from the true or expected.

bibliography. A list of references, either computer- or text-based.

bivariate analysis. Statistical procedures that involve the comparison of summary values from two groups of the same variable or of two variables within a group.

bivariate correlation. Analysis techniques that measure the extent of the linear relationship between two variables.

body of knowledge. Information, principles and theories that are organized by the beliefs accepted in a discipline at a given time.

borrowing. Appropriation and use of knowledge from other disciplines to guide nursing practice.

box-and-whisker plots. Exploratory data analysis technique to provide visualization of some of the major characteristics of the data, such as the spread, symmetry, and outliers.

bracketing. Qualitative research technique of suspending or laying aside what is known about an experience being studied.

breach of confidentiality. Accidental or direct action that allows an unauthorized person to have access to raw study data.

broad brush approach. An approach to searching the literature identified by Burnard (1995) and meaning searching the library indexes for any information that could be related to the topic area.

C

canonical correlation. Extension of multiple regression with more than one dependent variable.

case study design. Intensive exploration of a single unit of study, such as a person, family, group, community or institution.

catalogue. Identifies what is available in the library.

causal hypothesis or relationship. Identifies a cause-and-effect interaction between two or more variables, which are referred to as independent and dependent variables.

causal relationship. Relationship between two variables where one variable (independent variable) is thought to cause or determine the presence of the other variable (dependent variable).

causality. Includes three conditions: (1) must be a strong correlation between the proposed cause and effect, (2) proposed cause must precede the effect in time, and (3) cause has to be present whenever the effect occurs.

cell. Intersection between the row and column in a table where a specific numerical value is inserted.

census. A survey covering an entire population.

central limit theorem. States that even when statistics, such as means, come from a population with a skewed (asymmetrical) distribution, the sampling distribution developed from multiple means obtained from that skewed population will tend to fit the pattern of the normal curve.

central tendency. A statistical index of the 'typicalness' of a set of scores that come from the centre of the distribution of scores. The three most common indices of central tendency are the mode, the median, and the mean.

change agent. Professional outside a system who enters the system to promote adoption of an innovation.

chi-square (χ^2) test. Used to analyse nominal data to determine significance of differences between observed frequencies within the data and frequencies that were expected.

citation. A word that means that an author is being used to support the statement as in the sentence above. Burnard (1995) is being cited.

citation indexes. Written and computer indexes that cross reference the authors that writers are citing.

chronology. A type of unstructured observation that provides a detailed description of an individual's behaviour in a natural environment.

cleaning data. Checking raw data to determine errors in data recording, coding, or entry.

cluster sampling. A form of multistage sampling in which large groupings ('clusters') are selected first (e.g. nursing schools), with successive subsampling of smaller units (e.g. nursing students).

Cochran Q test. Nonparametric test that is an extension of the McNemar test for two related samples.

codebook. Identifies and defines each variable in a study and includes an abbreviated variable name (limited to 6–8 characters), a descriptive variable label, and the range of possible numerical values of every variable entered into a computer file.

coding. Process of transforming qualitative data into numerical symbols that can be computerized.

coercion. An overt threat of harm or excessive reward intentionally presented by one person to another in order to obtain compliance, such as offering subjects a large sum of money to participate in a dangerous research project.

coefficient of determination (R^2). Computed from a matrix of correlation coefficients and provides important information on multicollinearity. This value indicates the degree of linear dependencies among the variables.

cohorts. Samples in time-dimensional studies within the field of epidemiology.

comparative descriptive design. Used to describe differences in variables in two or more groups in a natural setting.

comparison group. The group not receiving a treatment or receiving the usual treatment (standard care) when non-random sampling methods are used.

complete observer. The researcher is passive and has no direct social interaction in the setting.

compatibility. The degree to which the innovation is perceived to be consistent with current values, past experience, and priority of needs.

complete participation. The researcher becomes a member of the group and conceals the researcher role.

complex hypothesis. Predicts the relationship (associative or causal) among three or more variables; thus, the hypothesis could include two (or more) independent and/or two (or more) dependent variables.

computerized database. A structured compilation of information that can be scanned, retrieved and analysed by computer and can be used for decisions, reports, and research.

computer searches. Conducted to scan the citations in different databases and identify sources relevant to a research problem.

concept. A term that abstractly describes and names an object or phenomenon, thus providing it with a separate identity or meaning.

conceptual definition. Provides a variable or concept with connotative (abstract, comprehensive, theoretical) meaning and is established through concept analysis, concept derivation, or concept synthesis.

conceptual framework. A set of highly abstract, related constructs that broadly explains phenomena of interest, expresses assumptions, and reflects a philosophical stance.

conclusions. Synthesis and clarification of the meaning of study findings.

concurrent validity. The degree to which scores on an instrument are correlated with some external criterion, measured at the same time.

confidence interval. A range where the value of the parameter is estimated to be.

confidentiality. Management of data in research so subjects' identities are not linked with their responses.

confounding variables. Variables recognized before the study is initiated but cannot be controlled, or variables not recognized until the study is in process, which may have an effect on the dependent variable.

consent form. A written form, tape-recording, or videotape used to document a subject's agreement to participate in a study.

consent rate. The percentage of people that indicate a willingness to participate in a study based on the total number of people approached.

constructs. Concepts at very high levels of abstraction that have general meanings.

construct validity. Examines the fit between conceptual and operational definitions of variables and determines if the instrument actually measures the theoretical construct it purports to measure.

content analysis. Qualitative analysis technique to classify words in a text into a few categories chosen because of their theoretical importance.

content validity. Examines the extent to which the method of measurement includes all the major elements relevant to the construct being measured.

context. The body, the world and the concerns unique to each person within which that person can be understood.

contingency tables. Cross-tabulation tables that allow visual comparison of summary data output related to two variables within a sample.

control. Imposing of rules by the researcher to decrease the possibility of error and increase the probability that the study's findings are an accurate reflection of reality.

control group. The group of elements or subjects not exposed to the experimental treatment.

convenience or accidental sampling. Subjects are included in the study because they happen to be in the right place at the right time; available subjects are simply entered into the study until the desired sample size is reached.

correlation. A tendency for variation in one variable to be related to variation in another variable.

correlation coefficient. Indicates the degree of relationship between two variables; the coefficients range in value from $+1.00$ (perfect positive relationship) to 0.00 (no relationship) to $+1.00$ (perfect negative or inverse relationship).

correlational analysis. Statistical procedure conducted to determine the direction (positive or negative) and magnitude (or strength) of the relationship between two variables.

correlational research. Systematic investigation of relationships between two or more variables to explain the nature of relationships in the world and not to examine cause and effect.

cost-benefit analysis. Analysis technique used in outcomes research that examines costs and benefits of alternative ways of using resources as assessed in monetary terms and the use that produces the greatest net benefit.

cost-effectiveness analyses. Type of outcomes research where the costs and benefits are compared for different ways of accomplishing a clinical goal, such as diagnosing a condition, treating an illness, or providing a service. The goal of cost-effectiveness analyses is to identify the strategy that provides the most value for the money.

covert data collection. Occurs when subjects are unaware that research data are being collected.

Cramer's V. Analysis technique for nominal data that is a modification of phi for contingency tables larger than 2×2.

criterion-referenced testing. Comparison of a subject's score with a criterion of achievement that includes the definition of target behaviours. When the behaviours are mastered, the subject is considered proficient in these behaviours.

critical analysis of studies. Minute examination of the merits, faults, meaning, and significance of studies.

critical incident technique. A method of obtaining data from study participants by in-depth exploration of specific incidents and behaviours related to the matter under investigation.

critical social theory. Qualitative research methodology guided by critical social theory; the researcher seeks to understand how people communicate and develop symbolic meanings in a society.

critique. An objective, critical and balanced appraisal of a research report's various dimensions (e.g. conceptual, methodological and ethical). It requires detailed critical analysis based on a fairly sophisticated level of knowledge about research.

crossover design. Includes the administration of more than one treatment to each subject with the treatments being provided sequentially, rather than concurrently, and comparisons are then made of the effects of the different treatments on the same subjects.

cross-sectional designs. Used to examine groups of subjects in various stages of development simultaneously with the intent of inferring trends over time.

cross-tabulation. A determination of the number of cases occurring when simultaneous consideration is given to the values of two or more variables (e.g., sex – male/female – cross-tabulated with smoking status – smoker/non-smoker). The results are typically presented in a table with rows and columns divided according to the values of the variables.

cultural immersion. Used in ethnographic research for gaining increased familiarity with such things as language, sociocultural norms, and traditions in a culture.

curvilinear relationship. The relationship between two variables varies depending on the relative values of the variables. The graph of the relationship is a curved line rather than a straight one.

D

data. Pieces of information that are collected during a study.

database. *See* computerized databases.

data analysis. Conducted to reduce, organize, and give meaning to data.

data coding sheet. A sheet for organizing and recording data for rapid entry into a computer.

data collection. Precise, systematic gathering of information relevant to the research purpose or the specific objectives, questions, or hypotheses of a study.

data entry. The process of entering data (usually in coded form) onto an input medium for computer analysis.

data reduction. Technique for analysing qualitative data that focuses on decreasing the volume of data to facilitate examination.

data transformation. A step often undertaken prior to the analysis of research data, to put the data in a form that can be meaningfully analysed (e.g., recoding of values).

data triangulation. Collection of data from multiple sources in the same study.

debriefing. Complete disclosure of the study purpose and results at the end of a study.

deception. Misinforming subjects for research purposes.

decision theory. Theory that is inductive in nature and is based on assumptions associated with the theoretical normal curve. The theory is applied when testing for differences between groups with the expectation that all of the groups are members of the same population.

decision trail. *See* auditability.

Declaration of Helsinki. Ethical code based on the Nuremberg code that differentiated therapeutic from non-therapeutic research.

deductive reasoning. Reasoning from the general to the specific or from a general premise to a particular situation.

degrees of freedom (*df*). The freedom of a score's value to vary given the other existing scores' values and the established sum of these scores ($df = N - 1$).

Delphi technique. A method of measuring the judgments of a group of experts for assessing priorities or making forecasts.

demographic variables. Characteristics or attributes of the subjects that are collected to describe the sample.

dependent variable. The response, behaviour, or outcome that is predicted or explained in research; changes in the dependent variable are presumed to be caused by the independent variable.

description. Involves identifying the nature and attributes of nursing phenomena and sometimes the relationships among these phenomena.

descriptive codes. Terms used to organize and classify qualitative data.

descriptive correlational design. Used to describe variables and examine relationships that exist in a situation.

descriptive design. Used to identify a phenomenon of interest, identify variables within the phenomenon, develop conceptual and operational definitions of variables, and describe variables.

descriptive research. Provides an accurate portrayal or account of characteristics of a particular individual, event, or group in real-life situations for the purpose of discovering new meaning, describing what exists, determining the frequency with which something occurs, and categorizing information.

descriptive statistics. Statistics that allow the researcher to organize the data in ways that give meaning and facilitate insight, such as frequency distributions and measures of central tendency and dispersion.

design. Blueprint for conducting a study that maximizes control over factors that could interfere with the validity of the findings.

dialectic reasoning. Involves the holistic perspective, where the whole is greater than the sum of the parts, and examining factors that are opposites and making sense of them by merging them into a single unit or idea, greater than either alone.

diary. Record of events kept by a subject over time that is collected and analysed by a researcher.

diffusion. Process of communicating research findings (innovations) through certain channels over time among the members of a discipline.

directional hypothesis. States the specific nature of the interaction or relationship between two or more variables.

discriminant analysis. Designed to allow the researcher to identify characteristics associated with group membership and to predict group membership.

disproportionate stratified sampling. A sampling strategy wherein the researcher samples differing proportions of subjects from different strata in the population to ensure adequate representation of subjects from strata that are comparatively smaller.

dissemination of research findings. The diffusion or communication of research findings.

double-blind experiment. An experiment in which neither the subjects nor those who administer the treatment know who is in the experimental or control group.

dummy variables. Categorical or dichotomous variables used in regression analysis.

E

early adopters of innovations. Opinion leaders in a social system who learn about new ideas rapidly, utilize them, and serve as role models for their use in nursing practice.

effect size. A statistical expression of the magnitude between two variables, or the magnitude of the difference between two groups, with regard to some attribute of interest.

eigen values. Numerical values generated with factor analysis that are the sum of the squared weights for each factor.

element of a study. A person (subject), event, behaviour, or any other single unit of a study.

emic approach. Anthropological research approach of studying behaviours from within the culture.

empirical generalization. Statements that have been repeatedly tested through research and have not been disproved. Scientific theories have empirical generalizations.

empirical literature. Includes relevant studies published in journals and books as well as unpublished studies, such as master's theses and doctoral dissertations.

empirical world. Experienced through our senses and is the concrete portion of our existence.

epistemology. The philosophical theory of knowledge. Epistemology seeks to define the nature, derivation, scope and reliability of the claims of knowledge.

equivalence. Type of reliability testing that involves comparing two versions of the same instrument or two observers measuring the same event.

error score. Amount of random error in the measurement process.

ethical inquiry. Intellectual analysis of ethical problems related to obligation, rights, duty, right and wrong, conscience, choice, intention, and responsibility to obtain desirable, rational ends.

ethical principles. Principles of respect for persons, beneficence, and justice relevant to the conduct of research.

ethical rigour. Requires recognition and discussion by the researcher of the ethical implications related to the conduct of the study.

ethics. The quality of research procedures with respect to their adherence to professional, legal, and social obligations to the research subjects.

ethnographic research. A qualitative research methodology for investigating cultures that involves collection, description, and analysis of data to develop a theory of cultural behaviour.

ethnomethodology. A research approach which aims to increase the understanding of taken-for-granted or implicit practices in a society, particularly in relation to social interaction. An ethnomethodological study usually uses documents and audio-visual taped materials that focus on everyday events as the source of the data.

etic approach. Anthropological research approach of studying behaviour from outside the culture and examining similarities and differences across cultures.

event sampling. In observational studies a sampling plan that involves the selection of integral behaviours or events.

exclusion criteria. Sampling requirements identified by the researcher that eliminate or exclude an element or subject from being in a sample. Exclusion criteria are exceptions to the inclusion sampling criteria.

execution errors. Errors that occur because of a defect in the data collection procedure.

experimental designs. Designs that provide the greatest amount of control possible in order to more closely examine causality.

experimental group. The subjects who are exposed to the experimental treatment.

experimental research. Objective, systematic, controlled investigation to examine probability and causality among selected variables for the purpose of predicting and controlling phenomena.

explanation. Achieved when research clarifies the relationships among phenomena and identifies why certain events occur.

explanatory codes. Developed late in the data collection process after theoretical ideas from the qualitative study have begun to emerge.

exploratory data analysis. Examining the data descriptively, to become as familiar as possible with the nature of the data.

exploratory factor analysis. Similar to stepwise regression in which the variance of the first factor is partialed out before analysis is begun on the second factor. It is performed when the researcher has few prior expectations about the factor structure.

exploratory regression analysis. Used when the researcher may not have sufficient information to determine which independent variables are effective predictors of the dependent variable; thus, many variables may be entered into the analysis simultaneously. This is the most commonly used regression analysis strategy in nursing studies.

external validity. The extent to which study findings can be generalized beyond the sample used in the study.

extraneous variables. Exist in all studies and can affect the measurement of study variables and the relationships among these variables.

F

face validity. Verifies that the instrument looked like or gave the appearance of measuring the content.

factor analysis. Analysis that examines inter-relationships among large numbers of variables and disentangles those relationships to identify clusters of variables that are most closely linked together. Two types of factor analysis are exploratory and confirmatory factor analysis.

factor rotation. An aspect of factor analysis where the factors are mathematically adjusted or rotated to reduce the factor structure and clarify the meaning.

factorial analysis of variance. Mathematically the analysis technique is simply a specialized version of multiple regression; a number of types of factorial ANOVAs have been developed to analyse data from specific experimental designs.

factorial design. Study design that includes two or more different characteristics, treatments, or events that are independently varied within a study.

fatigue effect. When a subject becomes tired or bored with a study.

feasibility of a study. Determined by examining the time and money commitment; the researcher's expertise; availability of subjects, facility, and equipment; cooperation of others; and the study's ethical considerations.

field research. The activity of collecting the data that requires taking extensive notes in ethnographic research.

findings. The translated and interpreted results from a study.

focus group interview. An interview in which the respondents are a group of individuals assembled to answer questions on a given topic.

forced choice. Response set for items in a scale that have an even number of choices, such as four or six, where the respondents cannot choose an uncertain or neutral response and must indicate support for or against the topic measured.

forward stepwise regression analysis. Type of stepwise regression analysis where the independent variables are entered into the analysis one at a time and an analysis is made of the effect of including that variable on R^2.

framework. The abstract, logical structure of meaning that guides the development of the study and enables the researcher to link the findings to a body of knowledge.

fraudulent publications. There is documentation or testimony from co-authors that the publication did not reflect what had actually been done.

frequency distribution. A statistical procedure that involves listing all possible measures of a variable and tallying each datum on the listing. There are two types of frequency distributions, ungrouped and grouped.

frequency polygon. Graphic display of a frequency distribution, in which dots connected by a straight line indicate the number of times a score value occurs in a set of data.

Friedman two-way analysis of variance by ranks. Non-parametric test used with matched samples or in repeated measures.

G

generalization. Extends the implications of the findings from the sample that was studied to the larger population or from the situation studied to a larger situation.

gestalt. Organization of knowledge about a particular phenomenon into a cluster of linked ideas. The clustering and interrelatedness enhances the meaning of the ideas.

going native. In ethnographic research, when the researcher becomes a part of the culture and loses all objectivity and, with it, the ability to observe clearly.

grounded theory research. An inductive research technique based on symbolic interaction theory, which is conducted to discover what problems exist in a social scene and the process persons use to handle them. The research process involves formulation, testing and redevelopment of propositions until a theory is developed.

Guttman scale. A method of measuring attitudes that makes use of a set of cumulative (monotone) items with which respondents are asked to agree or disagree.

H

hard copy. A written or typed paper copy of what is listed or written in a computer.

Hawthorne effect. A psychological response in which subjects change their behaviour simply because they are subjects in a study, not because of the research treatment.

heterogeneity. The researcher's attempt to obtain subjects with a wide variety of characteristics to reduce the risk of bias in studies not using random sampling.

historical research. A narrative description or analysis of events that occurred in the remote or recent past.

history effect. An event that is not related to the planned study but occurs during the time of the study and could influence the responses of subjects to the treatment.

homogeneity. The degree to which objects are similar or a form of equivalence, such as limiting subjects to only one level of an extraneous variable to reduce its impact on the study findings.

human rights. Claims and demands that have been justified in the eyes of an individual or by the consensus of a group of individuals and are protected in research.

hypothesis. Formal statement of the expected relationship between two or more variables in a specified population.

I

immersed in the culture. Involves gaining increasing familiarity with such things as language, sociocultural norms, traditions, communication patterns, religion, work patterns, and expression of emotion in a selected culture.

implications. The meaning of research conclusions for the body of knowledge, theory and practice.

inclusion criteria. Sampling requirements identified by the researcher that must be present for the element or subject to be included in the sample.

incomplete disclosure. Subjects are not completely informed about the purpose of a study because that knowledge might alter the subjects' actions. Following the study, the subjects must be debriefed.

incremental searching. A searching strategy identified by Burnard (1995) which suggests that a single piece of literature should be examined for its references. These references should then be found and examined for relevance and their references examined. This should occur until the searcher is satisfied that all the relevant pieces have been found.

independent groups. Groups where the selection of one subject is totally unrelated to the selection of other subjects. An example is when subjects are randomly assigned to the treatment and control groups.

independent variable. The treatment or experimental activity that is manipulated or varied by the researcher to create an effect on the dependent variable.

index. A list of references often to be found in a library. It can either be written or computer-based. Provides assistance in identifying journal articles and other publications relevant to a topic of interest.

indirect measurement. Used with abstract concepts, when the concepts are not measured directly but, rather, indicators or attributes of the concepts are used to represent the abstraction.

inductive reasoning. Reasoning from the specific to the general where particular instances are observed and then combined into a larger whole or general statement.

inferential statistics. Statistics designed to allow inference from a sample statistic to a population parameter; commonly used to test hypotheses of similarities and differences in subsets of the sample under study.

inferred causality. A cause-and-effect relationship is identified from numerous studies conducted over time to determine risk factors or causal factors in selected situations.

informed consent. The prospective subject's agreement to voluntarily participate in a study, which is reached after assimilation of essential information about the study.

innovation. An idea, practice, or object that is perceived as new by an individual or other unit of adoption.

innovators. Individuals who actively seek out new ideas.

institutional review. A process of examining studies for ethical concerns by a committee of peers.

instrumentation. A component of measurement that involves the application of specific rules to develop a measurement device or instrument.

interlibrary loan department. Department that locates books and articles in other libraries and provides the sources within a designated time.

internal validity. The extent to which the effects detected in the study are a true reflection on reality, rather than being the result of the effects of extraneous variables.

interpretative codes. Organizational system developed late in the qualitative data collection and analysis process as the researcher gains some insight into the processes occurring.

inter-rater reliability. The degree of consistency between two raters who are independently assigning ratings to a variable or attribute being investigated.

interrupted time-series designs. These designs are similar to descriptive time designs except that a treatment is applied at some point in the observations.

interval-scale measurement. Interval scales have equal numerical distances between intervals of the scale in addition to following rules of mutual exclusive categories, exhaustive categories, and rank ordering, such as temperature.

interviews. Structured or unstructured verbal communication between the researcher and subject, during which information is obtained for a study.

inverse linear relationship. Indicates that as one variable or concept changes, the other variable or concept changes in the opposite direction. Also referred to as a negative linear relationship.

investigator triangulation. Exists when two or more research-trained investigators with divergent backgrounds explore the same phenomenon.

J

justice, principle of. States that human subjects should be treated fairly.

K

Kendall's tau. Non-parametric test to determine correlation used when both variables have been measured at the ordinal level.

Kolmogorov–Smirnov two-sample test. Non-parametric test used to determine whether two independent samples have been drawn from the same population.

Kruskal–Wallis test. Most powerful nonparametric analysis technique for examining three independent groups for differences.

kurtosis. The degree of peakedness of the curve shape that is related to the spread or variance of scores.

L

laggards. Individuals who are security-oriented, tend to cling to the past, and are often isolated without a strong support system. Term used to describe persons who are reluctant or refuse to adopt innovations.

lambda. Analysis technique that measures the degree of association (or relationship) between two nominal level variables.

Likert scale. An instrument designed to determine the opinion or attitude of a subject; it contains a number of declarative statements with a scale after each statement.

limitations. Theoretical and methodological restrictions in a study that may decrease the generalizability of the findings.

linear relationship. The relationship between two variables or concepts will remain consistent regardless of the values of each of the variables or concepts.

logical positivism. The philosophy underlying the traditional scientific approach. The meaning of a proposition is in the method of its verification and any proposition which is not verified by observation is meaningless.

longitudinal study. A study designed to collect data at more than one point in time, in contrast to a cross-sectional study.

M

manipulation. To move around or to control the movement of a variable or treatment.

Mann–Whitney U test. Used to analyse ordinal data with 95% of the power of the t-test to detect differences between groups of normally distributed populations.

matching. This technique is used when an experimental subject is randomly selected and a subject similar in relation to important extraneous variables is randomly selected for inclusion in the control group.

maturation effect. Unplanned and unrecognized changes experienced during a study, such as growing older, wiser, stronger, hungrier, or more tired, that can influence the findings of a study.

McNemar test. Non-parametric test to analyse the changes that occur in dichotomous variables using a 2×2 table.

mean. The value obtained by summing all the scores and dividing that total by the number of scores being summed.

measurement. The process of assigning numbers to objects, events, or situations in accord with some rule.

measurement error. The difference between what exists in reality and what is measured by a research instrument.

measures of central tendency. Statistical procedures (mean, median and mode) for determining the centre of a distribution of scores or a typical value.

measures of dispersion. Statistical procedures (range, difference scores, sum of squares, variance and standard deviation) for examining how scores vary or are dispersed around the mean.

median. The score at the exact centre of the ungrouped frequency distribution.

memo. Developed by the researcher to record insights or ideas related to notes, transcripts, or codes during qualitative data analysis.

metaanalysis design. Merging of findings from several completed studies to determine what is known about a particular phenomenon.

method of least squares. Procedure in regression analysis for developing the line of best fit.

methodological limitations. Restrictions in the study design that limit the credibility of the findings and the population to which the findings can be generalized.

methodological triangulation. The use of two or more research methods or procedures, such as different designs, instruments and data collection procedures, in a study.

modal percentage. Appropriate for nominal data and indicates the relationship of a number of data scores represented by the mode to the total number of data scores.

mode. The numerical value or score that occurs with the greatest frequency in a distribution; but it does not necessarily indicate the centre of the data set.

mortality. Subjects drop out of a study before completion, which creates a threat to the internal validity.

multicausality. The recognition that a number of interrelating variables can be involved in causing a particular effect.

multilevel analysis. Used in epidemiology to study how environmental factors and individual attributes and behaviours interact to influence individual-level health behaviours and disease risks.

multiple regression analysis. Extension of simple linear regression with more than one independent variable entered into the analysis.

multivariate analysis techniques. Used to analyse data from complex research projects. *See also* multiple regression, factorial analysis of variance, analysis of covariance, factor analysis, discriminant analysis, canonical correlation, structural equation modelling, and time-series analysis.

N

natural settings. Field settings or uncontrolled, real-life situations examined in research.

negative linear relationship. *See* inverse linear relationship.

networking. A process of developing channels of communication between people with common interests throughout the country.

network sampling. Snowballing technique that takes advantage of social networks and the fact that friends tend to hold characteristics in common. Subjects meeting the sample criteria are asked to assist in locating others with similar characteristics.

nominal-scale measurement. Lowest level of measurement that is used when data can be organized into categories that are exclusive and exhaustive, but the categories cannot be compared, such as gender, race, marital status, and nursing diagnoses.

non-directional hypothesis. States that a relationship exists but does not predict the exact nature of the relationship.

non-equivalent control group designs. Designs in which the control group is not selected by random means, such as the one-group post-test-only design, post-test-only design with non-equivalent groups, and one-group pretest–post-test design.

non-parametric statistics. Statistical techniques used when the assumptions of parametric statistics are not met and most commonly used to analyse nominal- and ordinal-level data.

non-probability sampling. Not every element of the population has an opportunity for selection in the sample, such as convenience (accidental) sampling, quota sampling, purposive sampling, and network sampling.

non-therapeutic research. Research conducted to generate knowledge for a discipline, and the results from the study might benefit future patients but will probably not benefit those acting as research subjects.

normal curve. A symmetrical, unimodal bell-shaped curve that is a theoretical distribution of all possible scores, but no real distribution exactly fits the normal curve.

null hypothesis. States that there is no relationship between the variables being studied; a statistical hypothesis used for statistical testing and interpreting statistical outcomes.

Nuremberg Code. Ethical code of conduct to guide investigators in conducting research.

O

oblique rotation. A type of rotation in factor analysis used to accomplish the best fit (best factor solution) and the factors are allowed to be correlated.

observed score. The actual score or value obtained for a subject on a measurement tool.

observer-as-participant. The researcher's time is spent observing and interviewing subjects and less in the participation role.

one-tailed test of significance. An analysis used with directional hypotheses where extreme statistical values of interest are thought to occur in a single tail of the curve.

ontology. The theory of what really exists as opposed to what appears to exist. It is the primary element in metaphysics. It is contrasted with epistemology, the study of knowing, rather than being.

operational definition. Description of how variables or concepts will be measured or manipulated in a study.

operationalization. The process of translating research concepts into observable and/or measurable phenomena.

ordinal-scale measurement. Yields data that can be ranked but the intervals between the ranked data are not necessarily equal, such as levels of coping.

outcomes research. Important scientific methodology that was developed to examine the end results of patient care. The strategies used in outcomes research are a departure from the traditional scientific endeavours and incorporate evaluation research, epidemiology, and economic theory perspectives.

outliers. The extreme scores or values in a set of data.

P

p-value. In statistical testing, the probability that the obtained results result from chance alone.

paradigm. A way of looking at natural phenomena that encompasses a set of philosophical assumptions and that guides one's approach to inquiry.

parallel-forms reliability. *See* alternate forms reliability.

parameter. A measure or numerical value of a population.

parametric statistical analyses. Statistical techniques used when three assumptions are met: (1) the sample was drawn from a population for which the variance can be calculated, the distribution is expected to be normal or approximately normal; (2) the level of measurement should be interval or ratio with an approximately normal distribution; and (3) the data can be treated as random samples.

participant-as-observer. A special form of observation where researchers immerse themselves in the setting so they can hear, see, and experience the reality as the participants do. But the participants are aware of the dual roles of the researcher (participant and observer).

path coefficient. The effect of the independent variable on the dependent variable that is determined through path analysis.

Pearson's product-moment correlation coefficient. Parametric test used to determine the relationship between variables.

percent of variance. The value obtained by squaring the Pearson's correlation coefficient (r) and that is the amount of variability explained by the linear relationship.

phenomenology. An approach to human inquiry that emphasizes the complexity of human experience and the need to study that experience holistically as it is actually lived. In sociology, phenomenology is used to investigate people's assumptions involved in everyday social life.

phenomenological research. Inductive, descriptive qualitative methodology developed from phenomenological philosophy for the purpose of describing experiences as they are lived by the study participants.

phi coefficient. Analysis technique to determine relationships in dichotomous, nominal data.

philosophical inquiry. Research using intellectual analyses to clarify meanings, make values manifest, identify ethics, and study the nature of knowledge.

philosophy. A broad, global explanation of the world.

pilot study. A smaller version of a proposed study conducted to develop and/or refine the methodology, such as the treatment, instrument, or data collection process.

population. All elements (individuals, objects, or events) that meet sample criteria for inclusion in a study. Sometimes referred to as a target population.

positive linear relationship. Indicates that as one variable changes (value of the variable increases or decreases), the second variable will also change in the same direction.

poster session. Visual presentation of a study, using pictures, tables, and illustrations on a display board.

power. The probability that a statistical test will detect a significant difference that exists; power analysis is used to determine the power of a study.

power analysis. Used to determine the risk of a Type II error, so the study can be modified to decrease the risk if necessary.

practice effect. Occurs when subjects improve as they become more familiar with the experimental protocol.

precision. The accuracy with which the population parameters have been estimated within a study. Also used to describe the degree of consistency or reproducibility of measurements.

prediction. The ability to estimate the probability of a specific outcome in a given situation that can be achieved through research.

predictive validity. The degree to which an instrument can predict some criterion observed at a future time.

primary source. A source that is written by the person who originated or is responsible for generating the ideas published.

principal component analysis. The second step in exploratory factor analysis that provides preliminary information needed by the researcher in order for decisions to be made prior to the final factoring.

principal investigator (PI). In a research grant, the individual who will have primary responsibility for administering the grant and interacting with the funding agency.

probability sampling. Random sampling techniques in which each member (element) in the population should have a greater than zero opportunity to be selected for the sample; examples include simple random sampling, stratified random sampling, cluster sampling, and systematic sampling.

probability theory. Addresses statistical analysis from the perspective of the extent of a relationship or the probability of accurately predicting an event.

probing. Technique used by the interviewer to obtain more information in a specific area of the interview.

process-outcome matrix. Qualitative analysis technique that allows the researcher to trace the processes that led to differing outcomes.

proposal, research. Written plan identifying the major elements of a study, such as the problem, purpose, and framework, and outlining the methods to conduct the study. A formal way to communicate ideas about a proposed study to receive approval to conduct the study and to seek funding.

proposition. An abstract statement that further clarifies the relationship between two concepts.

prospective cohort study. An epidemiologic study in which a group of people are identified who are at risk for experiencing a particular event.

purposive sampling. Judgmental sampling that involves the conscious selection by the researcher of certain subjects or elements to include in a study.

Q

Q-sort methodology. A technique of comparative rating where a subject sorts cards with statements on them into designated piles (usually 7 to 10 piles in the distribution of a normal curve) that might range from best to worst.

qualitative research. A systematic, interactive, subjective approach used to describe life experiences and give them meaning.

quantitative research. A formal, objective, systematic process to describe, test relationships, and examine cause and effect interactions among variables.

quasi-experimental designs. Designs with limited control that were developed to provide alternate means for examining causality in situations not conducive to experimental controls.

quasi-experimental research. A type of quantitative research conducted to explain relationships, clarify why certain events happen, and examine causality between selected independent and dependent variables.

questionnaire. A printed self-report form designed to elicit information that can be obtained through written responses of the subject.

quota sampling. A convenience sampling technique with an added strategy to ensure the inclusion of subject types that are likely to be under-represented in the convenience sample, such as women, minority groups, and the under-educated.

R

R^2 **(coefficient of determination)**. Computed from a matrix of correlation coefficients and provides important information on multicollinearity. This value indicates the degree of linear dependencies among the variables.

random assignment to groups. (Also known as random allocation or randomization.) A procedure used to assign subjects to the treatment or control groups, where the subjects have an equal opportunity to be assigned to either group.

random error. An error that causes individuals' observed scores to vary haphazardly around their true score.

randomized controlled trials. Classic means of examining the effects of various treatments where the effects of a treatment are examined by comparing the treatment group with the no-treatment group.

random number table. A table of digits from 0 to 9 set up in such a way that each number is equally likely to follow any other. Used in randomization or random sampling.

random sampling. *See* probability sampling.

random variation. The expected difference in values that occurs when one examines different subjects from the same sample.

range. The simplest measure of dispersion obtained by subtracting the lowest score from the highest score.

rating scales. Crudest form of measure using scaling techniques that include a list of an ordered series of categories of a variable, assumed to be based on an underlying continuum.

ratio-level measurement. Highest measurement form that meets all the rules of other forms of measure: mutually exclusive categories, exhaustive categories, rank ordering, equal spacing between intervals, and a continuum of values and also has an absolute zero, such as weight.

refereed journal. Uses referees or expert reviewers to determine whether a manuscript will be accepted for publication.

references. This word has two meanings. (1) A list of the books and articles that have been referred to in the main body of writing. (2) A list of books and journals available in a library.

reflexive thought. Critically thinking through the dynamic interaction between the self and the data occurring during analysis of qualitative data. During this process, the researcher explores personal feelings and experiences that may influence the study and integrates this understanding into the study.

regression line. The line that best represents the values of the raw scores plotted on a scatter diagram and the procedure for developing the line of best fit is the method of least squares.

relational statement. Declares that a relationship of some kind exists between two or more concepts.

reliability. Represents the consistency of the measure obtained.

reliability testing. A measure of the amount of random error in the measurement technique.

replication. Reproducing or repeating a study to determine whether similar findings will be obtained.

representativeness of sample. A sample must be like the population in as many ways as possible.

research. Diligent, systematic inquiry or investigation to validate and refine existing knowledge and generate new knowledge.

research hypothesis. The alternative hypothesis to the null hypothesis that states there is a relationship between two or more variables.

research objectives. Clear, concise, declarative statements that are expressed to direct a study and are focused on identification and description of variables and/or determination of the relationships amongst variables.

research problem. A situation in need of a solution, improvement, or alteration, or a discrepancy between the way things are and the way they ought to be.

research proposal. *See* proposal, research.

research purpose. A concise, clear statement of the specific goal or aim of the study that is generated from the problem.

research questions. Concise, interrogative statements developed to direct studies that are focused on description of variables, examination of relationships among variables, and determination of differences between two or more groups.

research topics. Concepts or broad problem areas that provide the basis for generating numerous questions and research problems.

research tradition. A programme of research that is important for building a body of knowledge related to the phenomena explained by a particular conceptual model.

respect for persons, principle of. Indicates that persons have the right to self-determination and the freedom to participate or not participate in research.

response set. The parameters within which the question or item is to be answered in a questionnaire.

results. The outcomes from data analysis that are generated for each research objective, question, or hypothesis.

retrospective cohort study. An epidemiologic study in which a group of people are identified who have experienced a particular event; for example, studying occupational exposure to chemicals.

review of relevant literature. An analysis and synthesis of research sources to generate a picture of what is known about a particular situation and the knowledge gaps that exist in the situation.

rigour. The striving for excellence in research through the use of discipline, scrupulous adherence to detail, and strict accuracy.

risk-benefit ratio. Researchers and reviewers of research weigh potential benefits and risks in a study to promote the conduct of ethical research.

S

sample. A subset of the population that is selected for a study.

sampling. Includes selecting groups of people, events, behaviours, or other elements with which to conduct a study.

sampling criteria. A list of the characteristics essential for membership in the target population.

sampling distribution. Developed using statistical values (such as means) of many samples obtained from the same population.

sampling error. The difference between a sample statistic used to estimate a parameter and the actual but unknown value of the parameter.

sampling frame. Listing of every member of the population using the sampling criteria to define membership.

sampling method. The process of selecting a group of people, events, behaviours, or other elements that are representative of the population being studied.

sampling plan. Describes the strategies that will be used to obtain a sample for a study and may include either probability or nonprobability sampling methods.

scale. A self-report form of measurement that is composed of several items that are thought to measure the construct being studied; the subject responds to each item on the continuum or scale provided.

scatter plot. A graphic representation of the relationship between two variables.

science. A coherent body of knowledge composed of research findings, tested theories, scientific principles, and laws for a discipline.

scientific method. Incorporates all procedures that scientists have used, currently use, or may use in the future to pursue knowledge, such as quantitative research, qualitative research, and outcomes research.

secondary analysis design. Involves studying data previously collected in another study; data are re-examined using different organizations of the data and different statistical analyses.

secondary source. A source that summarizes or quotes content from primary sources.

selection bias (self-selection). A threat to the internal validity of the study resulting from pre-existing differences between the groups under study. The differences affect the dependent variable in ways extraneous to the effect of the independent variable.

self-determination. Based on the ethical principle of respect for persons, which states that humans are capable of controlling their own destiny. Right to self-determination is violated through the use of coercion, covert data collection, and deception.

semantic differential scale. An instrument that consists of two opposite adjectives with a seven-point scale between them. The subject selects one point on the scale that best describes his or her view of the concept being examined.

sensitivity. In measurement, the ability of the measuring tool to make fine discriminations between objects with differing amounts of the attribute being measured.

serendipity. The accidental discovery of something valuable or useful during the conduct of a study.

sets. A set of key words or words that can be associated with one topic area. This word is often used when searching for information on a computer.

setting. Location for conducting research, such as a natural, partially controlled, or highly controlled setting.

sign test. A non-parametric analysis technique developed for data that it is difficult to assign numerical values to, but where the data can be ranked on some dimension.

simple hypothesis. States the relationship (associative or causal) between two variables.

simple linear regression. Parametric analysis technique that provides a means to estimate the value of a dependent variable based on the value of an independent variable.

simple random sampling. Elements are selected at random from the sampling frame for inclusion in a study. Each study element has a probability greater than zero of being selected for inclusion in the study.

skewness. A curve that is asymmetrical (positively or negatively skewed) that is developed from an asymmetrical distribution of scores.

skim reading. A way of rapidly reading a piece of literature or a book to see if it is relevant to the topic area.

slope. Determines the direction and angle of the regression line within the graph. The value is represented by the letter b.

snowball sampling. The selection of subjects by means of nominations or referrals from earlier subjects.

Solomon four-group design. An experimental design that uses a before-after design for one pair of experimental/control groups, and an after-only design for a second pair.

Spearman rank-order correlation coefficient. A non-parametric analysis technique for ordinal data that is an adaptation of the Pearson's product-moment correlation used to examine relationships amongst variables in a study.

split-half reliability. Used to determine the homogeneity of an instrument's items, where the items are split in half, and a correlational procedure is performed between the two halves.

stability. Aspect of reliability testing that is concerned with the consistency of repeated measures.

standard deviation. A measure of dispersion that is calculated by taking the square root of the variance.

standard scores. Used to express deviations from the mean (difference scores) in terms of standard deviation units, such as Z scores where the mean is zero and the standard deviation is 1.

statistic. A numerical value obtained from a sample used to estimate the parameters of a population.

statistical regression. The movement or regression of extreme scores toward the mean in studies using a pretest–post-test design.

statistical significance. A term indicating that the results obtained in an analysis of sample data are unlikely to have been caused by chance, at some specified level of probability.

stem-and-leaf displays. Type of exploratory data analysis where the scores are visually presented to obtain insights.

stepwise regression analysis. Type of exploratory regression analysis where the independent variables are entered into or removed from the analysis one at a time.

stratified random sampling. Used when the researcher knows some of the variables in the population that are critical to achieving representativeness. The sample is divided into strata or groups using these identified variables.

strength of relationship. The amount of variation that is explained by the relationship.

structural equation modelling. Analysis technique designed to test theories.

structured interviews. Use of strategies that provide increasing amount of control by the researcher over the content of the interview.

structured observation. Clearly identifying what is to be observed and precisely defining how the observations are to be made, recorded, and coded.

subjects. Individuals participating in a study.

subject terms. A list of key words associated with a specific subject area. These words are often used when searching using a computer index.

substantive theory. A theory recognized within the discipline as useful for explaining important phenomena.

sum of squares. Mathematical manipulation that involves summing the squares of the difference scores and part of the analysis process for calculating the standard deviation.

survey. Technique of data collection using questionnaires or personal interviews to gather data about an identified population.

survey design. A design to describe a phenomenon by collecting data from a large sample using questionnaires or personal interviews.

symmetrical relationship. Complex relationship that consists of two statements: If A occurs (or changes), B will occur (or change); if B occurs (or changes), A will occur (or change); A × B.

systematic bias or variation. A consequence of selecting subjects whose measurement values are different or vary in some way from the population.

systematic error. Measurement error that is not random but occurs consistently, such as a scale that inaccurately weighs subjects three pounds heavy.

systematic sampling. Conducted when an ordered list of all members of the population is available and involves selecting every nth individual on the list, using a starting point that is selected randomly.

T

tails. Extremes of the normal curve where the significant statistical values exist.

target population. A group of individuals who meet the sampling criteria.

test–retest reliability. Determination of the stability or consistency of a measurement technique by correlating the scores obtained from repeated measures.

theoretical limitations. Weaknesses in the study framework and conceptual and operational definitions that restrict the abstract generalization of the findings.

theoretical literature. Includes concept analyses, maps, theories and conceptual frameworks that support a selected research problem and purpose.

theoretical triangulation. The use of two or more frameworks or theoretical perspectives in the same study; and the hypotheses are developed based on the different theoretical perspectives and tested using the same data set.

theory. Consists of an integrated set of defined concepts and relational statements that present a view of a phenomenon and can be used to describe, explain, predict and/or control that phenomenon.

theoretical notes. In field studies, notes about the observer's interpretations of observed activities.

therapeutic research. Research that provides the patient an opportunity to receive an experimental treatment that might have beneficial results.

thesaurus. A book or computer programme which groups together words that have similar meanings.

Thurstone scale. A type of attitude scale in which a panel of judges first rates the degree of favourability of a set of statements about some attitudinal object (e.g., abortion), and then subjects identify with the statements with which they agree.

time sampling. In observational research, the selection of time periods during which observations will take place.

time-series analysis. A technique designed to analyse changes in a variable across time and thus to uncover patterns in the data.

traditions. Truths or beliefs that are based on customs and past trends and provide a way of acquiring knowledge.

transformation of ideas. Movement of ideas across levels of abstraction to determine the existing knowledge base in an area of study.

translation. Involves transforming from one language to another to facilitate understanding and is part of the process of interpreting research outcomes where results are translated and interpreted into findings.

treatment. The independent variable that is manipulated in a study to produce an effect on the dependent variable. The treatment or independent variable is usually detailed in a protocol to ensure consistent implementation in the study.

trialability. The extent to which an individual or agency can try out the idea on a limited basis with the option of returning to previous practices.

trial and error. An approach with unknown outcomes used in a situation of uncertainty, where other sources of knowledge are unavailable.

triangulation. The use of two or more theories, methods, data sources, investigators, or analysis methods in a study.

true score. Score that would be obtained if there were no error in measurement but there is always some measurement error.

t-test. A parametric analysis technique used to determine significant differences between measures of two samples; t-test analysis techniques exist for dependent and independent groups.

two-tailed test of significance. The analysis used for a non-directional hypothesis where the researcher assumes that an extreme score can occur in either tail.

Type I error. Occurs when the researcher concludes that the samples tested are from different populations (there is a significant difference between groups) when, in fact, the samples are from the same population (there is no significant difference between groups). The null hypothesis is rejected when it is true.

Type II error. Occurs when the researcher concludes that there is no significant difference between the samples examined when, in fact, a difference exists. The null hypothesis is regarded as true when it is false.

U

unstructured interviews. Initiated with a broad question and subjects are usually encouraged to further elaborate on particular dimensions of a topic.

unstructured observations. Involve spontaneously observing and recording what is seen with a minimum of prior planning.

unsubstantiated statements. Statements that are argumentative and unsupported by the literature.

utilization of research findings. The use of knowledge generated through research to guide practice.

V

validity, design. The strength of a design to produce accurate results or findings may be determined by examining statistical conclusion validity, internal validity, construct validity, and external validity.

validity, instrument. Determining the extent to which the instrument actually reflects the abstract construct being examined.

variables. Qualities, properties, or characteristics of persons, things, or situations that change or vary and are manipulated or measured in research.

varimax rotation. A type of rotation in factor analysis used to accomplish the best fit (best factor solution) and the factors are uncorrelated.

vignette. A brief description of an event, person, or situation to which respondents are asked to react.

visual analogue scale. A line of 100 mm in length with right angle stops at each end, where subjects are asked to record their response to a study variable.

voluntary consent. The prospective subject has decided to take part in a study of his or her own volition without coercion or any undue influence.

W

weighting. A correction procedure used to arrive at population values when a disproportional sampling design has been used.

Wilcoxon matched-pairs signed-ranks test. Nonparametric analysis technique used to examine changes that occur in pretest/post-test measures or matched-pairs measures.

Z

z-scores. The standardized scores developed based on the normal curve.

Index

Please note that references to non-textual materials such as Boxes, Figures and Tables are in *italic* print. References to Glossary are in **bold** print.